T0383376

Anxiety Disorders

Guest Editors

MOIRA A. RYNN, MD
HILARY B. VIDAIR, PhD
JENNIFER URBANO BLACKFORD, PhD

CHILD AND ADOLESCENT PSYCHIATRIC CLINICS OF NORTH AMERICA

www.childpsych.theclinics.com

Consulting Editor
HARSH K. TRIVEDI, MD

July 2012 • Volume 21 • Number 3

SAUNDERS an imprint of ELSEVIER, Inc.

W.B. SAUNDERS COMPANY
A Division of Elsevier Inc.

Elsevier Inc. • 1600 John F. Kennedy Boulevard • Suite 1800 • Philadelphia, Pennsylvania 19103-2899

http://www.childpsych.theclinics.com

CHILD AND ADOLESCENT PSYCHIATRIC CLINICS OF NORTH AMERICA Volume 21, Number 3
July 2012 ISSN 1056–4993, ISBN-13: 978-1-4557-3841-0

Editor: Joanne Husovski

Child and Adolescent Psychiatric Clinics of North America (ISSN 1056-4993) is published quarterly by Elsevier Inc., 360 Park Avenue South, New York, NY 10010-1710. Months of issue are January, April, July, and October. Business and Editorial Offices: 1600 John F. Kennedy Boulevard, Suite 1800, Philadelphia, PA 19103-2899. Periodicals postage paid at New York, NY and additional mailing offices. Subscription prices are $297.00 per year (US individuals), $453.00 per year (US institutions), $150.00 per year (US students), $343.00 per year (Canadian individuals), $546.00 per year (Canadian institutions), $190.00 per year (Canadian students), $408.00 per year (international individuals), $546.00 per year (international institutions), and $190.00 per year (international students). International air speed delivery is included in all *Clinics* subscription prices. All prices are subject to change without notice. **POSTMASTER:** Send address changes to *Child and Adolescent Psychiatric Clinics of North America,* Elsevier Health Sciences Division, Subscription Customer Service, 3251 Riverport Lane, Maryland Heights, MO 63043. **Customer Service: 1-800-654-2452 (U.S. and Canada); 314-447-8871 (outside U.S. and Canada). Fax: 314-447-8029. E-mail: JournalsCustomerService-usa@elsevier.com (for print support) or journalsonlinesupport-usa@elsevier.com (for online support).**

Reprints. For copies of 100 or more of articles in this publication, please contact the Commercial Reprints Department, Elsevier Inc., 360 Park Avenue South, New York, New York 10010-1710 Tel.: (212) 633-3812; Fax: (212) 462-1935, e-mail: reprints@elsevier.com.

Child and Adolescent Psychiatric Clinics of North America is covered in *MEDLINE/PubMed (Index Medicus), ISI, SSCI, Research Alert, Social Search, Current Contents,* and *EMBASE/Excerpta Medica.*

Printed and bound by CPI Group (UK) Ltd, Croydon, CR0 4YY

Transferred to Digital Print 2012

Contributors

CONSULTING EDITOR

HARSH K. TRIVEDI, MD
Associate Professor of Psychiatry, Vanderbilt University School of Medicine; and
Executive Medical Director, and Chief of Staff, Vanderbilt Psychiatric Hospital, Nashville,
Tennessee

CONSULTING EDITOR EMERITUS

ANDRÉS MARTIN, MD, MPH

FOUNDING CONSULTING EDITOR

MELVIN LEWIS, MBBS, FRCPSYCH, DCH

GUEST EDITORS

MOIRA A. RYNN, MD
Associate Professor of Clinical Psychiatry, Division of Child and Adolescent Psychiatry,
Department of Psychiatry and New York State Psychiatric Institute (NYSPI), Columbia
University, New York, New York

HILARY B. VIDAIR, PhD
Assistant Professor, Clinical Psychology Doctoral Program, Co-Director of Clinical
Training, Long Island University, Post Campus, Brookville; Adjunct Assistant Professor
of Medical Psychology, Department of Psychiatry, Columbia University College of
Physicians and Surgeons, New York, New York

JENNIFER URBANO BLACKFORD, PhD
Assistant Professor of Psychiatry and Psychology, Vanderbilt University, Nashville,
Tennessee

AUTHORS

ANNE MARIE ALBANO, PhD, ABPP
Associate Professor of Clinical Psychology in Psychiatry, Columbia University/New York
State Psychiatric Institute; Director, Columbia University Clinic for Anxiety and Related
Disorders, New York, New York

KATJA BEESDO-BAUM, PhD
Professor, Institute of Clinical Psychology and Psychotherapy, Technische Universitaet
Dresden, Dresden, Germany

KRISTIN L. BENAVIDES, BA
Department of Psychiatry, University of Pennsylvania School of Medicine, Philadelphia, Pennsylvania

GAIL A. BERNSTEIN, MD
Endowed Professor in Child and Adolescent Anxiety Disorders; Head, Program in Child and Adolescent Anxiety and Mood Disorders, Division of Child and Adolescent Psychiatry, University of Minnesota Medical School, Minneapolis, Minnesota

JENNIFER URBANO BLACKFORD, PhD
Assistant Professor of Psychiatry and Psychology, Vanderbilt University, Nashville, Tennessee

ANGELO S. BOCCIA, MA
Doctoral Student, Doctoral Program in Clinical Psychology, Department of Psychology, Temple University, Philadelphia, Pennsylvania

MEGHAN CROSBY BUDINGER, MS, LCPC
Department of Psychiatry, Johns Hopkins University School of Medicine, Baltimore, Maryland

JOHN V. CAMPO, MD
Department of Psychiatry, The Ohio State University and Nationwide Children's Hospital, The Ohio State University Wexner Medical Center, OSU Harding Hospital, Columbus, Ohio

VICTOR G. CARRION, MD
Associate Professor, Department of Psychiatry and Behavioral Sciences, Division of Child and Adolescent Psychiatry, Stanford School of Medicine, Stanford University, Stanford, California

SHANNON CHEEK, MD
Department of Psychiatry, The Ohio State University and Nationwide Children's Hospital, Columbus, Ohio

DANIELA COLOGNORI, PsyD
Postdoctoral Fellow, Assistant Research Scientist, Anita Saltz Institute for Anxiety and Mood Disorders, NYU Child Study Center, Department of Child and Adolescent Psychiatry, NYU Langone Medical Center, New York, New York

JONATHAN S. COMER, PhD
Department of Psychology, Boston University, Center for Anxiety and Related Disorders, Boston, Massachusetts

CASSIE N. FICHTER, MS
Doctoral Candidate, Clinical Psychology Doctoral Program, Long Island University, Post Campus, Brookville, New York

JEREMY K. FOX, PhD
Postdoctoral Fellow, Assistant Research Scientist, Anita Saltz Institute for Anxiety and Mood Disorders, NYU Child Study Center, Department of Child and Adolescent Psychiatry, NYU Langone Medical Center, New York, New York

MARTIN E. FRANKLIN, PhD
Department of Psychiatry, University of Pennsylvania School of Medicine, Philadelphia, Pennsylvania

BELA GANDHI, MD
Department of Psychiatry, The Ohio State University and Nationwide Children's Hospital, Columbus, Ohio

JULIE P. HARRISON, BA
Department of Psychiatry, University of Pennsylvania School of Medicine, Philadelphia, Pennsylvania

BRYCE HELLA, PhD
Postdoctoral Fellow, Susan Myket, PhD and Associates, Naperville, Illinois

KATHLEEN HERZIG-ANDERSON, PhD
Postdoctoral Fellow, Assistant Research Scientist, Anita Saltz Institute for Anxiety and Mood Disorders, NYU Child Study Center, Department of Child and Adolescent Psychiatry, NYU Langone Medical Center, New York, New York

OLGA JABLONKA, BA
Senior Project Manager, Children's Day Unit, Department of Child and Adolescent Psychiatry, Columbia University/New York State Psychiatric Institute, New York, New York

COURTNEY P. KEETON, PhD
Assistant Professor of Psychiatry and Behavioral Sciences, Department of Psychiatry, Johns Hopkins University School of Medicine, Baltimore, Maryland

HILIT KLETTER, PhD
Clinical Researcher, Department of Psychiatry and Behavioral Sciences, Division of Child and Adolescent Psychiatry, Stanford School of Medicine, Stanford University, Stanford, California

SUSANNE KNAPPE, PhD
Research Assistant, Institute of Clinical Psychology and Psychotherapy, Technische Universitaet Dresden, Dresden, Germany

KRISTIN L. KUNKLE, MS
Doctoral Candidate, Clinical Psychology Doctoral Program, Long Island University, Post Campus, Brookville, New York

JAMES T. MCCRACKEN, MD
Joseph Campbell Professor of Psychiatry, Department of Psychiatry and Biobehavioral Sciences, David Geffen School of Medicine at University of California Los Angeles, Jane & Terry Semel Institute of Neuroscience and Human Behavior, Los Angeles, California

ERIKA L. NURMI, MD, PhD
Assistant Professor of Psychiatry, Division of Child and Adolescent Psychiatry, Department of Psychiatry and Biobehavioral Sciences, David Geffen School of Medicine at University of California Los Angeles, Jane & Terry Semel Institute of Neuroscience and Human Behavior, Los Angeles, California

DONNA B. PINCUS, PhD
Department of Psychology, Boston University, Center for Anxiety and Related Disorders, Boston, Massachusetts

DANIEL S. PINE, MD
Chief, Section on Development and Affective Neuroscience, Intramural Research Program, National Institutes of Mental Health, Bethesda, Maryland

ANTHONY C. PULIAFICO, PhD
Department of Psychiatry, Columbia University/New York State Psychiatric Institute, New York, New York

AMY M. RAPP, BA
Research Assistant, Children's Day Unit, Department of Child and Adolescent Psychiatry, Columbia University/New York State Psychiatric Institute, New York, New York

MOIRA A. RYNN, MD
Associate Professor of Clinical Psychiatry, Division of Child and Adolescent Psychiatry, Department of Psychiatry and New York State Psychiatric Institute (NYSPI), Columbia University, New York, New York

DARA J. SAKOLSKY, MD, PhD
Instructor of Psychiatry, Western Psychiatric Institute and Clinic, Department of Psychiatry, University of Pittsburgh Medical Center, Pittsburgh, Pennsylvania

ALIX SARUBBI, PsyD
Postdoctoral Fellow, Columbia University Clinic for Anxiety and Related Disorders, New York, New York

CATHERINE E. STEWART, BA
Project Assistant, Anita Saltz Institute for Anxiety and Mood Disorders, NYU Child Study Center, Department of Child and Adolescent Psychiatry, NYU Langone Medical Center, New York, New York

JEFFREY R. STRAWN, MD
Department of Psychiatry and Behavioral Neuroscience, University of Cincinnati, College of Medicine; Department of Psychiatry, Cincinnati Children's Hospital Medical Center, Cincinnati, Ohio

HILARY B. VIDAIR, PhD
Assistant Professor, Clinical Psychology Doctoral Program, Co-Director of Clinical Training, Long Island University, Post Campus, Brookville; Adjunct Assistant Professor of Medical Psychology, Department of Psychiatry, Columbia University College of Physicians and Surgeons, New York, New York

CARRIE MASIA WARNER, PhD
Associate Professor of Child and Adolescent Psychiatry and Pediatrics, Associate Director of the Anita Saltz Institute for Anxiety and Mood Disorders, NYU Child Study Center, Department of Child and Adolescent Psychiatry, NYU Langone Medical Center, New York; Research Scientist, Nathan S. Kline Institute for Psychiatric Research, Orangeburg, New York

Contents

SECTION 1: DEVELOPMENT AND NEUROBIOLOGY

> This review focuses on developmental aspects in the epidemiology of anxiety disorders including prevalence, onset, natural course, longitudinal outcome, and correlates and risk factors, with focus on childhood through young adulthood. Anxiety disorders are frequent and early-emerging conditions. They may remit spontaneously; however, the same or other mental disorders often recur. Although risk factors have been identified, more work is needed to identify the most powerful predictors for onset and the progression to more complex forms of psychopathology and to understand the underlying mechanisms and interactions. This identification is crucial to facilitate research prevention, early interventions, and treatment programs.

> This article reviews the familiality, linkage, candidate gene, and genomewide association studies of obsessive–compulsive disorder, panic disorder, posttraumatic stress disorder, and other anxiety disorders (ie, generalized anxiety disorder, separation anxiety disorder, social phobia, and specific phobia). Studies involving children and adolescents are highlighted. Clinical and research implications are discussed.

> The development of fear is a normative process, and significant progress has been made in identifying fear neurocircuitry. The normal development of fear goes awry in children who develop anxiety disorders, and dysfunction in fear circuitry is likely. In this article, the authors present current knowledge about the neural basis of normal fear development and reviews findings from structural and functional neuroimaging studies of childhood anxiety disorders.

development, and treatment outcomes are presented. A summary of current empirical interventions is provided. The authors present implications for future research and for clinical practice.

Panic Disorder and School Refusal

593

Bryce Hella and Gail A. Bernstein

This article provides clinical and research information about panic disorder, agoraphobia, and school refusal. Proposed changes to the definition of panic disorder and agoraphobia for the *Diagnostic and Statistical Manual of Mental Disorders, Fifth Edition* are outlined. Treatment of panic disorder, and school refusal in children and adolescents is also discussed.

Adapting Parent-Child Interaction Therapy to Treat Anxiety Disorders in Young Children

607

Anthony C. Puliafico, Jonathan S. Comer, and Donna B. Pincus

Anxiety disorders are prevalent in children 7 years and younger; however, these children generally do not possess developmental skills required in cognitive behavior treatment. Recent efforts have adapted parent-child interaction therapy (PCIT), originally developed for disruptive and noncompliant behavior, for young children with anxiety. This article reviews the principles underlying PCIT and the rationale for adapting it to target anxiety symptoms. The authors describe two related treatment approaches that have modified PCIT to treat anxiety: (1) Pincus and colleagues' treatment for separation anxiety, and (2) Puliafico, Comer, and Albano's CALM Program for the range of early child anxiety disorders.

Social Phobia and Selective Mutism

621

Courtney P. Keeton and Meghan Crosby Budinger

Social phobia (SOP) and selective mutism (SM) are related anxiety disorders characterized by distress and dysfunction in social situations. SOP typically onsets in adolescence and affects about 8% of the general population, whereas SM onsets before age 5 and is prevalent in up to 2% of youth. Prognosis includes a chronic course that confers risk for other disorders or ongoing social disability, but more favorable outcomes may be associated with young age and low symptom severity. SOP treatments are relatively more established, whereas dissemination of promising and innovative SM-treatment strategies is needed.

SECTION 3: TREATMENT IN OTHER SETTINGS AND PARENTAL IMPACT

Anxiety in the Pediatric Medical Setting

643

Bela Gandhi, Shannon Cheek, and John V. Campo

The relationship between pediatric anxiety disorders and physical health is not well-understood, but appreciation of the importance of this relationship is growing. Significant functional impairment may accompany a chronic physical health condition such as asthma, diabetes, or epilepsy, and anxiety may complicate the course. In addition, physical disease can present with symptoms of anxiety, and anxiety disorders may present or be associated with physical symptoms such as functional abdominal pain, headache, and fatigue. This article describes anxiety and its association with physical disease, outlines assessment, and presents a treatment overview including psychotherapy and pharmacotherapy.

Anxiety disorders are the most common class of psychopathology among youth, yet many of these youngsters do not receive treatment. This is particularly concerning given the chronic course of anxiety disorders, which often lead to mood disorders, substance abuse, and serious impairment. Schools are an optimal venue for identifying anxious students and delivering mental health treatment given access to youth and ability to overcome various barriers to treatment. This article reviews four school-based treatments for anxiety disorders that have been evaluated in controlled trials. Discussion centers on feasibility, challenges to school-based implementation, and future research directions for this critical area.

The increased risk of anxiety in children of parents with psychopathology is a significant public health problem, as early-onset is associated with a variety of difficulties later in life. The aim of this article is to determine if treating parents is associated with improvements in child anxiety through the review of both top-down (parent identified for treatment) and family-focused child anxiety treatment studies. The authors present conclusions based on the state of the current literature, discuss implications for research and clinical practice, and propose utilizing a family-based model for treating parental psychopathology, parental behavior, and child anxiety.

CHILD AND ADOLESCENT PSYCHIATRIC CLINICS

DOWNLOAD
Free App!

Review Articles
THE CLINICS

NOW AVAILABLE FOR YOUR iPhone and iPad

Preface

Childhood Anxiety: Lessons Learned

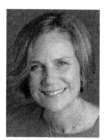 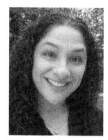 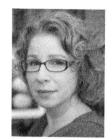

Moira A. Rynn, MD   Hilary B. Vidair, PhD   Jennifer Urbano Blackford, PhD

Guest Editors

It is an exciting time for clinicians and researchers who specialize in childhood anxiety disorders. Since the last coverage of this topic in 2005, significant advances have been made in both understanding the neurobiology of childhood anxiety and developing effective treatments for childhood anxiety. This issue is organized into three sections that cover a wide range of topics illustrating how far the field has progressed. In addition, each article highlights the areas in childhood anxiety that still require attention. Each of the articles reminds us how important it is to learn what causes pathological anxiety, how to identify it, and how to treat it effectively in order to prevent long-term adverse outcomes for children.

The first section focuses on the developmental epidemiology and the neurobiology of pediatric anxiety disorders to address the important issue of "What causes childhood anxiety?" The section begins with a review of the developmental epidemiology of childhood anxiety by Beeso and Knappe. Developmental epidemiology is a rapidly growing field where epidemiological methods are used to understand the origins and course of psychiatric disorders in large, representative samples. These studies have significantly contributed to the identification of biological and environmental factors that contribute to the origins of childhood anxiety, such as parental psychopathology, child temperament, and exposure to adverse environments. In addition, these studies have demonstrated that anxiety disorders start early and have a long course, including both continued anxiety as well as increased risk for other psychiatric disorders. In the second article, Sakolsky and colleagues review the current findings from genetic studies of anxiety. While rapid advances in genotyping technology have enabled large-scale psychiatric genetic studies, only recently have these studies focused on anxiety disorders. As with other psychiatric disorders, replications of genetic findings are few; however, there are several exciting and replicated findings in post-traumatic stress disorder, obsessive-compulsive disorder, and panic disorder. In the section's final article, Blackford and Pine review the normative development of fear, the neural circuitry involved in fear, and current neuroimaging findings in childhood anxiety disorders. Advances in neuroimaging technology and pediatric neuroimaging methods have enabled researchers

Child Adolesc Psychiatric Clin N Am 21 (2012) xiii–xv
http://dx.doi.org/10.1016/j.chc.2012.06.001   childpsych.theclinics.com

to examine the neural circuitry underlying childhood anxiety disorders. In generalized anxiety disorder and social phobia, dysfunction in amygdala-prefrontal cortex neurocircuitry is implicated, whereas in obsessive-compulsive disorder, structural and functional anomalies in the basal ganglia, orbitofrontal cortex, and anterior cingulate cortex are evident. Together these articles demonstrate that anxiety emerges relatively early in life and has a neurobiological basis. To prevent a long course of suffering, it is critical to both preempt the development of anxiety in high-risk children and intervene early with anxious children. Discovering the genetic and neural underpinnings of anxiety disorders will give insight into the underlying pathophysiology, leading to new targets for prevention, intervention, and treatment.

The second section provides the latest advances in treating pediatric anxiety disorders and related disorders from an evidence-based perspective. It begins with an article by Strawn and colleagues on pharmacotherapy for pediatric anxiety. The field of pediatric psychopharmacology for anxiety disorders has grown dramatically over the past 10 to 15 years. All this work has converged to recommend serotonin reuptake inhibitors as first-line medication treatment. However, even with adequate treatment with a medication there are still children who remain symptomatic, highlighting the need to develop new medication treatment options based on what is known about the underlying neurobiology. This section then takes a specific look at each anxiety disorder's diagnostic criteria, clinical presentation, differential diagnosis, evidence-based treatment and promising methods, and implications for research and clinical practice. First, Jablonka and colleagues begin by describing well-known and innovative cognitive-behavioral treatments for the child anxiety triad, a term that includes separation anxiety disorder, generalized anxiety disorder, and social phobia. Novel treatment approaches discussed include emotion-focused cognitive-behavioral therapy, mindfulness, and attention bias modification treatment. Second, Franklin and colleagues review phenomenological similarities, differences, and comorbidity between obsessive-compulsive disorder and tic-related disorders. They describe how to use exposure therapy and habit reversal techniques separately or in sequence to treat comorbid conditions. Clinical controversies surrounding these treatments' mechanism of action are addressed. Third, Carrion and colleagues review the presentation, treatment, and biology of childhood post-traumatic stress disorder. The field has advanced to appreciate that the presentation of this disorder in childhood is different from that seen in adults and may have to do with the timing and chronicity of the trauma. These advances have led to the development of psychotherapeutic techniques designed to target the inherent plasticity of the growing child's brain, for example, techniques that reduce stress-mediated inhibition and promote cortical neurogenesis. Fourth, Hella and Bernstein review the small but expanding literature base on the cognitive-behavioral and pharmacological treatment of childhood panic disorder and agoraphobia as well as the existing treatment literature on school refusal. They delineate the proposed DSM-V criteria for panic disorder. Ideas for collaboration between school professionals and clinicians to improve school attendance rates are also provided. Fifth, Puliafico and colleagues describe two modified versions of Parent-Child Interaction Therapy used to treat separation anxiety. This includes the newly developed CALM program, which incorporates parent-led, in vivo exposure. Finally, Keeton and colleagues focus on similarities, differences, and comorbidity between social phobia and selective mutism. Well-known cognitive-behavioral and pharmacological treatments for social phobia are reviewed. This is paired with an overview of emerging treatments for selective mutism, including internet-based CBT, developmentally modified CBT for preschoolers, and intensive summer camp programs. Together, these articles balance the impressive body of treatment research that has been conducted in the field of child anxiety disorders in the last two decades with their pitfalls and promising new interventions that have materialized to address these limitations.

The third section aims to address two cutting edge issues in our field: How can we effectively implement evidence-based treatments for child anxiety in real-world settings? and what are the best ways to address parental psychopathology in the context of managing child anxiety? First, Gandhi and colleagues describe the complexity of determining the presence of an anxiety disorder in children suffering from a chronic medical condition and the modification of present anxiety treatments delivered in the primary care setting. Second, Herzig and colleagues discuss advantages of and empirical evidence for school-based child anxiety interventions. Suggestions are made regarding future directions for schools as a venue that can provide children with access to mental health services they otherwise might not receive. Finally, Vidair and colleagues conducted the first comprehensive literature review aiming to understand the effects of treating parental psychopathology on child anxiety. They discuss research showing that parental psychopathology leads to worse outcomes for children suffering from anxiety disorders and the great need to develop treatment paradigms that equally treat the child and the parent.

In conclusion, during the past decade we have seen many important advances in both identifying some of the neurobiological underpinnings of childhood anxiety and developing effective treatments. We thank each of the authors for contributing to this issue—we could not have put together such an amazing collection of articles without them. We look forward to the advancements of new clinical and research directions in the field of child anxiety that are sure to come in the next decade.

Moira A. Rynn, MD
Department of Psychiatry New York State Psychiatric Institute & Columbia University
College of Physicians and Surgeons
1051 Riverside Drive, Mail Unit 74
New York, NY 10032, USA

Hilary B. Vidair, PhD
Clinical Psychology Doctoral Program
Long Island University, Post Campus
720 Northern Boulevard, Brookville
NY 11548, USA
Columbia University College of Physicians and Surgeons
1051 Riverside Drive, Unit 24
New York, NY 10032, USA

Jennifer Urbano Blackford, PhD
Departments of Psychiatry and Psychology
Vanderbilt University School of Medicine
1601 23rd Avenue South
Nashville, TN 37212, USA

E-mail addresses:
rynnm@nyspi.columbia.edu
hilary.vidair@liu.edu
Jennifer.Blackford@Vanderbilt.edu

Developmental Epidemiology of Anxiety Disorders

Katja Beesdo-Baum, PhD*, Susanne Knappe, PhD

KEYWORDS

- Anxiety • Prevalence • Onset • Course • Outcome • Risk factors

KEY POINTS

- Anxiety disorders are frequent and early-emerging conditions associated with considerable developmental, psychosocial, and psychopathologic complications.
- Early anxiety syndromes may remit spontaneously, but the vast majority of children and adolescents with an anxiety disorder suffer from either the same condition or other mental disorders throughout their life.
- Potential risk factors for the development of anxiety disorders have been identified, such as parental psychopathology, behaviorally inhibited temperament, and early life adversity.
- Effective treatments exist for anxiety disorders and related conditions, but the size of the problem cannot be resolved through treatment interventions alone; better strategies need to be identified for improved prevention and early intervention.

The period of childhood through adolescence is the core risk phase for the first occurrence of anxiety that may range from transient mild symptoms to full-blown persistent anxiety disorders. The clinically valid assessment of anxiety symptoms, syndromes, and disorders is crucial to determine the prevalence, incidence, and longitudinal course and outcome of anxiety disorders. Further, identification of risk factors and specific anxiety characteristics that could serve as solid predictors for malignant or more benign course patterns is important for improved early recognition as well as prevention and treatment in this age span.

Anxiety is a basic emotion already present in infancy and childhood, with expressions falling on a continuum from mild to severe. Anxiety is not typically pathologic but commonly adaptive when it facilitates avoidance of danger. The organisms' responses to danger and the underlying brain circuitry engaged by threats reflect these adaptive aspects of anxiety.[1] Read more in the article by Blackford and Pine elsewhere in this issue. Maladaptive and pathologic anxiety is characterized by

The authors have nothing to disclose.
Institute of Clinical Psychology and Psychotherapy, Technische Universitaet Dresden, Chemnitzer Strasse 46, 01187 Dresden, Germany
* Corresponding author.
E-mail address: Katja.Beesdo@tu-dresden.de

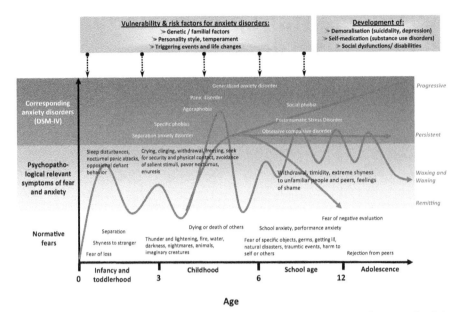

Fig. 1. Normative fears and pathological anxiety embedded in a heuristic framework of the evolution of anxiety disorders. Fears and anxieties manifest in childhood as part of typical development. In infancy, toddlerhood, and early childhood, children are fearful of immediate, concrete threats in the environment. As the child cognitively matures, these fears begin to incorporate anticipatory events and stimuli of an imaginary or abstract nature. Thus, normative fears are age-dependent and likely to be transient but may—if occurring intensively—be associated with psychopathologically relevant symptoms. These symptoms may develop into manifest anxiety disorders if they persist or occur exaggerated beyond normal developmental trends. The further natural course of anxiety disorders may be characterized by a progressing, chronic persistent, or recurrent (waxing and waning) form. Spontaneous remissions from an anxiety disorder are not rare, but syndromal shifts frequently occur. Note that the corresponding anxiety disorders in the figure are placed to reflect the earliest onset of these conditions. The peak incidence periods for these anxiety disorders are later in childhood and adolescence (see **Fig. 2**).

persisting or extensive degrees of anxiety and avoidance associated with subjective distress or impairment.[2] The differentiation between normal and pathologic anxiety can be difficult, particularly in children because many fears and anxieties manifest in childhood as part of typical development[3,4] (compare **Fig. 1**). Thus, these phenomena occur in most children, frequently acutely distressing, but typically transient.

Diagnostic criteria for anxiety disorders are described in the Diagnostic and Statistical Manual of Mental Disorders (DSM, currently version IV-TR, American Psychiatric Association[2]) and the International Classification of Diseases (ICD, currently version 10, World Health Organization[5]). Many anxiety disorders share common clinical features such as extensive anxiety, physiologic anxiety symptoms, behavioral disturbances such as extreme avoidance of feared objects, and associated distress or impairment.[2,6,7]

However, narrowly categorized, anxiety disorders such as panic disorder, agoraphobia, social phobia, and subtypes of specific phobias also exhibit a substantial degree of phenotypical diversity and heterogeneity (eg, Refs[6–10]). For example, even the various subtypes of specific phobias differ in terms of the focus of fear (eg, internal feelings such as disgust and fear of physical symptoms such as fainting in blood-injury-injection subtype versus fear of danger or harm in environmental subtype) and the physiologic fear response (eg, vasovagal fainting only in the blood-injury-injection subtype; different neural activation patterns across various specific phobia subtypes).[9,10] Further, the anxiety disorders might present differently in children and adolescents as compared with adults, which is crucial for assessment and diagnosis in this age span. The DSM-IV provides some, albeit few, differences in diagnostic criteria for children (vs adults), for example different requirements for duration or symptom type or count, or insight into the excessiveness/inadequacy of fear, within the same criteria set (**Box 1**). The exception is separation anxiety disorder, which is defined specifically for children. In the ICD-10, children receive diagnostic codings differing from adults for anxiety disorders that reflect exaggerations of normal developmental trends:

- Separation anxiety disorder
- Phobic anxiety disorder and social anxiety disorder of childhood
- Other childhood emotional disorders
- Childhood emotional disorder unspecified.

The development of explicit descriptive diagnostic criteria has facilitated the development of a range of diagnostic instruments for the assessment of anxiety symptoms, syndromes, and disorders. (For an overview see Ref.[11]) Also read the article by John Campo elsewhere in this issue. Diagnosticians and clinicians should be aware, however, of their limitations particularly related to obtaining self-reports from children and adolescents.[12–14] Young children may have difficulties in communicating relevant emotions, cognitions, and behaviors as well as the associated distress and impairments to the diagnostician[15] because of lack of cognitive capabilities, language skills, or emotional understanding. Assessments therefore require solicitation of information from multiple sources beyond the child, for example by parents or teachers, to reliably and validly distinguish among normal, subclinical, and pathologic anxiety. Clinicians should take into account these developmental differences when assessing anxiety in children in order to make a diagnostic decision[13] (see **Fig. 1**).

PREVALENCE OF ANXIETY DISORDERS IN CHILDHOOD AND ADOLESCENCE
Variance in Anxiety Estimates

Anxiety disorders are the most frequent class of mental disorders in childhood and adolescence. Prevalence estimates for anxiety disorders in community samples vary in part because of differences in the:

- Studied age groups
- Assessment instruments (eg, Composite International Diagnostic Interview, Kiddie-Schedule for Affective Disorders and Schizophrenia for school-aged children
- Information source (eg, self-report, parent/teacher report)
- Method of data aggregation (from multiple information sources or multiple assessment waves)
- Diagnostic systems used (ie, DSM-III-R, DSM-IV, ICD-10)
- Data aggregation from various assessment waves in prospective-longitudinal studies
- Number and type of diagnoses included in summary categories (eg, "any" anxiety disorder)
- Strictness of application of criteria in generating diagnoses (eg, impairment required or not).

Box 1
DSM-IV anxiety disorders and specific diagnostic criteria for children (vs adults)

DSM-IV Anxiety disorders and specific criteria for children

Anxiety disorders

Agoraphobia without history of panic disorder (no specific criteria for children)

Panic disorder with agoraphobia (no specific criteria for children)

Panic disorder without agoraphobia (no specific criteria for children)

Social phobia

Specific criteria for children:

B: Anxiety may be expressed by crying, tantrums, freezing, shrinking from social situations with unfamiliar people.

C: Recognizes that fear is excessive/unreasonable may be absent.

F: In individuals <18 years, duration is at least 6 months.

Specific phobia

Specific criteria for children:

B: Anxiety may be expressed by crying, tantrums, freezing, clinging.

C: Recognizes that fear is excessive/unreasonable may be absent.

F: In individuals <18 years, duration is at least 6 months.

Generalized anxiety disorder

Specific criteria for children:

C: 1 instead of 3 out of 6 symptoms is required.

Obsessive-compulsive disorder

Specific criteria for children:

B: Criterion does not apply to children.

Acute stress disorder (no specific criteria for children)

Posttraumatic stress disorder

Specific criteria for children:

A(2): Criterion may be expressed by disorganized behavior or agitated behavior.

B(1): Repetitive play may occur in which themes or aspects of the trauma are expressed.

B(2): Frightening dreams without recognizable content.

B(3): Trauma-specific reenactment may occur.

Residual category: **Anxiety disorder not otherwise specified** (no specific criteria for children)

Disorders usually first diagnosed in infancy, childhood, or adolescence

Separation anxiety disorder

Residual category: **Disorders usually first diagnosed in infancy, childhood, or adolescence not otherwise specified**

With the possible exception of posttraumatic stress disorder (PTSD),[16] differences in prevalence estimates from different countries are unlikely reflective of true regional differences, at least in Western, industrialized countries where most epidemiologic studies were conducted. As reviewed by Lewis-Fernández and colleagues,[17] however, there may be cross-cultural variability in prevalence rates for anxiety disorders with lower rates found among Asian and African American individuals.

Cumulative Prevalence of Anxiety Disorder

Despite some variation in prevalence rates due to method variance, the lifetime or cumulative prevalence of "any anxiety disorder" in children or adolescents from Western countries is about 15% to 20%[18–20] (see comprehensive overview in Ref[11]), and many affected youngsters are diagnosed with more than one anxiety disorder.[21] The cross-sectional adolescent supplement of the US National Comorbidity Survey (NCS-A) recently revealed among 13- to 18-year-olds a lifetime prevalence of 31.9% for any (pure or comorbid) anxiety disorder with some impairment or moderate symptom severity, and a rate of 8.3% when requiring severe distress or impairment (**Table 1**).[22] Given that period prevalence rates (eg, 1 year, 6 months, 1- month) are not considerably lower than the lifetime estimates for most anxiety conditions[19,23–25] (see comprehensive overview in Ref[11]), a considerable persistence in terms of chronicity or recurrence can be assumed.

Frequently Occurring Anxiety Disorders

The most frequent disorders among children and adolescents are

- Separation anxiety disorder with prevalence estimates ranging from 2.8% to 8%[22,26–28]
- Specific phobias with rates of approximately 15%[22,29,30]
- Social phobias with rates up to around 10%.[22,31,32]

In the NCS-A, separation anxiety disorder was found to be the anxiety disorder with drastically lower period prevalence rates (12-month: 1.6%, 30-day: .6%)[23] compared with the lifetime prevalence rate (7.6%),[22] which suggests that this condition rarely persists into adolescence.

Agoraphobia and panic disorder are low prevalence conditions in childhood (1% or lower)[33,34]; higher prevalence rates are found in adolescence (2% to 3% for panic and 3% to 4% for agoraphobia).[19,22,25,34]

A precise prevalence estimation for generalized anxiety disorder (GAD) in children and adolescents is difficult because prior to the introduction of DSM-IV in 1994, children presenting with worries about multiple events were given the diagnosis of overanxious disorder (OAD). Studies reveal lower prevalence rates for GAD than for OAD,[25,35] and it remains unclear whether the DSM-III-R criteria for OAD and the DSM-IV criteria for youth with GAD are identifying the same disorder.[36] The recent NCS-A reports a lifetime prevalence among US adolescents of 2.2%, with .9% being affected by severe GAD.[22] The prevalence was low (1%) among the youngest adolescents (12/13 years) and rates increased with age (3% among 17- to 18-year-olds). The cumulative incidence for GAD in the 10-year prospective-longitudinal Early Developmental Stages of Psychopathology (EDSP) study, which was conducted among adolescents and young adults from Munich, Germany, was 4.3% at age 34 with relatively few cases emerging in childhood and an incidence increase in adolescence.[37] These findings suggest that in contrast to OAD, DSM-IV–defined GAD is relatively rare in childhood and considerably more common among adolescents and young adults.

For PTSD, the NCS-A reports a total lifetime prevalence of 7.6%, which, however, is considerably lower (.6%) if requiring severe impairment/distress—a rate closer to estimates of other studies among adolescents.[18,19] Nevertheless, rates for PTSD may be higher in the United States than for example in European countries.[16]

Table 1
Prevalence estimates for anxiety disorders among US adolescents (NCS-A)

DSM-IV Disorder	Lifetime Prevalence by Sex %		Lifetime Prevalence by Age %				Lifetime Prevalence Total %	Lifetime Prevalence-Severe Impairment %	12-Month Prevalence %	1-Month Prevalence %
	Female	Male	13–14 y	15–16 y	17–18 y					
Agoraphobia	3.4	1.4	2.5	2.5	2.0		2.4	2.4	1.8	0.8
Generalized anxiety disorder	3.0	1.5	1.0	2.8	3.0		2.2	0.9	1.1	0.4
Social phobia	11.2	7.0	7.7	9.7	10.1		9.1	1.3	8.2	4.6
Specific phobia	22.1	16.7	21.6	18.3	17.7		19.3	0.6	15.8	9.5
Panic disorder	2.6	2.0	1.8	2.3	3.3		2.3	2.3	1.9	0.8
Posttraumatic stress disorder	8.0	2.3	3.7	5.1	7.0		5.0	1.5	3.9	1.6
Separation anxiety disorder	9.0	6.3	7.8	8.0	6.7		7.6	0.6	1.6	0.6
Any anxiety disorder	38.0	26.1	31.4	32.1	32.3		31.9	8.3	24.9	14.9

Data from Refs.[22,23]

The prevalence estimates for obsessive-compulsive disorder (OCD) in childhood and adolescence are low (.5% to 1%[38]), although some studies report higher rates among adolescents (eg, 1-year prevalence 4%[32]).

All anxiety disorders occur more frequently among females than among males with a ratio of approximately 2 to 1 to 3 to 1. Gender differences may emerge as early as childhood, and they increase with age.[39] This difference is exemplified by the lines in **Fig. 2**, which reflect the age-specific cumulative lifetime incidence rates for anxiety disorders up to age 33 among females and males as assessed in the EDSP study. In contrast to other anxiety disorders, for OCD some other studies report a male preponderance for the occurrence of first obsessions or compulsions in childhood, which turns into a female preponderance in adolescence (eg, Ref[40]).

ONSET OF ANXIETY DISORDERS

The onset for the first or any anxiety disorder is clearly in childhood.[22,37,41,42] There is, however, some noteworthy heterogeneity between the onset patterns of specific anxiety disorders. The bars in **Fig. 2** show the cumulative age of onset distribution for specific anxiety disorders in males and females assessed in the EDSP study. Separation anxiety disorder and specific phobia reveal the earliest onsets with 50% of cases emerging before the ages of 5 and 8, respectively, and almost all cases emerging until the age of 12. Social phobia and OCD show a steep increase in onset risk in early adolescence, followed by agoraphobia, panic disorder, and GAD that reveal core onset risk periods in later adolescent ages and into early adulthood, albeit first cases can emerge as early as childhood. PTSD was observed to emerge in adolescence and throughout early adulthood. For all the anxiety disorders, despite differences in prevalence, no remarkable gender differences in onset patterns occur. Slightly earlier onsets are seen for specific phobia in males, primarily due to natural environmental subtype (not shown in figure, compare Ref[11]), and for GAD and PTSD in females. Overall, these onset patterns are in line with findings from other studies.[41,43,44]

NATURAL COURSE AND OUTCOME OF ANXIETY DISORDERS

Findings from clinical adult populations[45,46] or cross-sectional studies that rely on retrospective information[23,47] suggest that anxiety disorders take a highly persistent course. The biases inherent in such studies, however, may lead to overestimations of the degree to which anxiety disorders typically appear chronic.[48] The natural course and outcome of anxiety disorders are therefore ideally assessed in prospective-longitudinal population–based studies conducted during the high-risk periods for manifestation of anxiety disorders, for example childhood and adolescence. Indeed, such studies only partially support the findings from clinical and cross-sectional retrospective studies.

Stability and Remission of Anxiety Disorders (Homotypic Continuity)

Whereas prospective-longitudinal population studies show that children or adolescents diagnosed with an anxiety disorder, compared with those without, are at statistically increased risk to have the same disorder[25,26,49] or signs and symptoms of the same disorder[48,50] at later points in time (*homotypic prediction*, Ref[51]), they also show that the proportion of youth diagnosed again with the same anxiety disorder (*stability rate*) is numerically rather low to moderate (for comprehensive review of studies see Refs[11,52]). For example, in the 15-year prospective multiwave Zurich Cohort-study[53] a low stability (4%) was found for pure (non-comorbid) anxiety disorders (defined as GAD or panic disorder). Last and colleagues[42,54] reported for

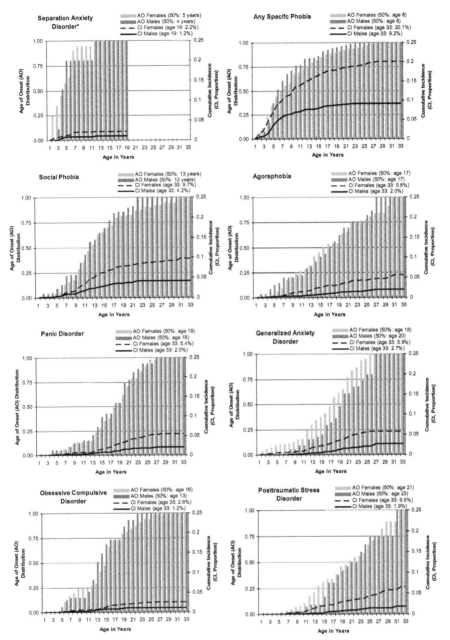

Fig. 2. Cumulative incidence (CI) and age of onset (AO) distribution of anxiety disorders by gender (EDSP; N = 3021). Bars show the cumulative age of onset distribution; lines show the age-dependent cumulative lifetime incidence; in phobias impairment was required among subjects aged 18 years or older. *Separation anxiety disorder was only assessed in the younger study cohort.

children and adolescents with anxiety disorders that 80% remitted from the anxiety shown initially over the 3- to 4-year follow-up. Similarly, in the prospective-longitudinal EDSP study, 19.7% of adolescents with threshold baseline anxiety disorder met threshold anxiety criteria again at 2-year follow-up.[50]

Stability of Diagnostic Status

The probability of a negative outcome increased as a function of severity of baseline anxiety diagnostic status. For specific anxiety diagnoses, a considerable variability in outcome can be observed. For example, in the EDSP study,[50] taking stable threshold and subthreshold diagnoses both at baseline and at follow-up, panic disorder (44%) and specific phobia (30.1%) were found to be most stable whereas other anxiety disorders showed lower stability rates, particularly agoraphobia (13.4%) and social phobia (15.8%). These stability rates may slightly increase, for example due to recurrences, when following up affected individuals for longer periods of time. For social phobia in the EDSP, for example, 15.1% of baseline threshold cases met threshold criteria again at least once during any of the follow-up assessments over up to 10 years, and further 21.2% had at least subthreshold social phobia.[48] Meeting continuously disorder criteria over long time periods, however, is rare. Based on higher 12-month to lifetime compared with 30-day to 12-month prevalence ratios in the cross-sectional NCS-A, Kessler and colleagues[23] recently concluded that persistence of anxiety disorders is more due to recurrences rather than chronicity. In the prospective Zurich cohort study, no individual with social phobia was diagnosed continuously at each follow-up assessment after the disorder had manifested.[55] Overall, among children and adolescents with an anxiety disorder, there is a considerable degree of fluctuation in diagnostic status of the specific anxiety disorder examined. Anxiety disorders have a strong tendency to naturally wax and wane over time, particularly in young age groups[50] (compare **Fig. 1**).

Predictors of Natural Course of Anxiety Disorders

Relatively little research exists on the correlates and predictors of the natural course of anxiety disorders among community youth. Kessler and colleagues[23] found, among US adolescents, female gender to be associated with a higher persistence of most anxiety disorders, whereas other demographic variables such as race/ethnicity, family income, and family composition were not consistently found as correlates. Consistent with the general notion of Noyes and colleagues[56] that "the past predicts the future," for example that the best prognostic indicators for the anxiety course are symptom severity and duration of illness, the prospective-longitudinal EDSP study revealed for social phobia several clinical features such as early age of onset, the generalized subtype, a high number of catastrophic anxiety cognitions, and severe avoidance and impairment as predictors for higher social phobia persistence and diagnostic stability.[48] Interestingly, comorbidity with other disorders was not found to predict the course of social phobia with the exception of co-occurring panic attacks that were associated with both higher persistence and diagnostic stability. In addition, established vulnerability characteristics for the onset of anxiety conditions such as parental history of social phobia and depression and a behavioral inhibited temperament (see later discussion) were related to poor prognosis. Thus, besides gender and clinical diagnostic information, familial and temperamental characteristics may inform about prognosis of anxiety disorders and seem useful to target treatment interventions.

Heterotypic Continuity

Despite the limited homotypic continuity of anxiety disorders observed in prospective-longitudinal community studies, children and adolescents whose specific anxiety disorder seems to improve or remit are usually not completely healthy in their further course of life. For example, in the EDSP

- Only 10% of children and adolescents with (pure or comorbid) specific phobias at baseline had no mental disorder at 10-year follow up (full diagnostic remission);
- 41% reported specific phobia again (strict homotypic continuity), and
- 73% overall were diagnosed with any anxiety and/or depressive disorder at subsequent assessments (heterotypic continuity).[57]

Similarly, for baseline social phobia cases

- Only 13% of baseline social phobia cases were free of any diagnosis during the 10-year follow-up;
- 35% reported the same disorder, and
- 64% reported any anxiety/depression.

For GAD and PTSD, all baseline cases revealed either homotypic or heterotypic continuity. Similar findings emerged from other multiwave, prospective-longitudinal studies.[26,42,53,58]

In childhood, after onset of the first (ie, pure) anxiety disorder emerged, a pattern with multiple anxiety disorders often develops by adolescence or early adulthood.[21] The "load" of anxiety seems to contribute to the development of secondary psychopathologic complications such as further anxiety disorders, major depression, substance dependence, and suicidality as well as to other adverse developmental outcomes such as educational underachievement and early parenthood.[59] Thus, for many anxiety cases even if strict homotypic continuity is moderate, there is a substantial degree of continuity of psychopathology as indicated by the later presence of other anxiety disorders (broad homotypic continuity) or other disorders (heterotypic continuity).

Development of Psychopathological Complications

The development of a cascade of psychopathologic complications is a frequent outcome of primary anxiety disorders.[6] Heterotypic predictions are found from childhood to adolescence, and from adolescence to early adulthood.[51] In particular, cross-sectional and longitudinal studies reveal strong associations between anxiety disorders and depressive disorders.[37,42,59–63] For example, prospective epidemiologic studies found that children and adolescents with specific fears and phobias (especially fear of darkness),[64] social phobia,[31,65,66] or other types of anxiety disorders (agoraphobia, panic disorder, GAD)[37,49,66] are at increased risk for a subsequent depressive disorder. Certain clinical characteristics of anxiety disorders, such as more severe impairment or co-occurring panic attacks, are associated with secondary depression risk.[31,66]

Besides depression, substance abuse or dependence often develops as heterotypic problem among individuals with primary anxiety disorders.[59,61,67–70] It has been suggested that alcohol, drug, or medication use is motivated possibly to deal with anxiety symptoms leading to substance-related problems over time.[71] Findings of no significant heterotypic predictions between specific anxiety disorders and later substance use disorders (eg, Refs[25,49]) may possibly be due to the fact that respondents have not been followed up long enough to develop this outcome.

CORRELATES AND RISK FACTORS FOR ANXIETY DISORDERS

A range of variables assessed in epidemiologic studies have been found to be associated with anxiety disorders. Cross-sectional studies merely allow us to identify correlates and to generate initial hypotheses about potential risk factors. Prospective-longitudinal studies are necessary to show that a factor precedes the outcome and can therefore be considered a risk factor.[72] Despite considerable overlap among the correlates and risk factors for specific anxiety disorders and for anxiety and depressive disorders, given the heterogeneity in terms of phenomenology, onset, and course, there are also important differences. Beyond the discussion here, further information on correlates and risk factors for anxiety disorders can be found in comprehensive reviews.[73–76]

Demographics

With the exception of urbanization (rural/urban),[18,22,77,78] various sociodemographic variables have been linked with anxiety disorders. Female gender is the most consistently found risk factor for the development of each of the specific anxiety conditions.[18,26,79] Gender differences are usually small in childhood and enhance with age to a ratio of approximately 2 to 1 to 3 to 1 for females versus males[39] (see also **Fig. 2**). The recent NCS-A found higher rates of anxiety disorders among non-Hispanic black compared with non-Hispanic white adolescents and among respondents with divorced or separated compared with married or cohabiting parents.[22] Anxiety disorders are frequently also found among individuals with lower compared with higher education,[18] whereby it remains unclear to which degree the lower educational performance is a predictor, correlate, or consequence of anxiety. In the NCS-A, low parental education was shown to be associated with adolescent anxiety disorders, but also with all other disorder classes assessed in the study. With some exceptions,[22,77,78] epidemiologic studies also evidence associations between low household income or unsatisfactory financial situations and anxiety disorders.[18] Consistent with the assumption that sociodemographic risks co-occur, Copeland and colleagues[80] identified a moderate risk class containing low parental education and poverty that was associated with offspring anxiety disorders as well as with depressive, but not externalizing, disorders. After controlling for comorbidity and a broad range of other putative risk factors, Shanahan and colleagues[81] found parental unemployment to be associated with anxiety and behavioral disorders, but not with depressive disorders in the offspring.

Familial Aggregation

Parental anxiety and depression

Family-based, clinical-epidemiologic, and twin studies revealed that anxiety disorders "run in families"—similar to depressive, substance, or other mental disorders. Family studies and epidemiologic studies with linked assessments of familial psychopathology consistently reveal a strong familial aggregation of anxiety disorders.[82–85] Children of parents with an anxiety disorder have a substantially increased risk to also develop an anxiety disorder.[86] A particular risk was evidenced for offspring with two affected parents[82,85] and for offspring of severely affected parents as indicated by impairment, number of anxiety disorders, and early onset of anxiety disorders.[87]

Besides parental anxiety disorders, parental depression was also found to be associated with offspring anxiety.[88,89] Investigations into the specificity of the familial aggregation of anxiety and other mental disorders revealed mixed findings with some evidence for specificity. For example, in the longitudinal Oregon study of youth, relatives of individuals with anxiety disorder alone and a depressive disorder alone more frequently also had an anxiety disorder alone and a depressive disorder alone, respectively. Relatives of adolescents with comorbid anxiety/depression were more likely to show pure anxiety, pure depression, or comorbid anxiety/depression.[90] In the Dunedin birth cohort, familial depression liability was associated with pure depression but not with pure GAD among offsprings.[91] In the EDSP study, parental GAD was associated with GAD and with pure panic/phobia conditions as well as with comorbid anxiety/depressive disorders among offspring but not with pure depressive disorders.[37] Parental pure depressive disorders were only associated with offspring pure depressive disorders, but not with pure panic/phobias or, after adjusting for comorbidity, with GAD. Thus, these findings indicate a familial transmission of anxiety that occurs at least partly independent from depression. Furthermore, some specificity seems to exist in the familial transmission of specific anxiety disorders.[37,92]

Transmission mechanisms
The exact mechanisms by which anxiety is transmitted from parents to offspring are complex and to date still poorly understood. The strong familial aggregation may be due to genetic factors, the family environment (eg, parental rearing, attachment), or both, for example in terms of gene-environment-interaction processes. Some research suggests that the familial transmission starts as early as during pregnancy[93] (see fetal programming[94]). The intrauterine development of the fetus is affected by multiple intertwined pregnancy processes, and recent findings provide strong support for associations of maternal perinatal anxiety and depressive disorders with a wide range of pregnancy and delivery complications, maternal postpartum disorders, and an increased risk for subsequent psychopathologically relevant childhood outcomes.[95] These outcomes (eg, high reactivity, behavioral inhibition, insecure attachment, regulation problems) might be diagnosis-specific, general vulnerability markers, or early antecedents, respectively, risk factors for later mental disorders in the offspring. Findings from twin studies that can disentangle genetic from shared and nonshared environmental contributions in the familial transmission of anxiety disorders (read more in the article by Smoller elsewhere in this issue) suggest a moderate genetic heritability (30% to 40%) for the range of anxiety disorders.[96] The considerable remaining variance in liability can be attributed primarily to individual (nonshared) rather than shared familial environmental factors. In terms of specificity, twin studies indicate that the genetic liability for specific anxiety disorders overlaps partly.[96,97] Furthermore, particularly GAD seems to share genetic liability with major depression, but both disorders can be differentiated based on environmental risk.[98,99] The identification of specific (single) genes underlying anxiety disorders is challenged by the etiologic and phenotypic heterogeneity, the use of different diagnostic systems or thresholds, and comorbidity.[100] So far, progress in identifying and replicating genes underlying mental disorders is still low.[101]

Personality and Temperament

Personality trait vulnerabilities such as neuroticism, trait-anxiety, and negative affect as well as temperamental styles such as behavioral inhibition are likely overlapping constructs that can be viewed as precursor conditions to anxiety disorders. The tripartite-model conceptualizes general distress or negative affectivity as general higher order vulnerability factor for anxiety and depression, whereas physiologic hyperarousal is specific to anxiety, and low positive affectivity is specific to depression.[102,103] Similarly, in a hierarchical model,[104] negative affectivity is the higher order factor relevant for anxiety and depression, but on a lower level each anxiety disorder contains an additional specific component. A number of studies support the tripartite and the hierarchical model for anxiety and depression symptoms (eg, Refs[105–107]). Twin studies consistently evidence high correlations between neuroticism and anxiety and depression as well as their co-occurrence.[108,109] It is estimated that about 50% of the genetic correlations between these disorders derives from the genetic factor for neuroticism. Epidemiologic studies are generally in support of these findings with few indications of specificity between anxiety and depression outcomes.[110,111]

Behavioral inhibition is conceptualized as the consistent tendency to display fear and withdrawal in unfamiliar situations,[112] which is under some genetic control, detectable early in life, and at least moderately stable across time.[113–115]

Temperamental extremes are often conceptualized as risk factors, but as noted by Angold and Costello,[116] there is also the possibility that "they already *are* the disorders of later life." Retaining the risk factor perspective here, with few exceptions,[117,118] behavioral inhibition was found to significantly increase the risk for the development of anxiety disorders[115,119,120] and social phobia in particular.[115,121,122] There are also indications for a specific link of behavioral inhibition with anxiety disorders in contrast to depression.[37,115]

Adverse Environment

A range of environmental factors have been examined as correlates and potential risk factors for anxiety disorders in epidemiologic research.

Childhood adversity
Most epidemiologic studies find associations between adverse experiences in childhood such as loss of parents, parental divorce, physical and sexual abuse, and almost all mental disorders, including anxiety disorders. For example, Kessler and colleagues[123] found in a large US community study of adults associations between retrospectively reported childhood adversities, including loss events (eg, parental divorce), parental psychopathologies (eg, maternal depression), interpersonal traumas (eg, rape), and the subsequent onset of anxiety disorders, mood disorders, addictive disorders, and acting out disorders.

A history of neglect or abuse was also found as a strong predictor of psychiatric morbidity (ie, anxiety disorders, depression, substance use disorders) in a large community study among adults in the Netherlands.[124] In a study among youth in New Zealand, individuals who reported childhood sexual abuse had higher rates of major depression, anxiety disorder, conduct disorder, substance use disorder, and suicidal behavior than those not reporting sexual abuse.[125] Furthermore, there were consistent relationships between the extent of childhood sexual abuse and the risk of mental disorders.

Only few studies examined whether the nonspecificity of the findings mainly emerges because of the frequent comorbidity among disorders. Moffitt and colleagues[91] found in the Dunedin birth cohort study that childhood maltreatment was associated with both pure GAD and pure major depression indicating in fact a nonspecific link between early adversities and mental disorders. Findings from the EDSP, in contrast, suggest some specificity. In this study, childhood separation events were associated with pure panic/phobias, with GAD and with comorbid anxiety/depression but not with pure depression.[37]

Negative life events

Negative life events have been consistently evidenced as risk factors for depressive disorders,[126,127] but several studies also found associations with anxiety disorders. For example, in the EDSP study, traumatic events predicted subsequent anxiety and depressive disorders.[128] It has been suggested that threat events tend to precede anxiety disorders, whereas loss events tend to precede depression.[129] Consistent with that result, Shanahan and colleagues[81] found, after controlling for comorbidity and a broad range of other putative risk factors, dangerous neighborhood was specifically associated with anxiety disorders. Loss events, in contrast, were associated with depressive disorders and with behavioral disorders. In a study that examined the relationship between parental loss before age 17 and adult pathology in female same-sex twins from a population-based registry, parental separation was associated with GAD and parental death with phobia.[130] Death of persons from the social network were more strongly associated with major depression than with GAD.[131] In a study contrasting pure disorder groups, loss and danger events were associated with the onset of GAD alone, whereas loss and humiliation events predicted the onset of pure depression and the onset of comorbid depression and GAD, suggesting a moderate level of specificity in the life event-psychopathology link.[132]

Parenting style

Several clinical but few epidemiologic studies examined parenting style as a risk factor for anxiety disorders (for an overview, see Ref[133]). In the EDSP study, parental overprotection and parental rejection were associated with increased rates of social phobia in offspring.[83,92] In the same study, overprotection was found to increase the risk for anxiety disorders but not pure depressive disorders, whereas depressive disorders were linked to parental rejection.[37]

After controlling for comorbidity and a broad range of other putative risk factors, Shanahan and colleagues[81] found among a range of emotional and behavioral outcomes harsh discipline to be specifically associated with GAD/OAD. Overintrusive parenting was revealed as a nonspecific risk factor for anxiety and behavioral disorders.

Kendler and colleagues[134] found in female adult twin pairs that high levels of parental coldness and authoritarianism were modestly associated with increased risk for nearly all disorders, whereas the impact of protectiveness was more variable. Any phobia, GAD, major depression, and panic disorder, but not bulimia, drug abuse, or alcohol dependence, were associated with protectiveness.

Interestingly, McLeod and colleagues[135] reviewed higher levels of parental rejection and control to account for only 4% and 6%, respectively, of the variance in child anxiety. The amount of explained variance in offspring anxiety increased to 42% when autonomy-granting as one particular facet of parenting was considered.

Overall, subdimensions of parenting behavior are likely differentially associated with offspring anxiety, with autonomy-granting and overinvolvement explaining the greatest proportion of variance.[135]

IMPLICATIONS FOR RESEARCH AND CLINICAL PRACTICE IN ANXIETY DISORDERS

As reviewed here, anxiety disorders are frequent and early-emerging conditions associated with considerable developmental, psychosocial, and psychopathologic complications. Early anxiety syndromes may remit spontaneously, but the vast majority of children and adolescents with an anxiety disorder will be suffering from either the same condition or other mental disorders (other anxiety disorders, depressive, and/or substance use disorders) throughout their life, causing tremendous burdens and costs for both the individual and society.[136,137] Although effective treatments exist for anxiety disorders and related conditions (see part II of this issue), the size of the problem cannot be resolved through treatment interventions alone. It is necessary to intensify research on causes to identify better strategies for improved prevention and early intervention. Several potential risk factors for the development of anxiety disorders have been identified, such as parental psychopathology, behaviorally inhibited temperament, and early life adversity. More work, however, is needed to identify the most powerful and specific risk factors for the onset and poor course of anxiety conditions and to understand the complex underlying biological and psychological mechanisms and interactions.

REFERENCES

1. Pine DS, Helfinstein SM, Bar-Haim Y, et al. Challenges in developing novel treatments for childhood disorders: lessons from research on anxiety. Neuropsychopharmacology 2009;34(1):213–28.
2. American Psychiatric Association. Diagnostic and Statistical Manual of Mental Disorders. 4th edition, Text Revision. Washington (DC): American Psychiatric Association; 2000.
3. Morris RJ, Kratochwill TR. Childhood fears and phobias. In: Kratochwill TR, Morris RJ, editors. The practice of child therapy.2nd edition. New York: Pergamon; 1991. p. 76–114.
4. Muris P, Merckelbach H, Mayer B, et al. Common fears and their relationship to anxiety disorders symptomatology in normal children. Pers Indiv Diff 1998;24(4): 575–8.
5. World Health Organization. The ICD-10 Classification of Mental and Behavioural Disorders: diagnostic criteria for research. Geneva (Switzerland): World Health Organization; 1993.
6. Shear MK, Bjelland I, Beesdo K, et al. Supplementary dimensional assessment in anxiety disorders. Int J Methods Psychiatr Res 2007;16(Suppl.1):S52–64.
7. Craske MG, Rauch SL, Ursano R, et al. What is an anxiety disorder? Depress Anxiety 2009;26(12):1066–85.
8. Burstein M, He JP, Kattan G, et al. Social phobia and subtypes in the national comorbidity survey-adolescent supplement: prevalence, correlates, and comorbidity. J Am Acad Child Adolesc Psychiatry 2011;50(9):870–80.
9. Lueken U, Kruschwitz JD, Muehlhan M, et al. How specific is specific phobia? Different neural response patterns in two subtypes of specific phobia. Neuroimage 2011;56:363–72.
10. LeBeau RT, Glenn D, Liao B, et al. Specific phobia: a review of DSM-IV specific phobia and preliminary recommendations for DSM-V. Depress Anxiety 2010;27(2): 148–67.
11. Beesdo K, Knappe S, Pine DS. Anxiety and anxiety disorders in children and adolescents: developmental issues and implications for DSM-V. Psychiatr Clin North Am 2009;32(3):483–524.
12. Schniering CA, Hudson JL, Rapee RM. Issues in the diagnosis and assessment of anxiety disorders in children and adolescents. Clin Psychol Rev 2000;20(4):453–78.
13. Campbell MA, Rapee RM, Spence SH. Developmental changes in the interpretation of rating format on a questionnaire measure of worry. Clinical Psychol 2000;5(2):49–59.
14. Kendall PC, Hedtke KA, Aschenbrand SG. Behavioral and emotional disorders in adolescents. Nature, assessment and treatment In: Wolfe DA, Mash EJ, editors. Anxiety disorders. New York: Guilford Press; 2006. p. 259–99.

15. McCathie H, Spence SH. What is the revised fear survey schedule for children measuring? Behav Res Ther 1991;29(5):495–502.

16. Wittchen H-U, Gloster AT, Beesdo K, et al. Posttraumatic stress disorder: diagnostic and epidemiological perspectives. CNS Spectr 2009;14(1 Suppl. 1):5–12.

17. Lewis-Fernández R, Hinton DE, Laria AJ, et al. Culture and the anxiety disorders: recommendations for DSM-V. Depress Anxiety 2010;27:212–29.

18. Wittchen H-U, Nelson CB, Lachner G. Prevalence of mental disorders and psychosocial impairments in adolescents and young adults. Psychol Med 1998;28:109–26.

19. Essau CA, Conradt J, Petermann F. Frequency, comorbidity, and psychosocial impairment of anxiety disorders in german adolescents. J Anxiety Disord 2000;14(3): 263–79.

20. Copeland W, Shanahan L, Costello EJ, et al. Cumulative prevalence of psychiatric disorders by young adulthood: a prospective cohort analysis from the Great Smoky Mountains study. J Am Acad Child Adolesc Psychiatry 2011;50(3):252–61.

21. Wittchen H-U, Lecrubier Y, Beesdo K, et al. Relationships among anxiety disorders: patterns and implications. In: Nutt DJ, Ballenger JC, editors. Anxiety disorders. Oxford (England): Wiley Blackwell; 2003:25–37.

22. Merikangas KR, He JP, Burstein M, et al. Lifetime Prevalence of mental disorders in U.S. adolescents: results from the National Comorbidity Survey Replication-Adolescent Supplement (NCS-A). J Am Acad Child Adolesc Psychiatry 2011;49(10):980–9.

23. Kessler RC, Avenevoli S, Costello EJ, et al. Prevalence, persistence, and sociodemographic correlates of DSM-IV disorders in the National Comorbidity Survey Replication-Adolescent Supplement. Arch Gen Psychiatry 2012;69:372–80.

24. Fergusson DM, Horwood LJ, Lynskey MT. Prevalence and comorbidity of DSM-III-R diagnoses in a birth cohort of 15 year olds. J Am Acad Child Adolesc Psychiatry 1993;32(6):1127–34.

25. Bittner A, Egger HL, Erkanli A, et al. What do childhood anxiety disorders predict? J Child Psychol Psychiatry 2007;48(12):1174–83.

26. Pine DS, Cohen P, Gurley D, et al. The risk for early-adulthood anxiety and depressive disorders in adolescents with anxiety and depressive disorders. Arch Gen Psychiatry 1998;55:56–64.

27. Bowen RC, Offord DR, Boyle MH. The prevalence of overanxious disorder and separation anxiety disorder: results from the Ontario Child Health Study. J Am Acad Child Adolesc Psychiatry 1990;29:753–8.

28. Bolton D, Eley TC, O'Connor TG, et al. Prevalence and genetic and environmental influences on anxiety disorders in 6-year-old twins. Psychol Med 2006;36(3): 335–44.

29. Breton J-J, Bergeron L, Valla J-P, et al. Quebec Child Mental Health Survey: prevalence of DSM-III-R mental health disorders. J Child Psychol Psychiatry 1999; 40:375–84.

30. Wittchen H-U, Lieb R, Schuster P , et al. When is onset? Investigations into early developmental stages of anxiety and depressive disorders. In: Rapoport JL, editor. Childhood onset of "adult" psychopathology, clinical and research advances. Washington (DC): American Psychiatric Press; 1999. p. 259–302.

31. Beesdo K, Bittner A, Pine DS, et al. Incidence of social anxiety disorder and the consistent risk for secondary depression in the first three decades of life. Arch Gen Psychiatry 2007;64(8):903–12.

32. Feehan M, McGee R, Raha SN, et al. DSM-III-R disorders in New Zealand 18-year-olds. Aust N Z J Psychiatry 1994;28:87–99.

33. Costello EJ, Angold A, Burns B, et al. The Great Smoky Mountains Study of Youth: goals, design, methods, and the prevalence of DSM-III-R disorders. Arch Gen Psychiatry 1996;53(12):1129–36.
34. Wittchen HU, Nocon A, Beesdo K, et al. Agoraphobia and panic: prospective-longitudinal relations suggest a rethinking of diagnostic concepts. Psychoth Psychosom 2008;77:147–57.
35. Romano E, Tremblay RE, Vitaro F, et al. Prevalence of psychiatric diagnoses and the role of perceived impairment: findings from and adolescent community sample. J Child Psychol Psychiatry 2001;42(4):451–61.
36. Andrews G, Hobbs MJ, Borkovec TD, et al. Generalized worry disorder: a review of DSM-IV generalized anxiety disorder and options for DSM-V. Depress Anxiety 2010;27:134–47.
37. Beesdo K, Pine DS, Lieb R, et al. Incidence and risk patterns of anxiety and depressive disorders and categorization of generalized anxiety disorder. Arch Gen Psychiatry 2010;67(1):47–57.
38. Lewinsohn PM, Hops H, Roberts RE, et al. Adolescents psychopathology: I. Prevalence and incidence of depression and other DSM-III-R disorders in high school students. J Abnorm Psychol 1993;102:133–44.
39. Craske MG. Origins of phobias and anxiety disorders: Why more women than men? Amsterdam (Netherlands): Elsevier; 2003.
40. Ruscio AM, Stein DJ, Chiu WT, et al. The epidemiology of obsessive-compulsive disorder in the National Comorbidity Survey Replication. Mol Psychiatry 2010;15(1): 53–63.
41. Kessler RC, Berglund P, Demler O, et al. Lifetime prevalence and age-of-onset distributions of DSM-IV disorders in the National Comorbidity Survey Replication. Arch Gen Psychiatry 2005;62:593–602.
42. Last CG, Perrin S, Hersen M, et al. A prospective study of childhood anxiety disorders. J Am Acad Child Adolesc Psychiatry 1996;35:1502–10.
43. Becker ES, Rinck M, Türke V, et al. Epidemiology of specific phobia subtypes: findings from the Dresden Mental Health Study. Eur Psychiatry 2007;22(2):69–74.
44. de Graaf R, Bijl R, Spijker J, et al. Temporal sequencing of lifetime mood disorders in relation to comorbid anxiety and substance use disorders. Soc Psychiatry Psychiatr Epidemiol 2003;38:1–11.
45. Yonkers KA, Bruce SE, Dyck IR, et al. Chronicity, relapse, and illness–course of panic disorder, social phobia, and generalized anxiety disorder: findings in men and women from 8 years of follow-up. Depress Anxiety 2003;17(3):173–9.
46. Bruce SE, Yonkers KA, Otto MW, et al. Influence of psychiatric comorbidity on recovery and recurrence in generalized anxiety disorder, social phobia, and panic disorder: a 12-year prospective study. Am J Psychiatry 2005;162:1179–87.
47. Blazer DG, Hughes D, George LK, et al. Generalized anxiety disorder. In: Robins LN, Regier DA, editors. Psychiatric disorders in America: the Epidemiologic Catchment Area Study. New York: The Free Press; 1991. p. 180–203.
48. Beesdo-Baum K, Knappe S, Fehm L, et al. The natural course of Social Anxiety Disorder among adolescents and young adults. Acta Psychiatr Scand, in press.
49. Copeland WE, Shanahan L, Costello J, et al. Childhood and adolescent psychiatric disorders as predictors of young adult disorders. Arch Gen Psychiatry 2009;66(7): 764–72.
50. Wittchen H-U, Lieb R, Pfister H, et al. The waxing and waning of mental disorders: evaluating the stability of syndromes of mental disorders in the population. Compr Psychiatry 2000;41(2 Suppl 1):122–32.

51. Costello EJ, Copeland W, Angold A. Trends in psychopathology across the adolescent years: what changes when children become adolescents, and when adolescents become adults? J Child Psychol Psychiatry 2011;52(10):1015–25.

52. Pine DS, Klein RG. Anxiety disorders. In: Rutter M, Bishop DVM, Pine DS, et al, editors. Rutter's child and adolescent psychiatry. 5th edition. Oxford (UK): Blackwell; 2009. [Chapter 39].

53. Angst J, Vollrath M. The natural history of anxiety disorders. Acta Psychiatr Scand 1991;84:446–52.

54. Last CG, Hansen C, Franco N. Anxious children in adulthood: a prospective study of adjustment. J Am Acad Child Adolesc Psychiatry 1997;36(5):645–52.

55. Merikangas KR, Avenevoli S, Acharyya S, et al. The spectrum of social phobia in the Zurich Cohort Study of young adults. Biol Psychiatry 2002;51:81–91.

56. Noyes RJ, Holt CS, Woodman CL. Natural course of anxiety disorders. In: Mavissakalian MR, Prien RF, editors. Long-term treatments of anxiety disorders. Washington (DC): American Psychiatric Press; 1996. p. 1–48.

57. Emmelkamp PM, Wittchen HU. Specific phobias. In: Andrews G, Charney DS, Sirovatka PJ, et al, editors. Stress-induced and fear circuitry disorders. Refining the research agenda for DSM-V. Arlington (VA): American Psychiatric Association; 2009. p. 77–101.

58. Wittchen H-U. Der Langzeitverlauf unbehandelter Angststörungen: wie häufig sind Spontanremissionen? Verhaltenstherapie 1991;1(4):273–82 [in German].

59. Woodward LJ, Fergusson DM. Life course outcomes of young people with anxiety disorders in adolescence. J Am Acad Child Adolesc Psychiatry 2001; 40(9):1086–93.

60. Fergusson DM, Woodward LJ. Mental health, educational, and social role outcomes of adolescents with depression. Arch Gen Psychiatry 2002;59:225–31.

61. Kessler RC, Nelson CB, McGonagle KA, et al. Comorbidity of DSM-III-R major depressive disorder in the general population: results from the US National Comorbidity Survey. Br J Psychiatry 1996;168:17–30.

62. Kessler RC, Stang P, Wittchen H-U, et al. Lifetime comorbidities between social phobia and mood disorders in the U.S. National Comorbidity Survey. Psychol Med 1999;29(3):555–67.

63. Kim-Cohen J, Caspi A, Moffitt TE, et al. Prior juvenile diagnoses in adults with mental disorder. Arch Gen Psychiatry 2003;60:709–17.

64. Pine DS, Cohen P, Brook J. Adolescent fears as predictors of depression. Biol Psychiatry 2001;50(9):721–4.

65. Stein MB, Fuetsch M, Müller N, et al. Social anxiety disorder and the risk of depression. A prospective community study of adolescents and young adults. Arch Gen Psychiatry 2001;58:251–6.

66. Bittner A, Goodwin RD, Wittchen H-U, et al. What characteristics of primary anxiety disorders predict subsequent major depressive disorder? J Clin Psychiatry 2004; 65(5):618–26.

67. Kessler RC, Crum RM, Warner LA, et al. Lifetime co-occurrence of DSM-III-R alcohol abuse and dependence with other psychiatric disorders in the National Comorbidity Survey. Arch Gen Psychiatry 1997;54:313–21.

68. Merikangas KR, Mehta RL, Molnar BE, et al. Comorbidity of substance use disorders with mood and anxiety disorders: results of the international consortium in psychiatric epidemiology. Addict Behav 1998;23:893–907.

69. Kessler RC, Chiu WT, Demler O, et al. Prevalence, severity, and comorbidity of 12-month DSM-IV disorders in the National Comorbidity Survey Replication. Arch Gen Psychiatry 2005;62:617–27.

70. Wittchen H-U, Frohlich C, Behrendt S, et al. Cannabis use and cannabis use disorders and their relationship to mental disorders: a 10-year prospective-longitudinal community study in adolescents. Drug Alcohol Depend 2007;88(Suppl 1):S60–70.
71. Zimmermann P, Wittchen H-U, Höfler M, et al. Primary anxiety disorders and the development of subsequent alcohol use disorders: a 4-year community study of adolescents and young adults. Psychological Medicine 2003;33:1211–22.
72. Kraemer HC, Kazdin AE, Offord DR, et al. Coming to terms with the terms of risk. Arch Gen Psychiatry 1997;54(4):337–43.
73. McLaughlin KA, Breslau J, Green JG, et al. Childhood socio-economic status and the onset, persistence, and severity of DSM-IV mental disorders in a US national sample. Soc Sci Med 2011;73(7):1088–96.
74. Stein DJ, Fineberg NA, Bienvenu OJ, et al. Should OCD be classified as an anxiety disorder in DSM-V? Depress Anxiety 2010;27(6):495–506.
75. Hettema JM. The nosological relationship between generalized anxiety disorder and major depression. Depress Anxiety 2008;25:300–16.
76. Goldberg DP, Krueger RF, Andrews G, et al. Emotional disorders: cluster 4 of the proposed meta-structure for DSM-V and ICD-11. Psychol Med 2009;39(12):2043–59.
77. Canino G, Shrout PE, Rubio-Stipec M, et al. The DSM-IV rates of child and adolescent disorders in Puerto Rico. Arch Gen Psychiatry 2004;61:85–93.
78. Vega WA, Kolody B, Aguilar-Gaxiola S, et al. Lifetime prevalence of DSM-III-R psychiatric disorders among urban and rural Mexican Americans in California. Arch Gen Psychiatry 1998;55:771–8.
79. Costello EJ, Mustillo S, Erkanli A, et al. Prevalence and development of psychiatric disorders in childhood and adolescence. Arch Gen Psychiatry 2003;60:837–44.
80. Copeland W, Shanahan L, Costello EJ, et al. Configurations of common childhood psychosocial risk factors. J Child Psychol Psychiatry 2009;50(4):451–9.
81. Shanahan L, Copeland W, Costello EJ, et al. Specificity of putative psychosocial risk factors for psychiatric disorders in children and adolescents. J Child Psychol Psychiatry 2008;49(1):34–42.
82. Merikangas KR, Avenevoli S, Dierker L, et al. Vulnerability factors among children at risk for anxiety disorders. Biol Psychiatry 1999;46(11):1523–35.
83. Lieb R, Wittchen H-U, Höfler M, et al. Parental psychopathology, parenting styles, and the risk for social phobia in offspring: a prospective-longitudinal community study. Arch Gen Psychiatry 2000;57:859–66.
84. Hettema JM, Neale MC, Kendler KS. A review and meta-analysis of the genetic epidemiology of anxiety disorders. Am J Psychiatry 2001;158(10):1568–78.
85. Johnson JG, Cohen P, Kasen S, et al. Parental concordance and offspring risk for anxiety, conduct, depressive, and substance use disorders. Psychopathology 2008;41:124–8.
86. Wittchen H-U, Kessler RC, Pfister H, et al. Why do people with anxiety disorders become depressed? A prospective-longitudinal community study. Acta Psychiatr Scand 2000;102(Suppl 406):14–23.
87. Schreier A, Wittchen HU, Höfler M, et al. Anxiety disorders in mothers and their children: prospective longitudinal community study. Br J Psychiatry 2008;129:308–9.
88. Lieb R, Isensee B, Höfler M, et al. Parental major depression and the risk of depressive and other mental disorders in offspring: a prospective-longitudinal community study. Arch Gen Psychiatry 2002;59:365–74.
89. Weissman MM, Wickramaratne P, Nomura Y, et al. Offspring of depressed parents: 20 years later. Am J Psychiatry 2006;163:1001–8.

90. Klein DN, Lewinsohn PM, Rohde P, et al. Family study of co-morbidity between major depressive disorder and anxiety disorders. Psychol Med 2003;33:703–14.
91. Moffitt TE, Caspi A, Harrington H, et al. Generalized anxiety disorder and depression: childhood risk factors in a birth cohort followed to age 32. Psychol Med 2007;37: 441–52.
92. Knappe S, Lieb R, Beesdo K, et al. The role of parental psychopathology and family environment for social phobia in the first three decades of life. Depress Anxiety 2009;26(4):363–70.
93. Martini J, Knappe S, Beesdo-Baum K, et al. Anxiety disorders before birth and self-perceived distress during pregnancy: associations with maternal depression and obstetric, neonatal and early childhood outcomes. Early Hum Dev 2010;86(5): 305–10.
94. Hodgson DM, Coe CL. Perinatal programming: early life determinants of adult health and disease. London: Taylor & Francis; 2006.
95. Alder J, Fink N, Bitzer J, et al. Depression and anxiety during pregnancy: a risk factor for obstetric, fetal and neonatal outcome? A critical review of the literature. J Matern Fetal Neonatal Med 2007;20(3):189–209.
96. Hettema JM, Prescott CA, Myers JM, et al. The structure of genetic and environmental risk factors for anxiety disorders in men and women. Arch Gen Psychiatry 2005;62:182–9.
97. Scherrer JF, True WR, Xian H, et al. Evidence for genetic influences common and specific to symptoms of generalized anxiety and panic. J Affect Disord 2000; 57(1–3):25–35.
98. Kendler KS. Major depression and generalised anxiety disorder. Same genes, (partly) different environments–revisited. Br J Psychiatry 1996;168(Suppl 30):68–75.
99. Kendler KS, Neale MC, Kessler RC, et al. Major depression and generalized anxiety disorder: Same genes, (partly) different environments? Arch Gen Psychiatry 1992; 49:716–22.
100. Merikangas KR, Low NC. Genetic epidemiology of anxiety disorders. Handb Exp Pharmacol 2005;169:163–79.
101. Low NC, Merikangas KR. Community versus clinic sampling: effect on the familial aggregation of anxiety disorders. Biol Psychiatry 2008;63:884–90.
102. Clark LA, Watson D. Tripartite model of anxiety and depression: psychometric evidence and taxonomic implications. J Abnorm Psychol 1991;100(3):316–36.
103. Clark DA, Steer RA, Beck AT. Common and specific dimensions of self-reported anxiety and depression: implications for the cognitive and tripartite models. J Abnorm Psychol 1994;103:645–54.
104. Zinbarg RE, Barlow DH. Structure of anxiety and the anxiety disorders: a hierarchical model. J Abnorm Psychol 1996;105(2):181–93.
105. Brown TA, Chorpita BF, Barlow DH. Structural relationships among dimensions of the DSM-IV anxiety and mood disorders and dimensions of negative affect, positive affect, and autonomic arousal. J Abnorm Psychol 1998;107(2):179–92.
106. Chorpita BF. The tripartite model and dimensions of anxiety and depression: an examination of structure in a large school sample. J Abnorm Child Psychol 2002; 30(2):177–90.
107. Mineka S, Watson D, Clark LA. Comorbidity of anxiety and unipolar mood disorders. Annu Rev Psychol 1998;49:377–412.
108. Hettema JM, Neale MC, Myers JM, et al. A population-based twin study of the relationship between neuroticism and internalizing disorders. Am J Psychiatry 2006; 163:857–64.

109. Khan AA, Jacobson KC, Gardner CO, et al. Personality and comorbidity of common psychiatric disorders. Br J Psychiatry 2005;186:190–6.
110. Hayward C, Killen JD, Kraemer HC, et al. Predictors of panic attacks in adolescents. J Am Acad Child Adolesc Psychiatry 2000;39(2):207–14.
111. de Graaf R, Bijl RV, Ravelli A, et al. Predictors of first incidence of DSM-III-R psychiatric disorders in the general population: findings from the Netherlands Mental Health Survey and Incidence Study. Acta Psychiatr Scand 2002;106:303–13.
112. Kagan J. Temperamental contributions to social behavior. Am Psychol 1989;44(4): 668–74.
113. Robinson JL, Kagan J, Reznick JS, et al. The heritability of inhibited and uninhibited behavior: a twin study. Dev Psychol 1992;28:1030–7.
114. Smoller JW, Rosenbaum JF, Biederman J, et al. Association of a genetic marker at the corticotropin-releasing hormone locus with behavioral inhibition. Biol Psychiatry 2003;54(12):1376–81.
115. Biederman J, Hirshfeld-Becker DR, Rosenbaum JF, et al. Further evidence of association between behavioral inhibition and social anxiety in children. Am J Psychiatry 2001;158(10):1673–9.
116. Angold A, Costello EJ. Nosology and measurement in child and adolescent psychiatry. J Child Psychol Psychiatry 2009;50(1–2):9–15.
117. Johnson SL, Turner RJ, Iwata N. BIS/BAS levels and psychiatric disorder: an epidemiological study. J Psychopathol Behav Assess 2003;25(1):25–36.
118. Caspi A, Moffitt TE, Newman DL, et al. Behavioral observations at age 3 years predict adult psychiatric disorders. Arch Gen Psychiatry 1996;53:1033–9.
119. Rohrbacher H, Hoyer J, Beesdo K, et al. Psychometric properties of the retrospective self report of inhibition (RSRI) in a representative German sample. Int J Methods Psychiatr Res 2008;17(2):80–8.
120. Hayward C, Killen JD, Kraemer HC, et al. Linking self-reported childhood behavioral inhibition to adolescent social phobia. J Am Acad Child Adolesc Psychiatry 1998; 37:1308–16.
121. Mick MA, Telch MJ. Social anxiety and history of behavioral inhibition in young adults. J Anxiety Disord 1998;12(1):1–20.
122. Schwartz CE, Snidman N, Kagan J. Adolescent social anxiety as an outcome of inhibited temperament in childhood. J Am Acad Child Adolesc Psychiatry 1999; 38(8):1008–15.
123. Kessler RC, Davis CG, Kendler KS. Childhood adversity and adult psychiatric disorder in the US National Comorbidity Survey. Psychol Med 1997;27:1101–19.
124. Bijl RV, Ravelli A, Van Zessen G. Prevalence of psychiatric disorder in the general population: results of the Netherlands Mental Health Survey and Incidence Study (NEMESIS). Soc Psychiatry Psychiatr Epidemiol 1998;33:587–95.
125. Fergusson DM, Horwood J, Lynskey MT. Childhood sexual abuse and psychiatric disorder in young adulthood. II. psychiatric outcomes of childhood sexual abuse. J Am Acad Child Adolesc Psychiatry 1996;35(10):1365–74.
126. Pine DS, Cohen P, Johnson J, et al. Adolescent life events as predictors of adult depression. J Affect Disord 2002;68:49–57.
127. Friis RH, Wittchen H-U, Pfister H, et al. Life events and changes in the course of depression in young adults. Eur Psychiatry 2002;17(5):241–53.
128. Perkonigg A, Kessler RC, Storz S, et al. Traumatic events and post-traumatic stress disorder in the community: prevalence, risk factors and comorbidity. Acta Psychiatr Scand 2000;101(1):46–59.
129. Finlay-Jones R, Brown GW. Types of stressful life event and the onset of anxiety and depressive disorders. Psychol Med 1981;11:803–15.

130. Kendler KS, Neale MC, Kessler RC, et al. Childhood parental loss and adult psychopathology in women. A twin study perspective. Arch Gen Psychiatry 1992; 49:109–16.
131. Kendler KS, Karkowski LM, Prescott CA. Stressful life events and major depression: risk period, long-term contextual threat, and diagnostic specificity. J Nerv Ment Dis 1998;186(11):661–9.
132. Kendler KS, Hettema JM, Butera F, et al. Life event dimensions of loss, humiliation, entrapment, and danger in the prediction of onsets of major depression and generalized anxiety. Arch Gen Psychiatry 2003;60:789–96.
133. Rapee RM. Potential role of childrearing practices in the development of anxiety and depression. Clin Psychol Rev 1997;17(1):47–67.
134. Kendler KS, Myers J, Prescott CA. Parenting and adult mood, anxiety and substance use disorders in female twins: an epidemiological, multi-informant, retrospective study. Psychol Med 2000;30:281–94.
135. McLeod BD, Wood JJ, Weisz JR. Examining the association between parenting and childhood anxiety: a meta-analysis. Clin Psychol Rev 2007;27(2):155–72.
136. Wittchen HU, Jacobi F, Rehm J, et al. The size and burden of mental disorders and other disorders of the brain in Europe 2010. Eur Neuropsychopharmacol 2011;21: 655–79.
137. Gustavsson A, Svensson M, Jacobi F, et al. Cost of disorders of the brain in Europe 2010. Eur Neuropsychopharmacol 2011;21(10):718–79.

Genetics of Pediatric Anxiety Disorders

Dara J. Sakolsky, MD, PhD[a,*], James T. McCracken, MD[b],
Erika L. Nurmi, MD, PhD[b]

KEYWORDS

- Pediatric anxiety • Genetics • Candidate genes • Obsessive–compulsive disorder
- Panic disorder • Posttraumatic stress disorder

KEY POINTS

- Heritability estimates for anxiety disorders range from 20% to 65%, indicating a substantial genetic basis.
- Early-onset anxiety represents a more genetically enriched population, ripe for investigation.
- Studies to identify susceptibility genes for anxiety disorders have relied on two established strategies, linkage and association analysis, but have been complicated by complex, multifactorial inheritance.
- Few candidate loci have been consistently replicated and supported by functional data.
- Identifying risk genes will require integrative approaches combining genetics, refined psychophysiologic assessments, functional studies, and computational and statistical creativity in large, adequately powered and carefully phenotyped populations.
- Unraveling the genetic basis of pediatric anxiety will improve our understanding of its pathophysiology and ability to diagnose and treat those affected with and at risk for anxiety-spectrum disorders.

INTRODUCTION

Anxiety disorders are the most common pediatric mental health disorders in community samples and often result in substantial distress and impairment.[1] The prognostic significance of childhood anxiety for adolescent and adult mental health is likewise substantial.[2] Awareness of pediatric anxiety disorders and strategies for

The authors have nothing to disclose.
[a] Department of Psychiatry, University of Pittsburgh, Western Psychiatric Institute and Clinic, University of Pittsburgh Medical Center, Bellefield Towers, Room 515, 100 North Bellefield Avenue, Pittsburgh, PA 15213, USA; [b] Department of Psychiatry and Biobehavioral Sciences, David Geffen School of Medicine at UCLA, Jane & Terry Semel Institute of Neuroscience and Human Behavior, 760 Westwood Plaza, Los Angeles, CA 90095, USA
* Corresponding author.
E-mail address: sakolskydj@upmc.edu

Child Adolesc Psychiatric Clin N Am 21 (2012) 479–500
http://dx.doi.org/10.1016/j.chc.2012.05.010
1056-4993/12/$ – see front matter © 2012 Elsevier Inc. All rights reserved.

successful treatments have advanced enormously in the past decade. As the clinical significance of childhood anxiety has been revealed, increasing efforts are underway to understand the biology, etiology, and risk markers of these disorders. Given that family history of anxiety is one of the major risk factors for the development of pediatric anxiety disorders, interest in examining the genetic basis of these disorders has also increased. This review provides a thorough update on genetic findings in the child and adolescent anxiety disorders, and attempts to synthesize their relevance to clinical practice and future research efforts. As will be seen, genetics advances are approaching potential application to risk assessment, to identification of relevant biological pathways leading to anxiety disorders, and to new and individualized interventions. Genetic discoveries are also raising questions about how we currently classify or diagnose these conditions.

Epidemiologic data, recently reviewed by Smoller and colleagues,[3] clearly demonstrate that genetic variation contributes to the risk of developing an anxiety disorder. Heritability estimates (ie, the proportion of variance in a population that is attributable to genetic factors) for anxiety disorders range from 20% to 65%,[4–6] similar to those of major depressive disorder, but less than of other, highly heritable pediatric mental health disorders (eg, attention deficit hyperactivity disorder, bipolar disorder, and autistic disorder).[3] The finding of moderate heritability supports the role of genetic variation in causation of childhood and adult anxiety disorders, but also underscores the likely interacting role for experiential and environmental factors.

FINDING RISK GENES

The goal of identifying individual gene variants that contribute to the risk of developing an anxiety disorder has proved challenging, likely because anxiety disorder risk arises from multiple genes, not single genes of major causative effect. Studies to localize and identify susceptibility genes for anxiety disorders have relied on two established strategies: linkage and association analysis.

1. **Linkage analysis** examines whether chromosomal segments are coinherited with the disorder among family members and is an appropriate strategy for finding genetic variants with moderate to large effects. Linkage analysis essentially asks: Where are the anxiety disorder genes located within the human genome?
2. **Association analysis** examines whether there is a correlation between a specific genetic variant and a disorder. Most association studies use a case-control design and test whether a genetic variant is more frequent among cases compared to controls. Association analysis essentially asks: Which genetic variants are more common in people with anxiety disorders?

The majority of association studies that have been conducted in anxiety disorder populations are known as candidate gene studies. These studies examine genetic variants that are proposed as candidates based on hypotheses about the biological pathways involved in the disorder (biological candidates) or based on their location within a chromosomal region implicated by a linkage study (positional candidates.) Candidate gene studies have often resulted in false-positive findings and nonreplication owing to limited knowledge of pathophysiology of anxiety disorders, heterogeneity of anxiety phenotypes, confounding by population stratification (ie, differences in genetic background of cases and controls), and lack of correction for multiple testing. Moreover, most candidate gene studies have been too small to provide definitive tests of the association of a gene with the disorder of interest. Because of these concerns, replication of findings in an adequately powered, independent sample has become critical to establishing the reliability of an initial

Table 1
Candidate genes with replicated association in anxiety disorders

Anxiety Disorder	Gene Name	Gene Symbol	Function
OCD	Glutamate transporter	SLC1A1	Neurotransmission
Panic disorder	Catechol-O-methyltransferase	COMT	Neurotransmission
	Neuropeptide S receptor gene	NPSR	Neuronal signaling
	Transmembrane protein 132D	TMEM132D	Unknown
PTSD	FK-506 binding protein	FKBP5	Glucocorticoid chaperone

positive study. **Table 1** summarizes the few candidate genes with variants that have shown compelling association with anxiety disorders in more than one sample. When available, in vitro or in vivo data demonstrating functional effects of associated variants helps to validate statistical findings.

Genotyping Advances

Advances in genotyping technology have facilitated our ability to efficiently assay DNA variation on a large scale. Millions of single-nucleotide polymorphisms (SNPs) can be genotyped rapidly and inexpensively. Rather than investigating a few SNPs, researchers can examine a large fraction of common variants across the entire genome. This is crucial, because individual genetic diversity is so enormous—on average every gene contains more than 50 common SNP variants, totaling millions of common variants genomewide. In addition, because nearby SNPs are often inherited together (a phenomenon known as linkage disequilibrium), all of the common variation across the genome can be captured by genotyping only a representative subset of markers (tag or tSNPs). By genotyping these tagging SNPs, genomewide association studies (GWAS) are able to survey the entire genome for association with a phenotype. Replication in independent samples and validation of functional effects remains key to establishing a convincing connection between genotype and phenotype. Such studies in the anxiety disorders, including many with children, are finally coming to fruition.

GENETICS OF OBSESSIVE–COMPULSIVE DISORDER

Lifetime prevalence of obsessive–compulsive disorder (OCD) ranges from 1% to 3% worldwide by adolescence and in adulthood,[7] and 80% of OCD cases have onset before age 18 years[8] so, in essence, OCD is a disorder of childhood. Persistence into adulthood is very high, although very early onset OCD may have a somewhat more variable course—the course of OCD has not been examined from a genetic perspective thus far.[9] Substantial impairment in vocational, academic, and social and family functioning is common.[10] Although the precise molecular pathophysiology of OCD remains elusive, dysfunction of the cortico-striato–thalamo–cortical circuitry is believed to play a central role, with glutamatergic dysfunction increasingly suspected.[11,12]

Familiality of OCD

Family aggregation and twins studies indicate a substantial genetic contribution to the etiology of OCD, and underscore the importance of a thorough family history as a part of clinical examination of suspected anxiety. The majority of published twin studies have been summarized in a comprehensive review.[5] Studies with sufficient sample sizes to estimate heritability and two more recent reports[13,14] support the major role of genetic factors in the development of OCD, especially for pediatric-onset OCD.[15,16] Heritability rates for pediatric-onset OCD have been estimated at 0.45 to 0.65.[5,6] OCD familiality has been demonstrated in both clinical and population studies.[17] OCD and OC symptoms occur at a significantly higher rate in relatives of OCD cases than in relatives of matched-controls.[15]

OCD subtypes

Many investigations have supported the clinical observations of characteristic symptom clustering, suggesting that there are distinct subtypes of OCD with different comorbidities and etiologic factors. Obsessive–compulsive symptom subtypes (contamination/cleaning, doubting/checking, symmetry/ordering, taboo thoughts and hoarding) have been proven to cluster and be transmitted in families.[18] Importantly, other anxiety disorders, OC-spectrum/habit disorders (body dysmorphic disorder, grooming disorders), tic disorders, attention deficit hyperactivity disorder (ADHD), and somatoform disorders have also shown substantial familial transmission in OCD families.[19–21] Many studies have demonstrated that significant shared genetic risk between OCD and other anxiety disorders appears to exist,[14] though environmental and cultural factors are also shared within families.[13] Notably, because the heritability and recurrence risk of childhood-onset OCD is substantially greater than that of adult-onset OCD,[5,15] it has been proposed that early-onset OCD represents a more heritable subtype of the disorder. Similarly, tic-related OCD is differentiated by common symptom clusters, comorbidities, and treatment response and appears to represent a subtype with even greater genetic loading.[22]

Mode of transmission

Although segregation analyses examining family patterns of disorders have supported a genetic etiology, the mode of transmission is unclear,[23–25] presumably due to complex genetic inheritance, with many genes of small effect and perhaps a few genes with greater contribution, further complicated by environmental factors. In other words, it remains unclear whether the inheritance patterns of OCD reflect dominant, recessive, or other modes of transmission. Nevertheless, the strong support for a role of genes underlying risk has led to a host of efforts to identify specific risk genes using modern genetic research methodology.

Linkage Studies of OCD

Four genetic linkage studies have been published. The largest study to date is the National Institute of Mental Health (NIMH) Obsessive–Compulsive Disorder Genetic Study (OCGS), which includes 219 multiplex families with at least two sibling pairs with early-onset OCD (before age 18).[26] Other linkage studies include three smaller samples of childhood-onset multigenerational and multiplex families[27,28] including a Costa Rican population isolate.[29]

Genomic regions

In the OCGS sample, several candidate genomic regions were highlighted, including 3q27–28, 7p, 1q, 15q15, 6q27.[26] Fine-mapping in the linkage intervals on chromosomes 1q and 15q localized signals to homeobox genes,[30] which are involved in neurodevelopment of the striatum, a brain region implicated in OCD pathophysiology. Within the OCGS study, even stronger evidence for linkage was reported for two different subsets of cases—males and an OCD-hoarding sub-type.[31,32] In male cases, an inherited region on chromosome 11p met genome-wide significance after fine-mapping.[32] In families with the OCD-hoarding sub-type, a region on chromosome 14q showed strong linkage.[31]

In the three other samples, the genomic regions with the strongest evidence for linkage were:

- 9p24—a region that showed linkage in two separate studies[27,33]
- 10q15—a region that had evidence for both linkage and association in one study[28]
- 15q14—a region identified in the Costa Rican sample that replicates a finding from the OCGS data set.[26]

Finally, a currently unpublished linkage scan was performed in 33 Caucasian US families with early-onset OCD. The strongest, genome-wide evidence for suggestive linkage was found on chromosome 1p36.33–p36.32 (HLOD = 3.77, after fine-mapping).[34] Other regions of linkage included 2p14, 5q13, 6p25, and 10p13.

Summary
While a number of candidate regions have been implicated by these linkage screens, regions of agreement across samples are few. What explains the apparent lack of convergence of these apparent significant findings? More than likely the lack of overlap represents differences in genetic background, given the diverse racial and ethnic origins of these samples. Thus, there may be risk genes for OCD that are unique to certain populations, but lead to similar phenotypes. These data also highlight the prospect that finer-grained analyses of the phenotype (hoarding vs non-hoarding) may reveal more homogeneous genetic pathways of risk.

Candidate Gene Studies of OCD

Candidate gene studies for OCD, like in other psychiatric disorders, have been largely conflicting and plagued by nonreplication, mainly again because of inadequate sample sizes where thousands rather than hundreds of subjects are necessary to prevent spurious results. However, such studies are of interest due to their testing of specific pathways or involvement of particular neurotransmitter systems, possibly relevant to current or hypothesized treatments.

Neurotransmitter candidate genes
Numerous studies, many in pediatric-onset cases (reviewed in Refs.[6,15] with an emphasis on childhood cases), have examined monoaminergic candidates suggested by systems involved in therapeutic drug action with mixed results, including:

- **Transporters** for serotonin (SLC6A4) and dopamine (SLC6A3), as well as the extraneuronal monoamine transporter (SLC22A3)
- **Receptors** for serotonin (HTR1B, HTR2A, HTR2B, HTR2C, HTR3A) and dopamine (DRD2, DRD3, DRD4)
- **Enzymes** involved in synthesis (TPH2) and degradation (monoamine oxidase A [MAOA], catechol-O-methyltransferase [COMT])

Enthusiasm for a role for glutamate signaling in OCD has evolved based on: increased cerebrospinal fluid (CSF) glutamate in OCD patients[35]; imaging data in both children and adults with OCD[36–38]; animal models with OC behavior[39,40]; and localization of the glutamate transporter gene (SLC1A1) within the 9p linkage interval. Support for variants in the glutamate system has emerged from studies in children and adults with OCD, with significant associations for polymorphisms in glutamate receptors involved in learning and memory (GRIN2B,[41–43] GRIK2[44,45]) and in glutamatergic synaptic protein SAPAP3 showing fluoxetine-responsive OC behaviors in mice.[46] The strongest evidence in OCD to date comes from 6 independent replications of *SLC1A1* haplotypes,[47–52] which were associated with differences in brain structure[43] and transporter expression.[48] The majority of the support for glutamate candidates, and especially *SCL1A1*, derives from childhood-onset samples.

Non-neurotransmitter candidate genes

A few non-neurotransmitter candidates have also demonstrated associations with pediatric and adult OCD. Several studies have examined growth factors (brain-derived neurotrophic factor [BDNF]) and their receptors (NTRK2, NTRK3), which have shown mixed evidence for association,[53–55] decreased serum levels in OCD,[37,56,57] and moderation of treatment response.[58] Although these studies were performed in adults, the majority of them included pediatric-onset cases. Interestingly, one positive study in a combined sample of both adult and childhood-onset cases showed strong effects in the childhood-onset sample and similar trends in the adult-onset sample.[54] The suggestion that identical genetic risk alleles contribute to both adult and childhood-onset OCD but are more robust in the early-onset sample is in line with the presumed greater genetic loading in early-onset OCD.

An examination of oligodendrocyte genes (*OLIG2*, *MOG*) was spurred by observations of white matter abnormalities in children[59,60] and adults[61,62] and possible immune system involvement.[63] Positive findings have been reported in childhood-onset cases of OCD.[64,65] Allelic variation in *MOG* was associated with greater white matter volume in adults with OCD.[66]

Summary

Despite the investigation of more than 80 genes for susceptibility to OCD, no study has been large enough to sufficiently test for convincing genomewide significance, and few genes are supported by consistent, replicated findings to yield confidence in their association. Furthermore, little evidence for the possible biological effects of the associated variants has been put forth. Candidate gene studies may be more successful when molecular pathways underlying OCD pathology are better understood, but currently have not revealed a consistent, coherent model of OCD etiology.

Genomewide Association Studies of OCD

Although most of the aforementioned studies have been too small to achieve definitive results in gene-finding efforts, research is advancing. Two major GWAS of OCD have been completed but remain unpublished at the time of this review.

International OCD foundation genetics collaborative

The International OCD Foundation (IOCDF) Genetics Collaborative conducted a GWAS on mixed adult and childhood-onset samples contributed from 21 different research sites from around the world, including 1739 trios (affected case and both parents) and 1817 singletons (only affected case) matched with more than 6000 control samples. The major findings from this study are the following:

- One SNP variant (rs6131295) which mapped downstream from the **BTB domain-containing 3 (***BTBD3***) gene** on chromosome 20p12.2 revealed genomewide significance in trios and is believed to regulate expression of several genes including *BTBD3*.[67]

- A SNP upstream from the **fas apoptotic inhibitory molecule 2 (***FAIM2***) gene** on chromosome 12q13.12 reached near genomewide significance in the combined trio-case-control data set, and many SNPs scored in the 10^{-6} range.

Among other top-ranked SNPs, many were associated with genes encoding glutamatergic postsynaptic density proteins and several tagged regions that had previously been linked to OCD subtypes, including chromosome 14 for compulsive hoarding and 19q for childhood-onset OCD.

NIMH obsessive–compulsive genetic association study

The NIMH Obsessive–Compulsive Genetic Association Study (OCGAS) is a second project by the OCGS collaborative with the aim of performing a GWAS for OCD in a carefully phenotyped sample of more than 1400 trios with childhood-onset probands and a similar number of matched controls.[68] The study is expected to report results in the coming years, and because of the rigorously characterized sample, can powerfully examine risk loci for OCD subtypes, cormorbidities, and other factors.

GENETICS OF PANIC DISORDER

The lifetime prevalence of panic disorder is 2.3% according to the National Comorbidity Survey Replication-Adolescent Supplement (NCS-A)[69] and shows a relatively unique pattern of onset versus other childhood anxiety disorders. Onset is uncommon in prepuberty, but then sharply increases later in development. Panic disorder can lead to substantial impairment in academic, social and family functioning, as well as serving as a risk factor for suicidal behavior. Although the pathogenesis is not fully understood, panic attacks are thought to originate from dysfunction in the brain's fear network involving the amygdala, brainstem, hypothalamus, hippocampus, and various cortical regions.[70]

Familiality of Panic Disorder

Data from twin and family studies suggest a substantial involvement of genetic factors in the familial transmission of panic disorder. An increased prevalence of panic disorder is seen among first-degree relatives of cases with panic disorder and also generalized anxiety disorder (GAD) and agoraphobia.[71] An even greater risk for panic disorder is observed in adult first-degree relatives when proband age at onset is younger than 20 years,[72] suggesting that early onset may be seen with higher genetic load. Heritability is estimated near 40%.[4] Segregation analyses support a complex genetic model of disease.

Linkage Studies of Panic Disorder

The largest and most recent linkage study included 120 extended families with panic disorder consisting of 1591 individuals of whom 992 were genotyped.[73] This study found genomewide evidence for linkage on chromosome 15q and suggestive evidence for linkage on chromosome 2q. Linkage analyses from other studies of panic disorder in adults have implicated several chromosomal regions including 1q32, 2p, 4q21.21–22.3, 4q31–34, 5q14.2–14.3, 7p15, 8p23.1, 9p, 9q31, 11p15, 13q32, 14q22.3-23.3, and 22q (for review see Ref.[74]); however, few are shared across samples.

If the risk for panic disorder results from many genes of modest effect, current linkage studies of panic disorder may not be adequately powered. Thus, future studies will require larger sample sizes or combination of multiple samples by meta-analysis. Current findings showing risk regions at 15q and 2q deserve more in-depth investigation.

Candidate Gene Studies of Panic Disorder

Numerous biological candidate gene studies have examined the association between one or more genetic variants and panic disorder. Selection of candidate genes has been guided by either:

1. Genes involved in the mechanism of action of panicogenic or panicolytic agents such as caffeine, yohimbine, benzodiazepines, and SSRIs; or
2. Anxiety phenotypes identified in transgenic mice.

COMT

Most candidate gene findings are limited to adult samples and few have been replicated.[75] The most promising results have been for the Val158Met (rs4680) variant of *COMT,* which encodes the enzyme *COMT.* The Val158Met variant has shown significant association with panic disorder in several studies.[76,77] Although one meta-analysis of these data found no conclusive association of this *COMT* variant with panic disorder,[78] a second meta-analysis clarified that a significant association was present in the Caucasian subset.[79] Thus, *COMT* variation may confer differential risk for panic disorder based on ethnicity.

Neuropeptide S receptor gene

Recently, variation in the neuropeptide S receptor gene (*NPSR*), a biological and positional candidate gene, has received greater study in panic disorder. *NPSR* encodes a G-protein–coupled receptor that modulates fear-like behaviors in rodents. A polymorphism in *NPSR* (rs324981) leads to an amino acid substitution from Asn to Ile, which increases expression of the neuropeptide S receptor.[80] This polymorphism was examined in a sample of Japanese men with panic disorder[81] and two large independent German adult case-control samples.[82] In both the Japanese male subjects and the female subgroup of the two German studies, the *T* allele of rs324981 was found to be associated with panic disorder. In the German study, the *T* allele of the neuropeptide S receptor was also related to multiple markers of anxiety, including elevated anxiety sensitivity, elevated heart rate, increased symptom endorsement during an avoidance task, and decreased brain activation in prefrontal cortical regions when viewing fear faces (a neuroimaging marker of anxiety). The results from this study illustrate the importance of converging evidence from genetics, psychophysiologic assessments, and functional imaging studies to develop a better understanding of the pathogenesis of anxiety disorders.

Other candidate genes

Several biological candidates, such as *NTRK3* and *ABCG1*, have been supported by single positive reports and a number of genes (eg, *CCK, CCKBR, COMT, HTR2A, MAOA, SLC6A4, SLC6A3, GABRB3, ADRA2A, DRD4, A2AR, BDNF,* and *TPH1*) have been evaluated in multiple studies with mixed results. However, the majority of candidate genes examined (eg, *NET, DRD2, HTR1A, HTR1D, ADRA2B, CCKRA, ESR1, CREM, POMC, CHRNA4,* and multiple γ-aminobutyric acid [GABA] receptor subunits) have failed to show any association.[75]

Genomewide Association Studies of Panic Disorder

Two GWAS screens have been performed using adult panic disorder samples. In a GWAS screen in 216 Caucasian patients with panic disorder and 222 controls,[83] no

SNPs were significantly associated with panic disorder after correction for multiple testing. The largest association was found for a polymorphism (rs7309727) in the *TMEM132D* gene, located on chromosome 12q24. *TMEM132D* encodes transmembrane protein 132D, a protein with unknown function expressed in oligodendrocytes. An associated between panic disorder and variation in *TMEM132D* was confirmed in three independent samples. In the combined sample (909 cases and 915 controls), a two-SNP haplotype (rs7309727 and rs11060369) reached near genomewide significance.[83] Furthermore, risk alleles correlated with increased *TMEM132D* expression in human frontal cortex[83] and with anxiety phenotypes in mice.[83]

Another GWAS was performed in 200 Japanese patients with panic disorder and 200 controls. Seven SNPs were associated with panic disorder with P-value of 1.0×10^{-6} or smaller.[84] Unfortunately, none of these SNPs were associated with panic disorder in a replication sample of 558 Japanese patients and 566 controls.[85]

To date, existing GWAS have been underpowered; much larger sample sizes, likely requiring large collaborative efforts, will be required to identify common genetic variants associated with panic disorder. Regardless, findings implicating *COMT*, *NPSR*, and *TMEM132D* appear to merit more research in relation to panic disorder.

GENETICS OF POSTTRAUMATIC STRESS DISORDER

Postraumatic stress disorder (PTSD) lifetime prevalence estimates range from 1.4% to 11.2%.[86] PTSD results in significant functional impairment and comorbidity for other mental and physical health conditions is common.[86] Although the traumatic events underlying PTSD often occur in childhood, few studies have been conducted in pediatric samples.

Genetic background is believed to influence those trauma-exposed individuals who will go on to manifest PTSD. Estimates of the familiality of PTSD are complicated by the lack of family members matched for trauma exposure[3] however, large-scale traumatic events, such as war, provide an opportunity to estimate genetic effects. In addition, genetic background may influence the likelihood of exposure to trauma, suggesting a complex relationship between genes and PTSD.

Familiality of PTSD

Twin studies in Vietnam combat and civilian populations have demonstrated heritability of PTSD symptoms up to 38%.[87,88] Studies of Holocaust-survivor and refugee populations have demonstrated that adult children of trauma survivors with PTSD were more likely to develop PTSD after a trauma compared to children of trauma-exposed individuals without PTSD.[89,90] The majority of genetic variance contributing to PTSD is shared with other comorbidities such as depression, anxiety, and substance dependence,[91] presumably due to shared risk factors, heightened PTSD vulnerability in psychiatric populations, and psychiatric sequelae of PTSD.

Familiality of trauma exposure

Twin studies in Vietnam combat and civilian populations have demonstrated heritability of exposure to trauma,[87,88] with an estimated 20% of the variance in trauma exposure attributable to genetic factors. Furthermore, the risk factors for exposure to trauma and PTSD symptoms appear to be shared.[87]

The genetic contribution to trauma exposure varies by trauma type. Genetic factors appear to play a role in exposure to assaultive (eg, sexual assault, robbery) and combat-related trauma, but not nonassaultive trauma (eg, motor vehicle accidents, natural disasters).[87,88,92] For example, in a sample of twins from the Vietnam Era Twin (VET) Registry, genetic effects on exposure to combat-related trauma were high (35%–47%), whereas shared environmental effects were nonsignificant[88] and factors predicting combat trauma exposure and combat-related PTSD symptoms were not shared.[88] These findings suggesting that trauma is a nonrandom event influenced by individual and familial risk factors.

Gene–environment interactions

Gene–environment interactions are critically important in PTSD etiology. As previously discussed, different types of PTSD appear to result from differential genetic and environmental contributions to risk. Underscoring this point, in a community sample of Canadian twin pairs, the number of traumatic events was linearly correlated with the severity of PTSD symptoms in nonassaultive trauma. In contrast, for assaultive trauma genetic factors moderated the relationship between number of traumatic events and PTSD symptom severity. Genetic effects only became less important than environmental effects after three or more traumatic events.[93] This framework is important in interpreting candidate gene studies, which have been performed in different populations and with or without examining gene × environment interactions.

Candidate Gene Studies of PTSD

Candidate genes in key pathways involved in stress have been examined for association with the development of PTSD after trauma.[94] Several systems have been highlighted by studies of gene expression in adult trauma survivors, including (1) neuroimmunoendocrine systems and (2) neural signaling systems.[91,95,96]

Neuroimmunoendocrine systems

The hypothalamic–pituitary–adrenal (HPA) axis—a major neuroendocrine system—is one brain pathway likely to be involved in the biological underpinnings of PTSD.[97] Genes involved in the HPA axis and glucocorticoid signaling have been the focus of many studies of PTSD genetic risk factors. One regulator of this pathway is the FK-506 binding protein FKBP5, which is a co-chaperone of the glucocorticoid receptor, thus regulating receptor sensitivity.[94] Polymorphisms in FKBP5 have been shown to impact gene expression in adults with PTSD and to correlate with: symptoms;[98] physiologic stress response in healthy adult subjects;[99] dissociative symptoms in medically-injured children;[100] and PTSD development in the context of past childhood sexual abuse.[101,102] In a study of PTSD among adult survivors of the World Trade Center attacks, homozygosity for any of four PTSD risk-related alleles at FKBP5 predicted FKBP5 expression, plasma cortisol, and PTSD severity.[103] Finally, a prospective study in adults showed that multiple inputs to glucocorticoid signaling pathway were independently associated with increased risk for a high level of PTSD symptoms in combat exposure. For example, PTSD symptoms were predicted by: predeployment high glucocorticoid receptor number; low FKBP5 mRNA expression; and high glucocorticoid-induced leucine zipper (GILZ) mRNA expression.[104]

Neural signaling systems: monoamines

Failure to successfully regulate amygdala activation likely plays a critical role in PTSD.[105] Monoamine regulation of amygdala activity derives from monoamine projections from the brainstem and top-down inputs from medial prefrontal cortex that are essential for fear extinction.[106] Monoaminergic involvement in PTSD is supported by (1) the association of norepinephrine release in limbic regions with emotional arousal,[107] (2) the role of norepinephrine and dopamine in fear memory consolidation,[108] (3) the influence of a common serotonin transporter polymorphism (5HTT-LPR) on extinction of fear conditioning,[109] and (4) the efficacy of serotonergic and adrenergic agents in anxiolysis and PTSD prevention after trauma exposure.[110]

Although several studies in adults and young adults have found interactions between both assaultive and nonassaultive trauma and the serotonin transporter gene (SLC6A4) on risk for PTSD, these effects vary across studies.[111–114] In Veterans with PTSD, a functional polymorphism in the catecholamine degradative enzyme (COMT Val158Met) was shown to moderate the observation of reduced anterior cingulate volume[115] and the dose–response relationship of trauma load to PTSD prevalence.[116]

Studies examining genes involved in neurotransmission and trauma-related phenotypes in adult populations have found mixed associations with the following genes: adrenergic synthetic enzyme (DBH), dopaminergic transporter (SLC6A3), dopamine receptors (DRD2 and DRD4), serotonin receptor (HTR2A), and synthetic enzyme (TPH).[111,117,118]

Neural signaling systems: other neurotransmitters

In addition to monoamines other signaling molecules—such as GABA, endocannabinoids, and G-protein signaling regulators—have been examined. GABAergic neurons within the amygdala receive inputs from the frontal cortex and appear to play a role in fear extinction in rats.[119] In a subset of subjects with childhood trauma with or without PTSD participating in a larger study of nicotine dependence, a block of GABA receptor (GABRA2) SNPs in strong linkage disequilibrium showed individual genotype by trauma interactions on risk for PTSD.[120] The endocannabinoid CB1 receptor is also expressed in the amygdala and involved in fear extinction in mice.[121,122] In a pediatric sample, a variant in the gene encoding this receptor (CNR1) was overtransmitted in trios segregating comorbid ADHD and PTSD.[123] Gene × environment analysis on risk for PTSD in adults revealed interaction between hurricane exposure and social support and regulator of G-protein signaling (RG2S) genotypes previously associated with anxious behavior in mice and anxiety in humans.[124]

Epigenetics

Epigenetic effects, which impact the expression of genes without altering the primary DNA sequence, may be of particular importance in PTSD.[125] Epigenetic marks occur often in the form of changes in DNA methylation and can be stable, enduring, and site-specific; specific to critical developmental periods; and intergenerationally transmitted. Environmental stress effects on epigenetic signatures have been shown in mice[126] and humans,[127] including the association of epigenetic changes with PTSD,[128–130] and provide a possible mechanism for the interaction of environmental trauma and genes.

Linkage and Genomewide Association Studies of PTSD

Linkage and GWAS screens in PTSD are lacking. These approaches are complicated by the fact that controls without equivalent environmental exposure to trauma may carry genetic risk alleles without manifesting the phenotype. Appropriate controls are those who have been exposed to similar trauma without progressing to a PTSD diagnosis, and represent a significant ascertainment challenge and barrier to large genetic screens. Future GWAS studies using appropriate controls can provide a comprehensive and unbiased approach to identifying genetic risk variants for PTSD.[131]

GENETICS OF OTHER ANXIETY DISORDERS (GENERALIZED ANXIETY DISORDER, SEPARATION ANXIETY DISORDER, SOCIAL PHOBIA AND SPECIFIC PHOBIA)

Generalized anxiety disorder (GAD), separation anxiety disorder (SAD), social phobia (SP), and specific phobia are common pediatric mental health disorders.[1] In both community and treatment seeking samples of youth, these disorders are highly comorbid. Because of the high comorbidity rate, many genetic studies have examined several anxiety disorders (eg, SP, SAD, GAD, specific phobia, and panic disorder) together as anxiety-spectrum disorders.

Familiality of Other Anxiety Disorders

Twin and family studies suggest a moderate level of familial transmission of SP, SAD, GAD, and specific phobia in youth (for review see Ref.[132]). Multivariate studies of anxiety disorders in children and adolescents have argued that both genetic and environmental effects are significant in shaping the co-occurrence of different anxiety disorders. For example, Eley and colleagues[133] showed that shared environmental factors explained the comorbidity between specific phobia and SAD, while familial (genetic or shared environmental) factors and nonshared environmental influences explained the comorbidity between specific phobia and SP. In a study of Italian twins (8–17 years old), genetic factors and nonshared environmental influences explained the comorbidity between SP, SAD, GAD, and panic disorder.[134] Furthermore, the effect of genetic factors may change across development, as evidenced by results from a large longitudinal twin study that measured heritability and genetic factors influencing specific phobia over four developmental time points between ages 8 and 20. In that study, heritability ranged from 50% to 69% at all time points; however, the contributory genetic factors were dynamic over time, arguing that different genes may have variable impact on anxiety phenotypes across the lifespan.[135]

Linkage Studies of Other Anxiety Disorders

While no linkage analyses have been performed with individuals meeting criteria for a single anxiety disorder (ie, SP, SAD, GAD, and specific phobia) owing to frequent comorbidity, three linkage screens have been performed in participants with multiple anxiety disorders. In a sample of families ascertained for panic disorder in which the majority of cases had pediatric onset, suggestive evidence for linkage with SP was found in a region of chromosome 16.[136] Similarly, evidence for linkage with specific phobia on chromosome 14 was reported in families ascertained for panic disorder with predominantly pediatric onset.[137] A linkage scan for SP, specific phobia, panic disorder, and agoraphobia in a sample with mixed adult and childhood-onset cases revealed strong evidence for linkage on chromosome 4q31–q34.[138] Because the risk for these common anxiety disorders is believed to result from many genes of modest effect, current linkage studies are likely underpowered.

Candidate Gene Studies of Other Anxiety Disorders

Candidate gene studies have examined the association between one or more genetic variants and anxiety disorders in youth, largely focusing on genes related to neurotransmitter (eg, serotonin, dopamine) or neuropeptide (eg, corticotrophin releasing hormone) signal transduction pathways (for review see Ref.[132]). Positive candidate gene findings in youth have not been replicated.

Serotonin transporter gene

The most extensively studied variant is a repeat polymorphism (ie, 5HTT-LPR, short vs long) in the linked promoter region (LPR) of the serotonin transporter gene

(SLC6A4). Four studies have examined the association of shyness (or the related construct, behavioral inhibition) with variation in 5HTT-LPR with conflicting results:

1. Association with the long allele was reported in second-grade children.[139]
2. The short allele predicted shyness in school-aged children.[140]
3. No effects were observed in a sample of preschool children.[141]
4. A gene–environment interaction between social support and 5HTT-LPR variation where children with both the short allele and low social support had increased risk for behavioral inhibition.[142]

Neurotrophic tyrosine kinase receptor type 2

Recent studies have examined candidate genes implicated by basic research using animal models of anxiety. For example, transgenic studies in mice have shown the overexpression of the BDNF receptor (TrkB) reduces anxiety,[143] while deletion in the forebrain leads to reduced explorative activity and impulsive reactions to novel stimuli.[144] In a longitudinal study, an 11-base-pair deletion in the promoter region of the human version of this gene (NTRK2) predicted anxious traits during childhood and the development of anxiety disorders (ie, GAD and panic disorder) in adulthood.

Contactin-associated protein-like 2

Other recent candidate gene studies have focused on genes involved in other childhood disorders with markedly elevated rates of comorbid anxiety disorders. For example, one study examined the association of a common genetic variant in the neurexin superfamily member, CNTNAP2, with selective mutism in childhood and social anxiety traits in young adults.[145] Polymorphisms in CNTNAP2 have been reliably associated with increased susceptibility to autism spectrum disorders.[146] A haplotype of rs2710102 and rs6944808 in CNTNAP2 was associated with selective mutism in a sample of children[145] and rs2710102 was associated with social anxiety in a sample of young adults.[145] Thus, candidate gene studies in anxiety often utilize broad phenotypes spanning Diagnostic and Statistical Manual of Mental Disorders (DSM) diagnoses (eg, shyness in children) and have been guided by animal models of anxiety and other disorders that share anxiety phenotypes.

Genomewide Association Studies of Other Anxiety Disorders

To date, no GWAS have been published in SP, SAD, GAD or specific phobia populations. However, a recent study has used a novel approach to examine genomewide association. Candidate genes associated with fear-related behaviors in mice were identified and then these candidate genes were ranked according to evidence from (1) linkage and knockout studies in mice; (2) a meta-analysis of human linkage scans (ie, eight GWAS of neuroticism and three GWAS of anxiety disorder); and (3) a preliminary human GWAS.[147] Then, top ranked regions were tested for association with human anxiety-spectrum disorders (ie, anxiety disorders, neuroticism, and major depression) in the Virginia Adult Twin Study of Psychiatric and Substance Use Disorders sample. In the end, multiple SNPs in the PPARGC1A gene demonstrated association for anxiety-related disorders. The PPARGC1A gene encodes the transcriptional coactivator, peroxisome proliferator-activated receptor gamma coactivator 1 alpha (PGC-1α), which plays a role in energy expenditure. In the brain, PGC-1α is contained in interneurons, and may provide neuroprotection by upregulating genes involved in the metabolism of reactive oxygen species.

IMPLICATIONS FOR CLINICAL PRACTICE AND RESEARCH

Although an understanding of the molecular basis of child and adolescent anxiety disorders is far from complete, the research findings described in the preceding text confirm several clinically important features of these conditions, and raise more research questions for future study. There is no question that genes play a significant role in child anxiety risk. Knowledge of the family history of anxiety disorders represents valuable clinical data to aid in the determination of anxiety diagnoses. Some subtypes, such as OCD-hoarding or tic-related OCD, carry large increases in risk for other family members. The presence of OCD should also encourage consideration of risk for other commonly associated OCD-spectrum conditions. The relationship between younger onset and increased heritability may suggest the need for earlier inclusion of biological treatments and more intensive, longer-term maintenance therapies. An emerging role for glutamate in OCD (and possibly other anxiety disorders) also should encourage more investigation of treatments involving glutamate-modulating agents, some of which have initial support in the literature. The surprisingly sparse research database on the genetics of child PTSD should spur more studies of risk and resiliency to the effects of early trauma, which could hold important implications for child and adult outcomes. Finally, the frequent comorbidity of different anxiety disorders, and even other mental illnesses, implies that genes driving risk for anxiety-spectrum phenotypes or overall psychiatric vulnerability may interact with those conferring risk for distinct disorders. In addition, the understanding of the moderating role of environmental influences on phenotypic expression of genetic risk will guide the development of early interventions.

SUMMARY

Strong evidence supports familial and genetic influences on pediatric anxiety disorders; however, identifying the specific genes that place children and adolescents at risk for anxiety disorders has been daunting. There are impressive data showing that early-onset anxiety represents a more genetically enriched set of conditions, ripe for additional studies of its molecular basis. Advances in molecular, statistical, and computational methods have made elucidating the genetic basis of complex disorders more feasible. Increased access of whole exome and genome sequencing approaches will expand the tools available in tackling this task. Further progress in identifying the genes underlying risk for pediatric anxiety disorders will require integrative approaches combining genetics, refined psychophysiologic assessments, functional imaging and molecular studies, and computational and statistical creativity in large, adequately powered and carefully phenotyped populations. Eventually, the identification of susceptibility genes will improve our understanding of the pathophysiology of anxiety and our ability to diagnose and treat those affected with and at risk for anxiety-spectrum disorders.

REFERENCES

1. Costello EJ, Egger HL, Angold A. The developmental epidemiology of anxiety disorders: phenomenology, prevalence, and comorbidity. Child Adolesc Psychiatr Clin N Am 2005;14(4):631–48, vii.
2. Pine DS, Cohen P, Gurley D, et al. The risk for early-adulthood anxiety and depressive disorders in adolescents with anxiety and depressive disorders. Arch Gen Psychiatry 1998;55(1):56–64.

3. Smoller JW, Block SR, Young MM. Genetics of anxiety disorders: the complex road from DSM to DNA. Depress Anxiety 2009;26(11):965–75.
4. Hettema JM, Neale MC, Kendler KS. A review and meta-analysis of the genetic epidemiology of anxiety disorders. Am J Psychiatry 2001;158(10):1568–78.
5. van Grootheest DS, Cath DC, Beekman AT, et al. Twin studies on obsessive-compulsive disorder: a review. Twin Res Hum Genet 2005;8(5):450–8.
6. Walitza S, Wendland JR, Gruenblatt E, et al. Genetics of early-onset obsessive-compulsive disorder. Eur Child Adolesc Psychiatry 2010;19(3):227–35.
7. Weissman MM, Bland RC, Canino GJ, et al. The cross national epidemiology of obsessive compulsive disorder. The Cross National Collaborative Group. J Clin Psychiatry 1994;55(Suppl):5–10.
8. Kessler RC, Berglund P, Demler O, et al. Lifetime prevalence and age-of-onset distributions of DSM-IV disorders in the National Comorbidity Survey Replication. Arch Gen Psychiatry 2005;62(6):593–602.
9. Stewart SE, Geller DA, Jenike M, et al. Long-term outcome of pediatric obsessive-compulsive disorder: a meta-analysis and qualitative review of the literature. Acta Psychiatr Scand 2004;110(1):4–13.
10. Piacentini J, Bergman RL, Keller M, et al. Functional impairment in children and adolescents with obsessive-compulsive disorder. J Child Adolesc Psychopharmacol. 2003;13(Suppl 1):S61–9.
11. Saxena S, Rauch SL. Functional neuroimaging and the neuroanatomy of obsessive-compulsive disorder. Psychiatr Clin North Am 2000;23(3):563–86.
12. Kalra SK, Swedo SE. Children with obsessive-compulsive disorder: are they just "little adults"? J Clin Invest 2009;119(4):737–46.
13. Bolton D, Rijsdijk F, O'Connor TG, et al. Obsessive-compulsive disorder, tics and anxiety in 6-year-old twins. Psychol Med 2007;37(1):39–48.
14. Tambs K, Czajkowsky N, Roysamb E, et al. Structure of genetic and environmental risk factors for dimensional representations of DSM-IV anxiety disorders. Br J Psychiatry 2009;195(4):301–7.
15. Pauls DL. The genetics of obsessive-compulsive disorder: a review. Dialog Clin Neurosci 2010;12(2):149–63.
16. Pinto A, Greenberg BD, Grados MA, et al. Further development of YBOCS dimensions in the OCD Collaborative Genetics study: symptoms vs. categories. Psychiatry Res 2008;160(1):83–93.
17. Grabe HJ, Ruhrmann S, Ettelt S, et al. Familiality of obsessive-compulsive disorder in nonclinical and clinical subjects. Am J Psychiatry 2006;163(11):1986–92.
18. Hasler G, Pinto A, Greenberg BD, et al. Familiality of factor analysis-derived YBOCS dimensions in OCD-affected sibling pairs from the OCD Collaborative Genetics Study. Biol Psychiatry 2007;61(5):617–25.
19. Bienvenu OJ, Samuels JF, Riddle MA, et al. The relationship of obsessive-compulsive disorder to possible spectrum disorders: results from a family study. Biol Psychiatry 2000;48(4):287–93.
20. Grados MA, Riddle MA, Samuels JF, et al. The familial phenotype of obsessive-compulsive disorder in relation to tic disorders: the Hopkins OCD family study. Biol Psychiatry 2001;50(8):559–65.
21. Black DW, Noyes R Jr, Goldstein RB, et al. A family study of obsessive-compulsive disorder. Arch Gen Psychiatry 1992;49(5):362–8.
22. Nestadt G, Di CZ, Riddle MA, et al. Obsessive-compulsive disorder: subclassification based on co-morbidity. Psychol Med 2009;39(9):1491–501.

23. Alsobrook IJ, Leckman JF, Goodman WK, et al. Segregation analysis of obsessive-compulsive disorder using symptom-based factor scores. Am J Med Genet 1999; 88(6):669–75.

24. Cavallini MC, Bertelli S, Chiapparino D, et al. Complex segregation analysis of obsessive-compulsive disorder in 141 families of eating disorder probands, with and without obsessive-compulsive disorder. Am J Med Genet 2000;96(3):384–91.

25. Nestadt G, Lan T, Samuels J, et al. Complex segregation analysis provides compelling evidence for a major gene underlying obsessive-compulsive disorder and for heterogeneity by sex. Am J Hum Genet 2000;67(6):1611–6.

26. Shugart YY, Samuels J, Willour VL, et al. Genomewide linkage scan for obsessive-compulsive disorder: evidence for susceptibility loci on chromosomes 3q, 7p, 1q, 15q, and 6q. Mol Psychiatry 2006;11(8):763–70.

27. Hanna GL, Veenstra-VanderWeele J, Cox NJ, et al. Genome-wide linkage analysis of families with obsessive-compulsive disorder ascertained through pediatric probands. Am J Med Genet 2002;114(5):541–52.

28. Hanna GL, Veenstra-Vanderweele J, Cox NJ, et al. Evidence for a susceptibility locus on chromosome 10p15 in early-onset obsessive-compulsive disorder. Biol Psychiatry 2007;62(8):856–62.

29. Ross J, Badner J, Garrido H, et al. Genomewide linkage analysis in Costa Rican families implicates chromosome 15q14 as a candidate region for OCD. Hum Genet 2011;130(6):795–805.

30. Nestadt G, Wang Y, Grados MA, et al. Homeobox genes in obsessive-compulsive disorder. Am J Med Genet B Neuropsychiatr Genet 2012;159B(1):53–60.

31. Samuels J, Shugart YY, Grados MA, et al. Significant linkage to compulsive hoarding on chromosome 14 in families with obsessive-compulsive disorder: results from the OCD Collaborative Genetics Study. Am J Psychiatry 2007;164(3):493–9.

32. Wang Y, Samuels JF, Chang YC, et al. Gender differences in genetic linkage and association on 11p15 in obsessive-compulsive disorder families. Am J Med Genet B Neuropsychiatr Genet 2009;150B(1):33–40.

33. Willour VL, Yao Shugart Y, Samuels J, et al. Replication study supports evidence for linkage to 9p24 in obsessive-compulsive disorder. Am J Hum Genet 2004;75(3): 508–13.

34. Mathews C, Badner J, Andresen J, et al. Genomewide linkage analysis of obsessive compulsive disorder implicates chromosome 1p36. Biol Psychiatry 2012. [Epub ahead of print].

35. Chakrabarty K, Bhattacharyya S, Christopher R, et al. Glutamatergic dysfunction in OCD. Neuropsychopharmacology 2005;30(9):1735–40.

36. MacMaster FP, O'Neill J, Rosenberg DR. Brain imaging in pediatric obsessive-compulsive disorder. J Am Acad Child Adolesc Psychiatry 2008;47(11):1262–72.

37. Maina G, Rosso G, Zanardini R, et al. Serum levels of brain-derived neurotrophic factor in drug-naive obsessive-compulsive patients: a case-control study. J Affect Disord 2010;122(1–2):174–8.

38. O'Neill J, Piacentini JC, Chang S, et al. MRSI correlates of cognitive-behavioral therapy in pediatric obsessive-compulsive disorder. Prog Neuropsychopharmacol Biol Psychiatry 2012;36(1):161–8.

39. Wu K, Hanna GL, Rosenberg DR, Arnold PD. The role of glutamate signaling in the pathogenesis and treatment of obsessive-compulsive disorder. Pharmacol Biochem Behav 2012;100(4):726–35.

40. Ting JT, Feng G. Neurobiology of obsessive-compulsive disorder: insights into neural circuitry dysfunction through mouse genetics. Curr Opin Neurobiol 2011; 21(6):842–8.

41. Arnold PD, Rosenberg DR, Mundo E, Tharmalingam S, Kennedy JL, Richter MA. Association of a glutamate (NMDA) subunit receptor gene (GRIN2B) with obsessive-compulsive disorder: a preliminary study. Psychopharmacology (Berl) 2004;174(4): 530–8.

42. Arnold PD, Macmaster FP, Richter MA, et al. Glutamate receptor gene (*GRIN2B*) associated with reduced anterior cingulate glutamatergic concentration in pediatric obsessive-compulsive disorder. Psychiatry Res 2009;172(2):136–9.

43. Arnold PD, Macmaster FP, Hanna GL, et al. Glutamate system genes associated with ventral prefrontal and thalamic volume in pediatric obsessive-compulsive disorder. Brain Imaging Behav 2009;3(1):64–76.

44. Delorme R, Krebs MO, Chabane N, et al. Frequency and transmission of glutamate receptors GRIK2 and GRIK3 polymorphisms in patients with obsessive compulsive disorder. NeuroReport 2004;15(4):699–702.

45. Sampaio AS, Fagerness J, Crane J, et al. Association between polymorphisms in GRIK2 gene and obsessive-compulsive disorder: a family-based study. CNS Neurosci Ther 2011;17(3):141–7.

46. Bienvenu OJ, Wang Y, Shugart YY, et al. Sapap3 and pathological grooming in humans: Results from the OCD collaborative genetics study. Am J Med Genet B Neuropsychiatr Genet 2009;150B(5):710–20.

47. Samuels J, Wang Y, Riddle MA, et al. Comprehensive family-based association study of the glutamate transporter gene *SLC1A1* in obsessive-compulsive disorder. Am J Med Genet B Neuropsychiatr Genet 2011;156B(4):472–7.

48. Wendland JR, Moya PR, Timpano KR, et al. A haplotype containing quantitative trait loci for SLC1A1 gene expression and its association with obsessive-compulsive disorder. Arch Gen Psychiatry 2009;66(4):408–16.

49. Shugart YY, Wang Y, Samuels JF, et al. A family-based association study of the glutamate transporter gene *SLC1A1* in obsessive-compulsive disorder in 378 families. Am J Med Genet B Neuropsychiatr Genet 2009;150B(6):886–92.

50. Stewart SE, Fagerness JA, Platko J, et al. Association of the SLC1A1 glutamate transporter gene and obsessive-compulsive disorder. Am J Med Genet B Neuropsychiatr Genet 2007;144B(8):1027–33.

51. Dickel DE, Veenstra-VanderWeele J, Cox NJ, et al. Association testing of the positional and functional candidate gene *SLC1A1/EAAC1* in early-onset obsessive-compulsive disorder. Arch Gen Psychiatry 2006;63(7):778–85.

52. Arnold PD, Sicard T, Burroughs E, et al. Glutamate transporter gene *SLC1A1* associated with obsessive-compulsive disorder. Arch Gen Psychiatry 2006;63(7): 769–76.

53. Alonso P, Gratacos M, Menchon JM, et al. Extensive genotyping of the *BDNF* and *NTRK2* genes define protective haplotypes against obsessive-compulsive disorder. Biol Psychiatry 2008;63(6):619–28.

54. Hall D, Dhilla A, Charalambous A, et al. Sequence variants of the brain-derived neurotrophic factor (*BDNF*) gene are strongly associated with obsessive-compulsive disorder. Am J Hum Genet 2003;73(2):370–6.

55. Wendland JR, Kruse MR, Cromer KR, et al. A large case-control study of common functional *SLC6A4* and *BDNF* variants in obsessive-compulsive disorder. Neuropsychopharmacology 2007;32(12):2543–51.

56. Wang Y, Mathews CA, Li Y, et al. Brain-derived neurotrophic factor (BDNF) plasma levels in drug-naive OCD patients are lower than those in healthy people, but are not lower than those in drug-treated OCD patients. J Affect Disord 2011;133(1–2):305–10.

57. Dos Santos IM, Ciulla L, Braga D, et al. Symptom dimensional approach and BDNF in unmedicated obsessive-compulsive patients: an exploratory study. CNS Spectr 2011. [Epub ahead of print].

58. Real E, Gratacos M, Soria V, et al. A brain-derived neurotrophic factor haplotype is associated with therapeutic response in obsessive-compulsive disorder. Biol Psychiatry 2009;66(7):674–80.

59. Jayarajan RN, Venkatasubramanian G, Viswanath B, et al. White matter abnormalities in children and adolescents with obsessive-compulsive disorder: a diffusion tensor imaging study. Depress Anxiety 2012. [Epub ahead of print].

60. Macmaster F, Vora A, Easter P, et al. Orbital frontal cortex in treatment-naive pediatric obsessive-compulsive disorder. Psychiatry Res 2010;181(2):97–100.

61. van den Heuvel OA, Remijnse PL, Mataix-Cols D, et al. The major symptom dimensions of obsessive-compulsive disorder are mediated by partially distinct neural systems. Brain. 2009;132(Pt 4):853–68.

62. Szeszko PR, Ardekani BA, Ashtari M, et al. White matter abnormalities in obsessive-compulsive disorder: a diffusion tensor imaging study. Arch Gen Psychiatry 2005; 62(7):782–90.

63. da Rocha FF, Correa H, Teixeira AL. Obsessive-compulsive disorder and immunology: a review. Prog Neuropsychopharmacol Biol Psychiatry 2008;32(5):1139–46.

64. Stewart SE, Platko J, Fagerness J, et al. A genetic family-based association study of OLIG2 in obsessive-compulsive disorder. Arch Gen Psychiatry 2007;64(2):209–14.

65. Zai G, Bezchlibnyk YB, Richter MA, et al. Myelin oligodendrocyte glycoprotein (MOG) gene is associated with obsessive-compulsive disorder. Am J Med Genet B Neuropsychiatr Genet 2004;129B(1):64–8.

66. Atmaca M, Onalan E, Yildirim H, et al. The association of myelin oligodendrocyte glycoprotein gene and white matter volume in obsessive-compulsive disorder. J Affect Disord 2010;124(3):309–13.

67. Stewart SE, Yu D, Scharf J, et al. IOCDF Genome-wide association study of obsessive-compulsive disorder. Paper presented at International Congress of Human Genetics 2011; Montreal, Canada.

68. Nestadt G. OCD Genetics: Progress Report from the OCD Collaborative Genetics Association (OCGAS) Study. Paper presented at International OCD Foundation. San Diego (CA):2011.

69. Merikangas KR, He JP, Burstein M, et al. Lifetime prevalence of mental disorders in U.S. adolescents: results from the National Comorbidity Survey Replication—Adolescent Supplement (NCS-A). J Am Acad Child Adolesc Psychiatry 2010;49(10): 980–9.

70. Gorman JM, Kent JM, Sullivan GM, et al. Neuroanatomical hypothesis of panic disorder, revised. Am J Psychiatry 2000;157(4):493–505.

71. Skre I, Onstad S, Edvardsen J, et al. A family study of anxiety disorders: familial transmission and relationship to mood disorder and psychoactive substance use disorder. Acta Psychiatr Scand 1994;90(5):366–74.

72. Goldstein RB, Wickramaratne PJ, Horwath E, et al. Familial aggregation and phenomenology of 'early'-onset (at or before age 20 years) panic disorder. Arch Gen Psychiatry 1997;54(3):271–8.

73. Fyer AJ, Hamilton SP, Durner M, et al. A third-pass genome scan in panic disorder: evidence for multiple susceptibility loci. Biol Psychiatry 2006;60(4):388–401.

74. Maron E, Hettema JM, Shlik J. Advances in molecular genetics of panic disorder. Mol Psychiatry 2010;15(7):681–701.

75. Gratacos M, Sahun I, Gallego X, et al. Candidate genes for panic disorder: insight from human and mouse genetic studies. Genes Brain Behav 6(Suppl 1):2–23.

76. Domschke K, Freitag CM, Kuhlenbaumer G, et al. Association of the functional V158M catechol-*O*-methyl-transferase polymorphism with panic disorder in women. Int J Neuropsychopharmacol 2004;7(2):183–8.
77. Rothe C, Koszycki D, Bradwejn J, et al. Association of the Val158Met catechol *O*-methyltransferase genetic polymorphism with panic disorder. Neuropsychopharmacology 2006;31(10):2237–42.
78. Zintzaras E, Sakelaridis N. Is 472G/A catechol-*O*-methyl-transferase gene polymorphism related to panic disorder? Psychiatr Genet 2007;17(5):267–73.
79. Domschke K, Deckert J, O'Donovan M C, et al. Meta-analysis of COMT val158met in panic disorder: ethnic heterogeneity and gender specificity. Am J Med Genet B Neuropsychiatr Genet 2007;144B(5):667–73.
80. Bernier V, Stocco R, Bogusky MJ, et al. Structure-function relationships in the neuropeptide S receptor: molecular consequences of the asthma-associated mutation N107I. J Biol Chem 2006;281(34):24704–12.
81. Okamura N, Hashimoto K, Iyo M, et al. Gender-specific association of a functional coding polymorphism in the neuropeptide S receptor gene with panic disorder but not with schizophrenia or attention-deficit/hyperactivity disorder. Prog Neuropsychopharmacol Biol Psychiatry 2007;31(7):1444–8.
82. Domschke K, Reif A, Weber H, et al. Neuropeptide S receptor gene—converging evidence for a role in panic disorder. Mol Psychiatry 2011;16(9):938–48.
83. Erhardt A, Czibere L, Roeske D, et al. *TMEM132D*, a new candidate for anxiety phenotypes: evidence from human and mouse studies. Mol Psychiatry 2011;16(6): 647–63.
84. Otowa T, Yoshida E, Sugaya N, et al. Genome-wide association study of panic disorder in the Japanese population. J Hum Genet 2009;54(2):122–6.
85. Otowa T, Tanii H, Sugaya N, et al. Replication of a genome-wide association study of panic disorder in a Japanese population. J Hum Genet 2010;55(2):91–6.
86. Afifi TO, Asmundson GJ, Taylor S, et al. The role of genes and environment on trauma exposure and posttraumatic stress disorder symptoms: a review of twin studies. Clin Psychol Rev 2010;30(1):101–12.
87. Stein MB, Jang KL, Taylor S, et al. Genetic and environmental influences on trauma exposure and posttraumatic stress disorder symptoms: a twin study. Am J Psychiatry 2002;159(10):1675–81.
88. Lyons MJ, Goldberg J, Eisen SA, et al. Do genes influence exposure to trauma? A twin study of combat. Am J Med Genet 1993;48(1):22–7.
89. Yehuda R, Halligan SL, Bierer LM. Relationship of parental trauma exposure and PTSD to PTSD, depressive and anxiety disorders in offspring. J Psychiatr Res 2001;35(5):261–70.
90. Sack WH, Clarke GN, Seeley J. Posttraumatic stress disorder across two generations of Cambodian refugees. J Am Acad Child Adolesc Psychiatry 1995;34(9): 1160–6.
91. Zieker J, Zieker D, Jatzko A, et al. Differential gene expression in peripheral blood of patients suffering from post-traumatic stress disorder. Mol Psychiatry 2007;12(2): 116–8.
92. Koenen KC. Genetics of posttraumatic stress disorder: review and recommendations for future studies. J Trauma Stress 2007;20(5):737–50.
93. Jang KL, Taylor S, Stein MB, et al. Trauma exposure and stress response: exploration of mechanisms of cause and effect. Twin Res Hum Genet 2007;10(4):564–72.
94. Hauger RL, Olivares-Reyes JA, Dautzenberg FM, et al. Molecular and cell signaling targets for PTSD pathophysiology and pharmacotherapy. Neuropharmacology 2012;62(2):705–14.

95. Segman RH, Shefi N, Goltser-Dubner T, et al. Peripheral blood mononuclear cell gene expression profiles identify emergent post-traumatic stress disorder among trauma survivors. Mol Psychiatry 2005;10(5):425, 500–13.

96. Yehuda R, Cai G, Golier JA, et al. Gene expression patterns associated with posttraumatic stress disorder following exposure to the World Trade Center attacks. Biol Psychiatry 2009;66(7):708–11.

97. Skelton K, Ressler KJ, Norrholm SD, et al. PTSD and gene variants: new pathways and new thinking. Neuropharmacology 2012;62(2):628–37.

98. Mehta D, Gonik M, Klengel T, et al. Using polymorphisms in FKBP5 to define biologically distinct subtypes of posttraumatic stress disorder: evidence from endocrine and gene expression studies. Arch Gen Psychiatry 2011;68(9):901–10.

99. Ising M, Depping AM, Siebertz A, et al. Polymorphisms in the *FKBP5* gene region modulate recovery from psychosocial stress in healthy controls. Eur J Neurosci 2008;28(2):389–98.

100. Koenen KC, Saxe G, Purcell S, et al. Polymorphisms in *FKBP5* are associated with peritraumatic dissociation in medically injured children. Mol Psychiatry 2005;10(12): 1058–9.

101. Binder EB, Bradley RG, Liu W, et al. Association of *FKBP5* polymorphisms and childhood abuse with risk of posttraumatic stress disorder symptoms in adults. JAMA 2008;299(11):1291–305.

102. Xie P, Kranzler HR, Poling J, et al. Interaction of *FKBP5* with childhood adversity on risk for post-traumatic stress disorder. Neuropsychopharmacology 2010;35(8): 1684–92.

103. Sarapas C, Cai G, Bierer LM, et al. Genetic markers for PTSD risk and resilience among survivors of the World Trade Center attacks. Dis Markers 2011;30(2–3): 101–10.

104. van Zuiden M, Geuze E, Willemen HL, et al. Glucocorticoid receptor pathway components predict posttraumatic stress disorder symptom development: a prospective study. Biol Psychiatry 2012;71(4):309–16.

105. Fanselow MS, LeDoux JE. Why we think plasticity underlying Pavlovian fear conditioning occurs in the basolateral amygdala. Neuron 1999;23(2):229–32.

106. Likhtik E, Pelletier JG, Paz R, et al. Prefrontal control of the amygdala. J Neurosci 2005;25(32):7429–37.

107. Cahill L, Prins B, Weber M, et al. Beta-adrenergic activation and memory for emotional events. Nature 1994;371(6499):702–4.

108. Ouyang M, Young MB, Lestini MM, et al. Redundant catecholamine signaling consolidates fear memory via phospholipase C. J Neurosci 2012;32(6):1932–41.

109. Pezawas L, Meyer-Lindenberg A, Drabant EM, et al. 5-HTTLPR polymorphism impacts human cingulate-amygdala interactions: a genetic susceptibility mechanism for depression. Nat Neurosci 2005;8(6):828–34.

110. Cukor J, Spitalnick J, Difede J, et al. Emerging treatments for PTSD. Clin Psychol Rev 2009;29(8):715–26.

111. Kilpatrick DG, Koenen KC, Ruggiero KJ, et al. The serotonin transporter genotype and social support and moderation of posttraumatic stress disorder and depression in hurricane-exposed adults. Am J Psychiatry 2007;164(11):1693–9.

112. Koenen KC, Aiello AE, Bakshis E, et al. Modification of the association between serotonin transporter genotype and risk of posttraumatic stress disorder in adults by county-level social environment. Am J Epidemiol 2009;169(6):704–11.

113. Kolassa IT, Ertl V, Eckart C, et al. Association study of trauma load and *SLC6A4* promoter polymorphism in posttraumatic stress disorder: evidence from survivors of the Rwandan genocide. J Clin Psychiatry 2010;71(5):543–7.

114. Mercer KB, Orcutt HK, Quinn JF, et al. Acute and posttraumatic stress symptoms in a prospective gene × environment study of a university campus shooting. Arch Gen Psychiatry 2012;69(1):89–97.

115. Schulz-Heik RJ, Schaer M, Eliez S, et al. Catechol-*O*-methyltransferase Val158Met polymorphism moderates anterior cingulate volume in posttraumatic stress disorder. Biol Psychiatry 2011;70(11):1091–6.

116. Kolassa IT, Kolassa S, Ertl V, et al. The risk of posttraumatic stress disorder after trauma depends on traumatic load and the catechol-*O*-methyltransferase Val(158)Met polymorphism. Biol Psychiatry 2010;67(4):304–8.

117. Amstadter AB, Nugent NR, Koenen KC. Genetics of PTSD: fear conditioning as a model for future research. Psychiatr Ann 2009;39(6):358–67.

118. Bailey JN, Goenjian AK, Noble EP, et al. PTSD and dopaminergic genes, *DRD2* and *DAT*, in multigenerational families exposed to the Spitak earthquake. Psychiatry Res 2010;178(3):507–10.

119. Amano T, Unal CT, Pare D. Synaptic correlates of fear extinction in the amygdala. Nat Neurosci 2010;13(4):489–94.

120. Nelson EC, Agrawal A, Pergadia ML, et al. Association of childhood trauma exposure and *GABRA2* polymorphisms with risk of posttraumatic stress disorder in adults. Mol Psychiatry 2009;14(3):234–5.

121. Kamprath K, Marsicano G, Tang J, et al. Cannabinoid CB1 receptor mediates fear extinction via habituation-like processes. J Neurosci 2006;26(25):6677–86.

122. Kamprath K, Romo-Parra H, Haring M, et al. Short-term adaptation of conditioned fear responses through endocannabinoid signaling in the central amygdala. Neuropsychopharmacology 2011;36(3):652–63.

123. Lu AT, Ogdie MN, Jarvelin MR, et al. Association of the cannabinoid receptor gene (*CNR1*) with ADHD and post-traumatic stress disorder. Am J Med Genet B Neuropsychiatr Genet 2008;147B(8):1488–94.

124. Amstadter AB, Koenen KC, Ruggiero KJ, et al. Variant in RGS2 moderates posttraumatic stress symptoms following potentially traumatic event exposure. J Anxiety Disord 2009;23(3):369–73.

125. Yehuda R, Bierer LM. The relevance of epigenetics to PTSD: implications for the DSM-V. J Trauma Stress 2009;22(5):427–34.

126. Weaver IC, Cervoni N, Champagne FA, et al. Epigenetic programming by maternal behavior. Nat Neurosci 2004;7(8):847–54.

127. McGowan PO, Sasaki A, D'Alessio AC, et al. Epigenetic regulation of the glucocorticoid receptor in human brain associates with childhood abuse. Nat Neurosci 2009;12(3):342–8.

128. Ressler KJ, Mercer KB, Bradley B, et al. Post-traumatic stress disorder is associated with PACAP and the PAC1 receptor. Nature 2011;470(7335):492–7.

129. Uddin M, Aiello AE, Wildman DE, et al. Epigenetic and immune function profiles associated with posttraumatic stress disorder. Proc Natl Acad Sci U S A 2010; 107(20):9470–5.

130. Rusiecki JA, Chen L, Srikantan V, et al. DNA methylation in repetitive elements and post-traumatic stress disorder: a case-control study of US military service members. Epigenomics 2012;4(1):29–40.

131. Cornelis MC, Nugent NR, Amstadter AB, et al. Genetics of post-traumatic stress disorder: review and recommendations for genome-wide association studies. Curr Psychiatry Rep 2010;12(4):313–26.

132. Gregory AM, Eley TC. Genetic influences on anxiety in children: what we've learned and where we're heading. Clin Child Fam Psychol Rev 2007;10(3):199–212.

133. Eley TC, Rijsdijk FV, Perrin S, et al. A multivariate genetic analysis of specific phobia, separation anxiety and social phobia in early childhood. J Abnorm Child Psychol. 2008;36(6):839–48.

134. Ogliari A, Spatola CA, Pesenti-Gritti P, et al. The role of genes and environment in shaping co-occurrence of DSM-IV defined anxiety dimensions among Italian twins aged 8–17. J Anxiety Disord 2010;24(4):433–9.

135. Kendler KS, Gardner CO, Annas P, et al. The development of fears from early adolesence to young adulthood: a multivariate study. Psychol Med 2008;38(12): 1759–69.

136. Gelernter J, Page GP, Stein MB, et al. Genome-wide linkage scan for loci predisposing to social phobia: evidence for a chromosome 16 risk locus. Am J Psychiatry. 2004;161(1):59–66.

137. Gelernter J, Page GP, Bonvicini K, et al. A chromosome 14 risk locus for simple phobia: results from a genomewide linkage scan. Mol Psychiatry 2003;8(1): 71–82.

138. Kaabi B, Gelernter J, Woods SW, et al. Genome scan for loci predisposing to anxiety disorders using a novel multivariate approach: strong evidence for a chromosome 4 risk locus. Am J Hum Genet 2006;78(4):543–53.

139. Arbelle S, Benjamin J, Golin M, et al. Relation of shyness in grade school children to the genotype for the long form of the serotonin transporter promoter region polymorphism. Am J Psychiatry 2003;160(4):671–6.

140. Battaglia M, Ogliari A, Zanoni A, et al. Influence of the serotonin transporter promoter gene and shyness on children's cerebral responses to facial expressions. Arch Gen Psychiatry 2005;62(1):85–94.

141. Schmidt LA, Fox NA, Rubin KH, et al. Molecular genetics of shyness and aggression in preschoolers. Pers Individ Dif 2002;33(2):227–38.

142. Fox NA, Nichols KE, Henderson HA, et al. Evidence for a gene-environment interaction in predicting behavioral inhibition in middle childhood. Psychol Sci 2005;16(12):921–6.

143. Koponen E, Voikar V, Riekki R, et al. Transgenic mice overexpressing the full-length neurotrophin receptor trkB exhibit increased activation of the trkB-PLCgamma pathway, reduced anxiety, and facilitated learning. Mol Cell Neurosci 2004;26(1): 166–81.

144. Zorner B, Wolfer DP, Brandis D, et al. Forebrain-specific trkB-receptor knockout mice: behaviorally more hyperactive than "depressive." Biol Psychiatry. 2003;54(10): 972–82.

145. Stein MB, Yang BZ, Chavira DA, et al. A common genetic variant in the neurexin superfamily member *CNTNAP2* is associated with increased risk for selective mutism and social anxiety-related traits. Biol Psychiatry 2011;69(9):825–31.

146. Alarcon M, Abrahams BS, Stone JL, et al. Linkage, association, and gene-expression analyses identify *CNTNAP2* as an autism-susceptibility gene. Am J Hum Genet 2008;82(1):150–9.

147. Hettema JM, Webb BT, Guo AY, et al. Prioritization and association analysis of murine-derived candidate genes in anxiety-spectrum disorders. Biol Psychiatry 2011;70(9):888–96.

Neural Substrates of Childhood Anxiety Disorders
A Review of Neuroimaging Findings

Jennifer Urbano Blackford, PhD[a,b,]*, Daniel S. Pine, MD[c]

KEYWORDS

- Anxiety disorders • Neuroimaging • Functional magnetic resonance imaging
- Children • Adolescents

KEY POINTS

- Development of fear is a normative process; normal development of the fear system goes awry in children who develop anxiety disorders and dysfunction in the amygdala-prefrontal cortex fear circuitry is likely.
- In the fear-based anxiety disorders, neuroimaging studies have reported brain dysfunction in both the amygdala and multiple regions of the PFC.
- In OCD, neuroimaging studies have reported functional and/or structural anomalies in the basal ganglia, orbitofrontal cortex and anterior cingulate cortex.
- Functional and structural neuroimaging studies have contributed to the significant progress made in identifying possible neural substrates of childhood anxiety disorders.

INTRODUCTION

Anxiety disorders are the most common group of childhood psychiatric disorders, with almost one in three children having suffered from an anxiety disorder at some point during childhood or adolescence.[1] Most anxiety disorders begin early in development, with a median age at onset of 12 years.[1] Although significant advances have been made in

The preparation of this manuscript was partially supported by Award No. K01-MH083052 to Jennifer Urbano Blackford from the National Institute of Mental Health. The content is solely the responsibility of the authors and does not necessarily represent the official views of the National Institutes of Mental Health or the National Institutes of Health.
The authors have nothing else to disclose.
[a] Psychiatric Neuroimaging Program, Department of Psychiatry, Vanderbilt University School of Medicine, 1601 23rd Avenue South, Nashville, TN 37212, USA; [b] Department of Psychology, Vanderbilt University, 301 Wilson Hall, 111 21st Avenue South, Nashville, TN 37240, USA; [c] Section on Development and Affective Neuroscience, Intramural Research Program, National Institutes of Mental Health, Building 1, Room B310-0135, 1 Center Drive MSC 0135, Bethesda, MD 20895, USA
* Corresponding author. Psychiatric Neuroimaging Program, Department of Psychiatry, Vanderbilt University School of Medicine, 1601 23rd Avenue South, Nashville, TN 37212.
E-mail address: Jennifer.Blackford@Vanderbilt.edu

identifying the best treatments for anxious children,[2] little is known about the neural underpinnings of anxiety disorders. Identifying the neural basis of childhood anxiety disorders can guide development of prevention programs, a critical step in reducing these early-onset and highly prevalent disorders. This article reviews the available literature to provide a current understanding of the neural basis of childhood anxiety disorders. It reviews the development of normative fear and the development of the brain regions that subserve fear and anxiety. It further provides a comprehensive summary of relevant functional and structural neuroimaging studies, including studies examining children with anxiety disorders and children at-risk for developing anxiety disorders.

NORMATIVE DEVELOPMENT OF FEAR
Development of Fear

Fear is a normal and adaptive response to potential threat. Key components of the fear system mature early in development,[3] and multiple periods of child development are marked by normative fears[4] (see Ref.[3] for a review). For example, most infants experience a period of stranger anxiety around 8 to 12 months of age, marked by wariness or distress around new people.[5-8] Stranger anxiety is often followed by separation anxiety, typically evident around 10 to 18 months, and characterized by distress about being separated from the mother or father.[6] Stranger and separation fears are thought to be protective, preventing the child from encountering harm during developmental periods marked by the onset of walking and increased exploration away from caregivers. For most children, these normative fears vanish by 2 to 3 years of age; however, for some, childhood is marked by the persistence of these fears and the development of new fears. Increases in the prevalence of anxiety disorders parallel decreases in normal fear, such that separation anxiety disorder typically arises relatively early in life, shortly after the age-typical diminution in normal separation anxiety. Similarly, social phobia typically arises in adolescence, around the time of age-typical decreases in normal social anxieties.

These normative fears are observed in most children and manifest across cultures,[3] suggesting that fundamental aspects of human brain development sculpt developmental changes in fear. The universality of the development of early fears raises questions about the nature of relationships between brain development and fear. Although we expect that developmental changes in brain function relate to developmental changes in both normal and abnormal fears, the nature of these relationships largely remains unknown.

Fear Neurocircuitry

Research on rodents and nonhuman primates has identified the key components of fear circuitry.[9-14] Using fear conditioning tasks in rodents, researchers have identified that the amygdala—a small subcortical collection of nuclei in the medial temporal lobe—is critical for the production of fear behaviors.[9] In nonhuman primates, amygdala lesions result in significantly reduced fear behaviors,[11,15] providing further support for the amygdala's role in the production of fear behaviors. However, some debate persists concerning the precise role of the amygdala in fear. Findings appear most consistent for stimulus-reinforcement learning, as it relates to fear in classical conditioning, in which the amygdala is necessary for such forms of learning. But the amygdala also supports stimulus-reinforcement learning as it relates to positive stimuli.[16-18] Moreover, animals that suffer amygdala lesions still are capable of manifesting fear. In fact, under some circumstances, amygdala lesions actually can lead to increases in fear.[19] Thus, the amygdala's role in fear may represent one prototypical function of a broader role in emotional processing.

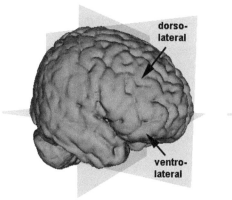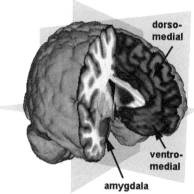

Fig. 1. Illustration of the amygdala and the major divisions of the PFC. The planes (*in blue*) show the major dorsal/ventral and anterior/posterior divisions of the brain. The lateral PFC is shown on the left and the medial PFC and amygdala are shown on the right. Brain images and surface constructions were created using Mango (Research Imaging Center, UTHSCSA; http://ric.uthscsa.edu/mango/mango.html) and a Montreal Neurological Institute standard brain.

The amygdala has received substantial attention as a core component of fear circuitry; however, other brain regions are also involved in fear and anxiety. For example, the bed nucleus of the stria terminalas (BNST)—a part of the "extended amygdala"—is involved in sustained fear reactions (in contrast to short-term or phasic fear responses) in rodents.[10] These sustained reactions, which are elicited by less specific and less predictable threats, are maintained over time and are considered akin to anxiety in humans.[20]

Another major component of the fear circuit is the prefrontal cortex (PFC), a brain region involved in both the automatic and effortful regulation of emotion. Within the prefrontal cortex, multiple regions are engaged during emotion processing and emotion regulation; however, as with research on the amygdala, debate persists about the nature of specific PFC contributions. Most current theories divide the primate PFC using two axes, one separating the medial from lateral PFC and another separating the dorsal from ventral PFC (**Fig. 1**).

Of the multiple PFC brain regions, the ventromedial PFC (vmPFC) is most strongly implicated in anxiety. The vmPFC plays a critical role in the inhibition of conditioned fear expression[14,21] and extinction of conditioned fear,[22–24] which can be viewed as two instances of emotion regulation.[23,25] Evidence also exists showing that vmPFC activity in some specific locales correlates positively with negative emotions,[26,27] suggesting that at least some particular portions of the vmPFC may drive negative emotions. These multiple roles may reflect different functions of subregions of the vmPFC. For example, some research suggests that in rodents the prelimbic component of vmPFC supports fear-related behaviors whereas the infralimbic component of vmPFC suppresses fear-related behaviors. However, because the majority of this research has examined rodents, issues of cross-species differences in PFC function preclude firm conclusions in humans.

In humans, other research focuses on lateral and dorsal regions of the PFC. The ventrolateral PFC (vlPFC) has been implicated in emotion regulation,[28,29] which may reflect the role of this region in attention control. The dorsomedial PFC (dmPFC) is engaged during the intentional control of emotional reactions,[23,30–33] which may reflect the broader role of the dmPFC in monitoring. Finally, the dorsolateral PFC (dlPFC) is implicated in intentional emotion regulation,[33–35] which may relate to the dlPFC's role in cognitive control and executive function.

Neuronal tracer studies in nonhuman primates provide evidence of anatomic connections between the amygdala and multiple regions of the PFC (for reviews see Ref.[35–37]). The amygdala has strong, bidirectional connections to medial prefrontal regions along the anterior cingulate cortex surrounding the corpus callosum, extending from ventral regions (subgenual cingulate) (**Fig. 2**) to rostral (pregenual cingulate) and dorsal (supragenual cingulate) regions (**Fig. 2**). The amygdala also has dense projections to the vlPFC,[38–40] but these connections are more unilateral and are mostly ascending from vlPFC to the amygdala.[38–42] In contrast, the amygdala appears to have relatively few connections to frontal regions of the PFC (frontal pole) or dlPFC regions.[38,40–42] Ongoing research continues to refine understandings of these connections, both from anatomic and functional perspectives. Given that the majority of this research has focused on mature organisms and that connections continue to change across development, understandings of these connections remain even less precisely specified in immature organisms. For example, although it is clear that children and adolescents are capable of utilizing all portions of the PFC to perform at least some of the functions for which adults utilize the PFC, the precise timing when specific PFC functions and associated connections mature in humans remains unclear.

PFC connections to the amygdala synapse in multiple regions. However, interest focuses primarily on γ-aminobutyric acid-ergic (GABAergic) neurons, emphasizing an inhibitory role for the PFC over amygdala function.[41,43,44] At least in some contexts, neuroimaging studies in humans show an inverse relationship between the amygdala and multiple PFC regions including vmPFC,[45,46] vlPFC,[32,47,48] dmPFC,[23,34,49–54] and dlPFC.[25,34] Particularly for the vlPFC and vmPFC, in which PFC–amygdala connections have been mapped, these findings suggest inhibitory input; however, such findings remain indirect.

In summary, the amygdala and PFC are key components of human fear neurocircuitry. The amygdala and PFC are interconnected with the PFC modulating amygdala responses. To date, the majority of our knowledge about the neural bases of anxiety comes from functional neuroimaging studies in adults (for a meta-analysis see Ref.[55]). Results from these studies suggest that adult anxiety disorders may be characterized by brain dysfunction resulting in "too much gas and not enough brakes"; that is, the fear production system is too strong and the fear regulation system is too weak.

Development of Fear Circuitry

The developmental trajectories of both the amygdala and PFC are consistent with this idea of an imbalance between the fear production and fear regulation systems. The amygdala is functional early in development,[56] shortly after birth in humans.[57] Studies of amygdala lesions occurring early versus late in development provide critical information about the development of amygdala function. In rhesus monkeys, early lesions (2 weeks) result in a decreased fear to threatening objects during multiple stages of development,[19,58,59] demonstrating that early damage to the amygdala has an early and sustained impact on nonsocial fear processing. In contrast, amygdala lesions in neonatal rhesus monkeys result in increased fear during nonthreatening social interactions at both 6 to 8 months of age[19] and 12 months of age,[60] suggesting a different early role for the amygdala in social processing. In adult rhesus monkeys, amygdala lesions produce decreased fear to threatening objects[11] and decreased fear during both nonthreatening and threatening social interactions.[11,15] Thus, the

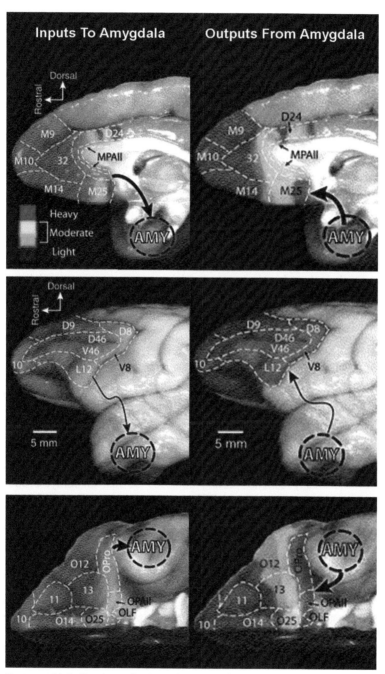

Fig. 2. Degree of labeling intensity in PFC neurons for both inputs to the amygdala (*left column*) and outputs from the amygdala (*right column*). Rows show different surface views: medial surface (*top*), lateral surface (*middle*), and ventral surface (*bottom*). (*Adapted from* Ghashghaei H, Hilgetag CC, Barbas H. Sequence of information processing for emotions based on the anatomic dialogue between prefrontal cortex and amygdala. NeuroImage 2007;34:905–23; with permission.)

amygdala's role in nonsocial fear is consistent across development, with both early and late amygdala lesions similarly decreasing fear to threatening objects. However, the role of the amygdala in the development of social fear is more complex, pointing to possible developmental differences in the contribution of the amygdala to social behaviors.

Evidence from human studies of amygdala lesions also indicates developmental effects; for example, individuals with early amygdala lesions fail to show the normal emotional enhancement of memory and understanding of others' emotional states.[61,62] Developmental functional magnetic resonance imaging (fMRI) studies of amygdala responses to human expressions of fear ("fear faces") may provide clues about amygdala development (see Ref.[63] for a review). When viewing fear faces, adult humans show an increase in amygdala activation relative to amygdala activation during a baseline condition, such as viewing a fixation cross or blank screen.[16–18] Increased amygdala activation likely represents the salience of the stimulus[64–66] because the amygdala responds robustly to negative and positive stimuli,[16] as well as novel[67] stimuli. Preliminary studies in children and adolescents suggest that amygdala activation to fear faces in children is similar to adults, but intriguingly is heightened in adolescents[45,68,69] (although not all studies find this developmental effect[70]). This heightened fear response in adolescence is consistent with heightened emotion recognition accuracy during this period.[70] Together, findings from lesion and neuroimaging studies demonstrate that the amygdala is critical for the normal development of the fear system.

Both the ventral and dorsal regions of the PFC are among the last brain regions to mature, undergoing significant structural and functional changes during development.[71–76] fMRI studies comparing different age groups provide evidence of differences across between children, adolescents, and adults in activation in the vlPFC,[69,77] vmPFC,[78,79] dmPFC,[70,79–81] and dlPFC.[72,79,82,83] These findings are consistent with behavioral data showing increasing skill with age for both emotional tasks[45,84] and cognitive tasks.[84–87] PFC development is relatively linear with age, and the development of the PFC provides a mechanism for dampening amygdala hyper-responsivity through increased emotion regulation abilities. Casey and colleagues[88,89] provide an integrative developmental theory that postulates that the increased emotionality common during adolescence results from the imbalance between patterns of amygdala and PFC development (**Fig. 3**). According to this model, during adolescence amygdala function is enhanced relative to PFC function, resulting in an overcontribution of the amygdala to adolescent emotions and behavior. As PFC development catches up during early adulthood, emotions and behavior are stabilized. This amygdala–PFC imbalance may contribute to the increased prevalence of anxiety disorders during early adolescence.

Attentional Modulation of the Amygdala

Attention contributes to fear processing and the amygdala's response to stimuli is modulated by attention. Multiple studies have demonstrated that amygdala activity varies as a function of task demands.[34,68,90–93] Neuroimaging studies using a passive viewing task—in which attention is not specifically constrained by the task—show greater amygdala activation than studies that use a specific task, such as gender discrimination or emotion rating.[16,17] Reduced amygdala activation during tasks likely reflects the effects of emotion regulation brain regions that are engaged during the tasks.[34,90–93] However, it should also be noted that attention is not required in all circumstances for amygdala response to emotional stimuli—for example, amygdala activation to fearful faces can occur in the absence of attention, potentially when the

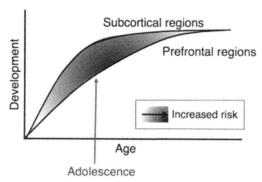

Fig. 3. Model illustrating the imbalance between the early maturation of subcortical regions, such as the amygdala, and late maturation of PFC regions during adolescence. The shaded areas indicate degree of amygdala–PFC imbalance. (*From* Somerville LH, Jones RM, Casey B. A time of change: behavioral and neural correlates of adolescent sensitivity to appetitive and aversive environmental cues. Brain Cogn 2010;72:124–33; with permission.)

fearful faces are masked and not consciously detected[94]—although debate remains surrounding this point.[95]

The modulating role of attention is especially important for understanding anxiety disorders, given that attentional processes are altered in children and adults with anxiety disorders.[96,97] In anxiety disorders, a commonly studied attentional process is attentional bias. Attentional bias is often measured using the "dot probe task." In that task, individuals fixate on a central point on the screen and are then shown a threatening and a neutral image on opposite sides of the screen. After the brief stimulus presentation, a dot is presented on one side of the screen and individuals must press a button as soon as they detect the dot. A shorter latency to detect the dot that appears in the same position as the threatening stimulus is evidence of attentional vigilance to threat. Anxious individuals are more likely to show attentional bias to threat, such as aversive images, fear faces, or angry faces (see Refs.[96,98] for reviews).

In fMRI studies of anxiety, a limitation of passive viewing studies (studies that do not require the subject to perform a task) is that observed amygdala differences may be a consequence of differences in attention. Controlling for attentional differences using a task can help to dissect differences in amygdala activation caused by anxiety from those caused by attention. Thus, neuroimaging findings need to be considered within the context of the attention requirements of various study designs.

NEUROIMAGING STUDIES OF FEAR-BASED ANXIETY DISORDERS: GENERALIZED ANXIETY DISORDER, SOCIAL PHOBIA, SEPARATION ANXIETY DISORDER

Although we assume that differences in brain function underlie childhood anxiety, little research has focused on identifying the underlying neural causes. Studies of adult anxiety have provided critical information about possible brain dysfunction in childhood anxiety disorders; however, we do not know whether the differences found in adults reflect the underlying causes of anxiety or are the consequence of anxiety. Thus, studies in children with anxiety or at high-risk for developing anxiety are critical for uncovering the neural causes of anxiety.

Findings from fMRI studies of adults with anxiety disorders[55] provide the initial candidate brain regions for studies of childhood anxiety—the amygdala and PFC.

Most neuroimaging studies of child anxiety have used the same experimental tasks previously used to study anxious adults. However, several groups are developing new tasks that are especially valid for studying children and adolescents, such as the "chat room" task (see section on Social Phobia). While this is an exciting time in the evolution of our understanding of the neural bases of childhood anxiety disorders, we still have much to discover.

Studies of children with anxiety disorders provide a direct approach to identifying the neural bases of anxiety disorders. An equally important approach is to study traits that are associated with high-risk for developing anxiety.[99] Advances in neuroscience methods, such as neuroimaging and genetics, provide new opportunities to link neurobiological measures to dimensional traits in individuals with and without anxiety disorders. Among various high-risk traits, a commonly studied trait is behavioral inhibition—or inhibited temperament—a trait characterized by wary or avoidant responses to novel people, places, or things.[100] Behavioral inhibition emerges in infancy,[101,102] is heritable,[103] and is associated with a distinct physiologic profile.[104–107] Inhibited children have a four-fold increase in risk for developing any anxiety disorder, with specific risk for social phobia.[108–110] Studies of young adults who were inhibited as children provide evidence for amygdala dysfunction[111–114] which is best characterized as a failure of the amygdala to habituate normally to repeated presentations of faces,[114,115] resulting in a sustained amygdala response.[112] Recent studies provide initial evidence for both structural[116] and functional differences in the PFC.[117] Thus, studying traits associated with anxiety provide a promising approach to identifying the structural and functional correlates of anxiety.

This section reviews and integrates functional and structural neuroimaging findings in generalized anxiety disorder, social phobia, and separation anxiety disorder, as well as the associated high-risk traits.

Generalized Anxiety Disorder

Functional MRI

Childhood generalized anxiety disorder (GAD) is characterized by excessive anxiety and worry about a variety of events and situations, difficulty controlling the anxiety, and presence of one or more physical symptoms.[118] To date, the majority of studies in GAD have focused on the amygdala. The most consistent finding in childhood GAD is increased amygdala activation during viewing of negative emotional expressions. Increased amygdala activation has been reported across multiple study designs including passive viewing of fear faces,[119] subjective ratings of fear,[120,121] viewing masked angry faces during a dot-probe task,[122] and viewing both subsequently remembered and forgotten faces during a face memory task.[123] In one of the studies, amygdala activation to fear faces also correlated with anxiety severity,[119] suggesting a direct link between amygdala response and anxiety. It should be noted that one study failed to find differences in amygdala activation when viewing masked angry faces during the dot-probe task.[124]

Multiple studies also report differences in PFC activation to negative emotions in GAD. For example, anxious children had increased activation during subjective ratings of fear, relative to healthy controls, in the vlPFC[120,121] and dmPFC.[120] In another study, adolescents with GAD showed increased activation in the vlPFC relative to healthy controls when viewing masked angry faces in a dot-probe task; but, within the GAD adolescents, degree of vlPFC activation correlated negatively with anxiety severity, suggesting a regulatory role.[124] However, not all studies report PFC differences.[122]

Children with GAD also show differences in functional connectivity between the amygdala and other brain regions. For example, when making subjective ratings of fear faces, anxious children showed increased functional connectivity between the amygdala and insula, relative to healthy controls,[120] and the degree of connectivity correlated positively with anxiety symptoms. In another study, healthy controls showed an inverse functional connectivity between the amygdala and vlPFC that was diminished in the children with GAD.[122]

Several studies have examined the neural correlates of treatment effects in childhood GAD. A preliminary study examined the association between pretreatment differences in brain function with symptom improvement following treatment with medication or cognitive behavior therapy in adolescents with GAD.[125] Pretreatment amygdala activation was associated with less clinical improvement after treatment. A second study examined the neural correlates of treatment response in adolescents with GAD.[126] Successful treatment with either cognitive behavioral therapy (CBT) or fluoxetine was associated with increased activation to angry faces in the right vlPFC, a region associated with emotion regulation.

In summary, children with GAD consistently show increased amygdala activation across a variety of tasks. Although several studies reported PFC differences, the direction of the effect was not consistent. It is important to note that task differences likely impact the direction of the PFC effect (increase vs decrease) when comparing individuals with anxiety relative to healthy controls. For example, because healthy controls do not typically show an attentional bias, it is unlikely that they will engage attentional or regulatory regions. In this case, PFC activation should be higher in the anxious group because they have an attentional bias, but increased activation should not be interpreted as "better" function. To understand how PFC dysfunction relates to anxiety, it is critical to examine the association between PFC activation and anxiety severity or symptom improvement. Relatively lower vlPFC activation was associated with higher anxiety severity and lower symptom improvement with treatment, suggesting dysfunction in vlPFC regulation of the amygdala contributes to GAD anxiety symptoms.

Structural MRI

Findings of structural differences in the amygdala are less consistent. A study of adolescents with GAD showed larger right amygdala volume relative to controls[127]; however, another study of adolescents with anxiety disorders (predominantly GAD) found smaller left amygdala volume.[128] Sample sizes in both studies were relatively small; moreover, methods in the two studies also were quite different. Therefore, larger samples studied comprehensively will be useful in resolving the conflicting amygdala results. To date, only one study has examined PFC volume and found no differences in adolescents with GAD compared to controls in PFC gray matter volume or white matter volume.[129] Thus, support for structural differences in childhood GAD remains weak.

At-risk children

Trait anxiety reflects a temperamental trait characterized by persistent anxiety and worry and is therefore very similar to GAD. Generally, higher trait anxiety is associated with increased risk for GAD; however, a child can have high trait anxiety but not meet diagnostic criteria for GAD. Telzer and colleagues[130] demonstrated that trait anxiety in healthy children and adolescents corresponded to both a behavioral attentional bias toward angry faces and increased activation in the right dlPFC. When viewing all faces (regardless of emotion), higher trait anxiety was associated with increased vlPFC activation.

Krain and colleagues[131] examined intolerance of uncertainty—the tendency to react negatively to situations that are uncertain—a major symptom of GAD.[132,133] In healthy adolescents and anxious adolescents (GAD, social phobia, or both), higher intolerance of uncertainty was associated with increased activation in the amygdala, vmPFC and dmPFC during decision making in the context of absolute uncertainty (50/50 chance of being right). Within only the anxious adolescents, there was substantial variability in both intolerance of uncertainty and brain function. Anxious adolescents with high intolerance of uncertainty had increased amygdala and orbitofrontal cortex activation, whereas anxious adolescents with low intolerance of uncertainty had decreased activation in these same brain regions. These findings point to the importance of examining specific traits or symptoms of anxiety even within individuals with an anxiety diagnosis.

Social Phobia

Functional MRI

Among the anxiety disorders, social phobia (SP) is very common, second in prevalence only to specific phobias.[1] Blair and colleagues[134] explored brain function differences in adolescents with SP relative to healthy controls during an emotional face processing task. Adolescents with SP had increased activation in the amygdala and vmPFC when viewing fear faces. In addition, social anxiety severity correlated with vmPFC activation to both angry and fearful faces in the anxious group. The findings in adolescents were similar to results in adults with SP compared to controls, suggesting that the neural substrates of adult SP are already present in adolescence.

The emotion processing tasks commonly used to study brain function in anxiety disorders use both human faces and negative emotional expressions—both of which are particularly salient for SP—however, emotion processing tasks may not tap into other key factors that elicit SP, such as social-evaluative processes. Recently, several groups have begun to develop ecologically valid experimental tasks. Guyer and colleagues[135] have developed a "chat room" task to engage concerns about peer evaluation. In this task, adolescents rate pictures of other adolescents based on their desire to chat with them in a future encounter. During a second visit, adolescents rate how much they think the other adolescents want to chat with them. Anxious adolescents showed increased activation in the amygdala and vmPFC when rating how much the other adolescents would want to chat with them; interestingly, activation was increased only when viewing the adolescents that the subjects had previously rated as low desirability. Anxious adolescents, but not healthy controls, showed functional connectivity between the amygdala and vlPFC, with higher anxiety associated with stronger functional connectivity.

At-risk children

Several studies in children and adolescents have examined traits relevant to SP, such as behavioral inhibition. Inhibited children and adolescents are typically shy, cautious, and reserved and are at significantly increased risk for developing social phobia.[108,110,136] Behavioral inhibition is observable across development and can be measured using a variety of methods including direct observation, parent report, current self-report, and retrospective self-report. The most commonly used method for identifying behavioral inhibition in children is direct observation of behavior and using measured with laboratory assessments consisting of unfamiliar objects, unfamiliar peers, and unfamiliar adults.[100,101,106,137] Laboratory assessments are considered by many to be the gold standard because they provide objective assessments of behavior; but, behavioral assessments are time-consuming, expensive, and may not reflect real-world behaviors. Parent-report and self-report questionnaires provide efficient and economical assessments of behavior across a wide variety of situations; but, questionnaires are subject to a variety of reporter biases, including over-reporting and under-reporting. Although there is evidence for moderate convergence across the two methods,[138] it is important to consider methodologic issues when interpreting study results.

Studies of young adults who were inhibited as children demonstrate that behavioral inhibition is associated with amygdala hyperactivity[111–114,117] and dmPFC hypoactivity[117]; however, only a handful of studies have examined brain function in inhibited children and adolescents. Perez-Edgar and colleagues[139] compared neural responses during emotion processing in adolescents who were either characterized as inhibited or noninhibited as young children. The emotion processing task included a passive viewing (no task) condition and several attention conditions in which subjects subjectively rated emotional or nonemotional characteristics of the faces. In the inhibited adolescents, amygdala activation to fear faces was increased, relative to the noninhibited adolescents, when attention was focused on rating the emotion but decreased when the fear faces were passively viewed. These results suggest that inhibited adolescents have different neural responses to emotional faces and that the neural responses are modulated by attention and emotional state.

An important contribution of high-risk trait studies is the discovery that behaviorally inhibited adolescents are not only sensitive to threatening stimuli, but are also sensitive to reward. In an initial behavioral study, shy (inhibited) adolescents had faster reaction times during reward conditions in the Monetary Incentive Delay (MID) task, suggesting increased reward sensitivity.[140] Using fMRI, Guyer and colleagues[141] compared neural responses in the striatum (including the nucleus accumbens, caudate, and putamen) during the MID task in inhibited, relative to noninhibited, adolescents. Inhibited adolescents showed significantly greater striatal activation to increasing amounts of incentives (gain or loss) relative to the noninhibited adolescents. In a subsequent fMRI study, Bar-Haim and colleagues[142] tested the effects of reward while controlling for possible effects due to performance evaluation by including a noncontingent motor task. Inhibited adolescents showed increased activation in the nucleus accumbens when reward outcome was contingent on their response but did not show differences in the noncontingent condition. These studies demonstrate that behaviorally inhibited adolescents have increased sensitivity during performance-dependent rewarding tasks, in addition to increased sensitivity to threat. This pattern of increased sensitivity to both threatening and rewarding stimuli is remarkably similar to increases seen normally during adolescence, consistent with an imbalance between development of the amygdala and PFC.

In summary, studies of children with SP or children at-risk for developing SP demonstrate increased amygdala activation to anxiogenic stimuli and demonstrate increased striatal activation to rewarding stimuli, suggesting a general heightened reactivity. In the PFC, childhood SP was associated with increased vmPFC activation. Although more studies of PFC function are needed, increased the observed vmPFC activation may result from specific regions of the vmPFC that drive amygdala activation and negative emotions.

Separation Anxiety Disorder

Separation anxiety disorder (SAD) is characterized by anxiety caused by separation from the child's home or caretakers that causes impairment because it leads to avoidance of separation. School refusal and difficulty sleeping alone are common symptoms of SAD. Although no study to date has used neuroimaging methods to probe brain structure or function in SAD, one study included a continuous measure of separation anxiety. In that study, amygdala activation to fear faces was examined in healthy children.[143] Continuous measures of anxiety symptoms were assessed using

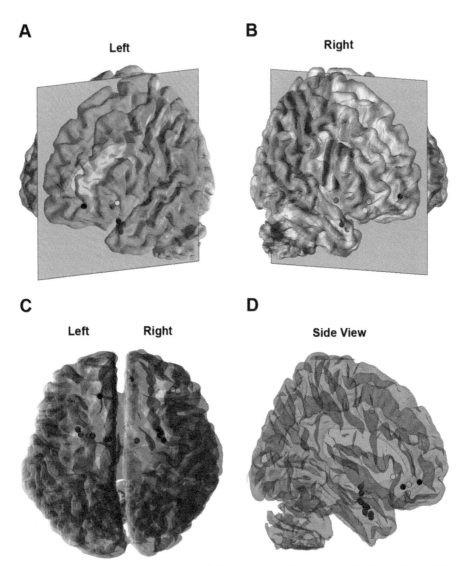

Fig. 4. Peak activations from studies of children and adolescents with GAD, SP, or SAD (relative to healthy controls). Seventeen peaks from nine studies are illustrated on a 3-D transparent brain. Four perspectives are shown: (A) left lateral view, (B) right lateral view, (C) top view, and (D) side view. Dot colors represent different brain regions: red = amygdala (n = 11); dark blue = vmPFC (n = 2); light blue = vlPFC (n = 3); green = dmPFC (n = 1). Images were created using the plot_points_on_suface Matlab script included in the Multilevel Kernel Density Analysis toolbox (Tor Wager; http://wagerlab.colorado.edu/tools/).

the Multidimensional Anxiety Scale for Children (MASC[144]). Higher separation anxiety symptoms were associated with increased amygdala activation to fear faces, providing preliminary evidence for the amygdala as one neural basis of separation anxiety disorder.

Summary

In summary, children and adolescents with GAD, SP, SAD, or high-risk traits show dysfunction in the amygdala and multiple PFC brain regions during experimental tasks probing fear neurocircuitry (**Fig. 4**). These findings are consistent with the results of a recent meta-analysis that reports that childhood anxiety (GAD, OCD, PTSD) is associated with alterations in the amygdala, vlPFC, and dmPFC.[145] Across the studies, amygdala activation was increased in anxious children and adolescents, consistent with findings in anxious adults. Increased amygdala activation was also demonstrated in high-risk individuals, suggesting that amygdala hyper-reactivity is a heritable trait that confers risk for developing anxiety. In the PFC, the most common finding was increased activation, not a lack of PFC activation as predicted by developmental evidence for increasing emotion regulation and PFC activation with age. These preliminary findings are intriguing and suggest several possibilities. Group differences in PFC activation may reflect differential effects of the tasks on the two groups; examination of the relationship between anxiety severity and PFC function is important for understanding the role of the PFC. Also, increased PFC activation in anxious children may reflect differences in the duration of amygdala–PFC processing. Whereas both anxious and nonanxious children may initially engage the PFC during emotional tasks, the PFC may effectively inhibit amygdala activation quickly in nonanxious children, but not in the anxious children. Thus, anxious children may continue to engage the PFC in an attempt to inhibit amygdala response, with the effect of greater activation over the task. Alternatively, increased PFC activation could be driving increased amygdala activation, as suggested by some findings of coactivation of these regions in adults.[26] Functional differences may be caused by underlying structural differences, but to date there are too few structural studies to draw any conclusions. Thus, although the foundation has been laid, much research is needed to understand the precise nature of the brain dysfunction that gives raise to childhood anxiety.

NEUROIMAGING STUDIES OF OBSESSIVE–COMPULSIVE DISORDER

Childhood-onset obsessive–compulsive disorder (OCD) can be considered to be distinct from the other childhood anxiety disorders.[146] Instead of having fear at its core, childhood OCD is defined by recurrent obsessions and compulsions that are time consuming or cause marked distress or significant impairments in daily function.[118] Childhood-onset OCD, relative to adult-onset OCD, is characterized more by motor and vocal tics and the presence of comorbid diagnoses such as Tourette syndrome and attention-deficit/hyperactivity disorder.[147,148] In addition, the prevalence of OCD is substantially lower than for the other anxiety disorders (see the article by Franklin and colleagues elsewhere in this issue for further exploration of this topic).[149]

Although fear is not a defining feature of OCD, some early theories about the neural substrates of OCD posited amygdala deficits[150,151] with the amygdala having a role in maintaining compulsive behaviors. Like the other anxiety disorders, OCD has been conceptualized as an imbalance between a subcortical hyper-responsivity and cortical hyporesponsivity. In the case of OCD, the hyper-responsivity has been hypothesized to arise from the basal ganglia, with hyporesponsivity in multiple PFC regions, including the orbitofrontal cortex (OFC) and the anterior cingulate cortex (ACC). Deficits in these regions support the notion of OCD as a disorder of overmonitoring and difficulty inhibiting responses. Neuroimaging findings to date suggest that dysfunction in cortico–striato–thalamic circuit may underlie OCD.[152,153]

Relative to the other childhood anxiety disorders, OCD has received significantly more neuroimaging research attention. A relatively large and growing number of neuroimaging studies have examined both functional and structural correlates of childhood OCD. In light of this volume and the broad focus of the current review, only general conclusions can be provided. Despite the many challenges of studying childhood OCD—including small sample sizes, different experimental tasks, and medication status—some common trends are emerging (for extensive review please see Refs.[154–158]).

Functional MRI

Early neuroimaging research in childhood OCD has not shown evidence of increased amygdala activation in response to either contamination or symmetry provocations.[159] A common probe of amygdala function used to study other anxiety disorders is the presentation of pictures of human emotional expressions. As reviewed earlier, anxious children often show increased amygdala activation when viewing fear faces; however, in children with OCD, amygdala activation is decreased, relative to healthy controls.[160] This result is in contrast to other studies in the other childhood anxiety disorders, providing further evidence for a distinction between OCD and the other disorders.

To examine cortico–striato–thalamic dysfunction Woolley and colleagues[161] tested response inhibition. During successful response inhibition, OCD was associated with decreased activation in the OFC, thalamus, and basal ganglia (caudate head, putamen, globus pallidus). During unsuccessful response inhibition OCD was associated with decreased medial PFC activation. To isolate the contributions of cognitive flexibility deficits to OCD, Britton and colleagues[162] tested cognitive inflexibility while controlling for motor behavior. Children with OCD, relative to controls, had decreased OFC activation during set shifting, but there were no differences in the striatum, dmPFC, or dlPFC. Caudate activation was positively correlated with a behavioral measure cognitive flexibility in healthy controls, but negatively correlated in OCD. Findings from these studies are consistent with a meta-analysis of functional brain differences found that childhood OCD was associated with functional differences in the frontal and parietal cortices, striatum, and thalamus.[145] Together, these fMRI studies provide preliminary evidence that children with OCD have dysfunction in the OFC, thalamus, and basal ganglia.

The first neuroimaging studies to examine the effect of treatment on brain function in children with OCD used regional cerebral blood flow (rCBF) measures. Diler and colleagues[163] compared rCBF at baseline and after 12 weeks of treatment with paroxetine. At baseline, children with OCD had increased blood flow in the caudate, dlPFC, and ACC; blood flow in these regions was reduced following treatment. A subsequent study failed to find changes in rCBF using clomipramine.[164] Using fMRI, Lazaro and colleagues[165] examined the effect of treatment on brain activation during a serial reaction time task in treatment-naïve children with OCD. At baseline, the serial reaction time task produced increased activation in the caudate, middle frontal gyrus, and inferior parietal lobe; total OCD scores correlated with activation in the nucleus accumbens and superior parietal lobe and obsession scores correlated with activation in the ACC. After 6 months of fluoxetine treatment and significant clinical improvement, activation in the insula and putamen were decreased during performance of the serial reaction time task.

Structural MRI

Investigations of differences in amygdala volume have been inconsistent. An initial study found no amygdala volume differences in medication-naïve children with OCD[152]; however, a later study reported an initial amygdala asymmetry in OCD (left larger than right) relative to controls.[151]

Several structural studies have found evidence that children with OCD have larger volumes in the putamen[166–168]; however, two studies reported either smaller volumes or no differences in the putamen[169,170] and another study reported smaller volume in the globus pallidus.[170] Other structural differences include larger volume in the thalamus,[171] caudate,[168] and cerebellum.[172] In the PFC, the most consistent structural finding to date is that childhood OCD is associated with larger gray-matter volume in the ACC, a finding that has been replicated in multiple samples using both manual tracing[152,166,170] and voxel-based morphometry[162] methods. However, one study reported areas of smaller gray matter volume in the ACC.[167] Larger gray-matter volume has also been reported in the OFC[162,166] and larger gray matter volume correlated with higher symptom severity.[166] Other PFC areas that show differences in OCD include the medial frontal gyrus[162,167] and inferior frontal gyrus.[162]

Several studies have examined treatment effects on brain structure. For the amygdala, one study reported that an initial amygdala asymmetry was normalized with selective serotonin reuptake inhibitor (SSRI) treatment.[151] In another study, thalamic volume normalized with treatment and decreased volume with treatment was associated with reduced OCD symptom severity.[171] However, in another study no changes in thalamic volume were seen with CBT, even though symptom severity reduced with treatment.[173]

IMPLICATIONS FOR RESEARCH AND CLINICAL PRACTICE

Using functional and structural neuroimaging methods to isolate the neural underpinnings of childhood anxiety disorders is still in its infancy, with the first childhood anxiety fMRI study conducted a little over a decade ago. Given this relatively short period of time, significant progress has been made in identifying possible sources of brain dysfunction contributing to childhood anxiety. In the fear-based anxiety disorders (GAD, SP, SAD), neuroimaging studies have reported brain dysfunction in both the amygdala and multiple regions of the PFC. In OCD, the basal ganglia, orbitofrontal cortex, and anterior cingulate cortex are emerging as key regions of structural and functional deficits.

Studies of children and adolescents at high-risk for developing an anxiety disorder have contributed substantially to our current knowledge of possible neural substrates of anxiety disorders. Given the National Institute of Mental Health's new emphasis on dimensional traits—the Research Domain Criteria (RDoC)—we expect that more neuroimaging studies will begin to study high-risk traits, such as behavioral inhibition. The use of dimensional approaches may be especially useful for childhood anxiety disorders given that many children have subsyndromal symptoms or symptoms across multiple anxiety disorders.[174]

Although progress has been made, many important questions remain. Some important future areas for research include:

1. Measure individual differences in developmental brain trajectories to identify the neural underpinnings of trajectories that result in childhood anxiety.

2. Study the developmental brain trajectories of children with anxiety disorders, because not all anxious children become anxious adults. Identifying the brain and behavioral trajectories associated with reduction in anxiety may inform novel targets for treatment.
3. Increase focus on isolating the neural bases of dimensional traits associated with risk for developing anxiety, such as behavioral inhibition, trait anxiety, and intolerance of uncertainty.
4. Collect measures of behavior and arousal, in addition to functional neuroimaging measures, to provide greater clarity about the meaning of differences in brain activation in anxious children.
5. Develop new functional tasks to examine the relative contributions of the amygdala and the PFC to anxiety and to identify the sequelae of individual differences in the amygdala–PFC imbalance.
6. Test the effects of pharmacologic and nonpharmacologic treatments on the developing brain. Research is greatly needed to identify whether treatment success is associated with changes in brain function and/or development.

The current findings from the functional and structural neuroimaging studies reviewed in this article suggest that anxious children and adolescents have dysfunction in amygdala–PFC neurocircuitry. While it is likely that common treatments for childhood anxiety—such as CBT and selective serotonin reuptake inhibitors (SSRIs)—act on this circuit, empirical evidence is still needed. Importantly, identification of dysfunction in the amygdala–PFC neurocircuitry may suggest new avenues for the development of novel therapies. For example, evidence of dysfunction in PFC-dependent attentional processes has led to the development and testing of attention retraining therapies.[97,175] In addition, new pharmacotherapies or behavioral therapies can capitalize on neuroscience findings by targeting emotion regulation abilities in anxious children.

REFERENCES

1. Merikangas KR, He Jp, Burstein M, et al. Lifetime prevalence of mental disorders in U.S. adolescents: results from the National Comorbidity Survey Replication—Adolescent Supplement (NCS-A). J Am Acad Child Adolesc Psychiatry 2010;49(10): 980–9.
2. Walkup JT, Albano AM, Piacentini J, et al. Cognitive behavioral therapy, sertraline, or a combination in childhood anxiety. N Engl J Med 2008;359(26):2753–66.
3. Gullone E. The development of normal fear: a century of research. Clin Psychol Rev 2000;20(4):429–51.
4. Scarr S, Salapatek P. Patterns of fear development during infancy. Merrill Palmer Q 1970;16(1):53–90.
5. Waters E, Matas L, Sroufe LA. Infants' reactions to an approaching stranger: description, validation, and functional significance of wariness. Child Dev 1975;46(2): 348–56.
6. Thompson RA, Limber SP. Social anxiety in infancy: stranger and separation reactions. In: Leitenberg H, editor. Handbook of social and evaluation anxiety. New York: Plenum Press; 1992. p. 85–137.
7. Campos JJ, Emde RN, Gaensbauer T, et al. Cardiac and behavioral interrelationships in the reactions of infants to strangers. Dev Psychol 1975;11(5):589–601.
8. Gaensbauer TJ, Emde RN, Campos JJ. Stranger distress: confirmation of a developmental shift in a longitudinal sample. Percept Mot Skills 1976;43(1):99–106.
9. Davis M. The role of the amygdala in fear and anxiety. Annu Rev Neurosci 1992;15: 353–75.

10. Davis M, Walker DL, Lee Y. Amygdala and bed nucleus of the stria terminalis: differential roles in fear and anxiety measured with the acoustic startle reflex. Philos Trans Biol Sci 1997;352(1362):1675–87.
11. Kalin NH, Shelton SE, Davidson RJ. The role of the central nucleus of the amygdala in mediating fear and anxiety in the primate. J Neurosci 2004;24(24):5506–15.
12. Kalin NH, Shelton SE, Davidson RJ. Role of the primate orbitofrontal cortex in mediating anxious temperament. Biol Psychiatry 2007;62:1134–9.
13. Phelps EA, LeDoux JE. Contributions of the amygdala to emotion processing: from animal models to human behavior. Neuron 2005;48(2):175–87.
14. Quirk GJ, Beer JS. Prefrontal involvement in the regulation of emotion: convergence of rat and human studies. Curr Opin Neurobiol 2006;16(6):723–7.
15. Emery NJ, Capitanio JP, Mason WA, et al. The effects of bilateral lesions of the amygdala on dyadic social interactions in rhesus monkeys (Macaca mulatta). Behav Neurosci 2001;115(3):515–44.
16. Costafreda SG, Brammer MJ, David AS, et al. Predictors of amygdala activation during the processing of emotional stimuli: a meta-analysis of 385 PET and fMRI studies. Brain Res Rev 2008;58(1):57–70.
17. Sergerie K, Chochol C, Armony JL. The role of the amygdala in emotional processing: a quantitative meta-analysis of functional neuroimaging studies. Neurosci Biobehav Rev 2008;32(4):811–30.
18. Zald DH. The human amygdala and the emotional evaluation of sensory stimuli. Brain Res Rev 2003;41(1):88–123.
19. Prather MD, Lavenex P, Mauldin-Jourdain ML, et al. Increased social fear and decreased fear of objects in monkeys with neonatal amygdala lesions. Neuroscience 2001;106(4):653–8.
20. Davis M, Walker DL, Miles L, et al. Phasic vs sustained fear in rats and humans: role of the extended amygdala in fear vs anxiety. Neuropsychopharmacology 2010;35(1): 105–35.
21. Quirk GJ, Likhtik E, Pelletier JG, et al. Stimulation of medial prefrontal cortex decreases the responsiveness of central amygdala output neurons. J Neurosci 2003;23(25):8800–7.
22. Quirk GJ, Garcia R, Gonzalez-Lima F. Prefrontal mechanisms in extinction of conditioned fear. Biol Psychiatry 2006;60(4):337–43.
23. Diekhof EK, Geier K, Falkai P, et al. Fear is only as deep as the mind allows: a coordinate-based meta-analysis of neuroimaging studies on the regulation of negative affect. NeuroImage 2011;58(1):275–85.
24. Phelps EA, Delgado MR, Nearing KI, et al. Extinction learning in humans: role of the amygdala and vmPFC. Neuron 2004;43(6):897–905.
25. Urry HL, van Reekum CM, Johnstone T, et al. Amygdala and ventromedial prefrontal cortex are inversely coupled during regulation of negative affect and predict the diurnal pattern of cortisol secretion among older adults. J Neurosci 2006;26(16): 4415–25.
26. Myers-Schulz B, Koenigs M. Functional anatomy of ventromedial prefrontal cortex: implications for mood and anxiety disorders. Mol Psychiatry 2012;17:132–41.
27. Morgan MA, LeDoux JE. Differential contribution of dorsal and ventral medial prefrontal cortex to the acquisition and extinction of conditioned fear in rats. Behav Neurosci 1995;109(4):681–8.
28. Phan KL, Fitzgerald DA, Nathan PJ, et al. Neural substrates for voluntary suppression of negative affect: a functional magnetic resonance imaging study. Biol Psychiatry 2005;57(3):210–9.

29. Goldin PR, McRae K, Ramel W, et al. The neural bases of emotion regulation: reappraisal and suppression of negative emotion. Biol Psychiatry 2008;63(6):577–86.

30. Bush G, Luu P, Posner MI. Cognitive and emotional influences in anterior cingulate cortex. Trends Cogn Sci 2000;4(6):215–22.

31. Kober H, Barrett LF, Joseph J, et al. Functional grouping and cortical-subcortical interactions in emotion: a meta-analysis of neuroimaging studies. NeuroImage 2008;42(2):998–1031.

32. Ochsner KN, Ray RD, Cooper JC, et al. For better or for worse: neural systems supporting the cognitive down- and up-regulation of negative emotion. NeuroImage 2004;23(2):483–99.

33. Phillips ML, Drevets WC, Rauch SL, et al. Neurobiology of emotion perception I: The neural basis of normal emotion perception. Biol Psychiatry 2003;54(5):504–14.

34. Ochsner KN, Bunge SA, Gross JJ, et al. Rethinking feelings: an fMRI study of the cognitive regulation of emotion. J Cogn Neurosci 2002;14(8):1215–29.

35. Ray RD, Zald DH. Anatomical insights into the interaction of emotion and cognition in the prefrontal cortex. Neurosci Biobehav Rev 2012;36:479–501.

36. Price JL, Drevets WC. Neurocircuitry of mood disorders. Neuropsychopharmacology 2010;35(1):192–216.

37. Price JL, Drevets WC. Neural circuits underlying the pathophysiology of mood disorders. Trends Cogn Sci 2012;16(1):61–71.

38. Amaral DG, Price JL, Pitkanen A, et al. Anatomical organization of the primate amygdaloid complex. In: Aggleton JP, editor. The amygdala: neurobiological aspects of emotion, memory, and mental dysfunction. New York: Wiley-Liss; 1992. p. 1–66.

39. Carmichael ST, Price JL. Limbic connections of the orbital and medial prefrontal cortex in macaque monkeys. J Comp Neurol 1995;363(4):615–41.

40. Ghashghaei H, Hilgetag CC, Barbas H. Sequence of information processing for emotions based on the anatomic dialogue between prefrontal cortex and amygdala. NeuroImage 2007;34(3):905–23.

41. Ghashghaei HT, Barbas H. Pathways for emotion: interactions of prefrontal and anterior temporal pathways in the amygdala of the rhesus monkey. Neuroscience 2002;115(4):1261–79.

42. Porrino LJ, Crane AM, Goldmanrakic PS. Direct and indirect pathways from the amygdala to the frontal-lobe in rhesus-monkeys. J Comp Neurol 1981;198(1):121–36.

43. Amano T, Unal CT, Pare D. Synaptic correlates of fear extinction in the amygdala. Nat Neurosci 2010;13(4):489–U112.

44. McDonald AJ, Mascagni F, Guo L. Projections of the medial and lateral prefrontal cortices to the amygdala: a *Phaseolus vulgaris* leucoagglutinin study in the rat. Neuroscience 1996;71(1):55–75.

45. Hare TA, Tottenham N, Galvan A, et al. Biological substrates of emotional reactivity and regulation in adolescence during an emotional go-nogo task. Biol Psychiatry 2008;63(10):927–34.

46. Johnstone T, van Reekum CM, Urry HL, et al. Failure to regulate: counterproductive recruitment of top-down prefrontal-subcortical circuitry in major depression. J Neurosci 2007;27(33):8877–84.

47. Delgado MR, Nearing KI, LeDoux JE, et al. Neural circuitry underlying the regulation of conditioned fear and its relation to extinction. Neuron 2008;59(5):829–38.

48. Banks SJ, Eddy KT, Angstadt M, et al. Amygdala–frontal connectivity during emotion regulation. Soc Cogn Affect Neurosci 2007;2(4):303–12.

49. Etkin A, Egner T, Peraza DM, et al. Resolving emotional conflict: a role for the rostral anterior cingulate cortex in modulating activity in the amygdala. Neuron 2006;51(6):871–82.

50. Hariri AR, Mattay VS, Tessitore A, et al. Neocortical modulation of the amygdala response to fearful stimuli. Biol Psychiatry 2003;53(6):494–501.
51. Sarinopoulos I, Grupe DW, Mackiewicz KL, et al. Uncertainty during anticipation modulates neural responses to aversion in human insula and amygdala. Cereb Cortex 2010;20(4):929–40.
52. Killgore WDS, Yurgelun-Todd DA. Cerebral correlates of amygdala responses during non-conscious perception of facial affect in adolescent and pre-adolescent children. Cogn Neurosci 2010;1(1):33–43.
53. Schlund MW, Siegle GJ, Ladouceur CD, et al. Nothing to fear? Neural systems supporting avoidance behavior in healthy youths. NeuroImage 2010;52(2):710–9.
54. Stein JL, Wiedholz LM, Bassett DS, et al. A validated network of effective amygdala connectivity. NeuroImage 2007;36(3):736–45.
55. Etkin A, Wager TD. Functional neuroimaging of anxiety: a meta-analysis of emotional processing in PTSD, social anxiety disorder, and specific phobia. Am J Psychiatry 2007;164(10):1476–88.
56. Benes FM. Development of the corticolimbic system. In: Dawson G, Fischer K, editors. Human behavior and the developing brain. New York: Guilford Press; 1994. p. 176–206.
57. Clancy B, Finlay BL, Darlington RB, et al. Extrapolating brain development from experimental species to humans. Neurotoxicology 2007;28(5):931–7.
58. Bliss-Moreau E, Toscano JE, Bauman MD, et al. Neonatal amygdala or hippocampus lesions influence responsiveness to objects. Dev Psychobiol 2010;52(5):487–503.
59. Bliss-Moreau E, Toscano JE, Bauman MD, et al. Neonatal amygdala lesions alter responsiveness to objects in juvenile macaques. Neuroscience 2011;178:123–32.
60. Bauman MD, Lavenex P, Mason WA, et al. The development of social behavior following neonatal amygdala lesions in rhesus monkeys. J Cogn Neurosci 2004; 16(8):1388–411.
61. Shaw P, Lawrence EJ, Radbourne C, et al. The impact of early and late damage to the human amygdala on 'theory of mind' reasoning. Brain 2004;127:1535–48.
62. Shaw P, Brierley B, David AS. A critical period for the impact of amygdala damage on the emotional enhancement of memory? Neurology 2005;65(2):326–8.
63. Somerville LH, Fani N, Clure-Tone EB. Behavioral and neural representation of emotional facial expressions across the lifespan. Dev Neuropsychol 2011;36(4): 408–28.
64. Ewbank MP, Barnard PJ, Croucher CJ, et al. The amygdala response to images with impact. Soc Cogn Affect Neurosci 2009;4(2):127–33.
65. Santos A, Mier D, Kirsch P, et al. Evidence for a general face salience signal in human amygdala. NeuroImage 2011;54(4):3111–6.
66. Sander D, Grafman J, Zalla T. The human amygdala: an evolved system for relevance detection. Rev Neurosci 2003;14(4):303–16.
67. Blackford JU, Buckholtz JW, Avery SN, et al. A unique role for the amygdala in novelty detection. NeuroImage 2010;50(3):1188–93.
68. Guyer AE, Monk CS, Clure-Tone EB, et al. A developmental examination of amygdala response to facial expressions. J Cogn Neurosci 2008;20(9):1565–82.
69. Monk CS, McClure EB, Nelson EE, et al. Adolescent immaturity in attention-related brain engagement to emotional facial expressions. NeuroImage 2003;20(1):420–8.
70. Williams LM, Brown KJ, Palmer D, et al. The mellow years? Neural basis of improving emotional stability over age. J Neurosci 2006;26(24):6422–30.

71. Gogtay N, Giedd JN, Lusk L, et al. Dynamic mapping of human cortical development during childhood through early adulthood. Proc Natl Acad Sci U S A 2004;101(21): 8174–9.
72. Luna B, Thulborn KR, Munoz DP, et al. Maturation of widely distributed brain function subserves cognitive development. NeuroImage 2001;13(5):786–93.
73. Casey BJ, Giedd JN, Thomas KM. Structural and functional brain development and its relation to cognitive development. Biol Psychol 2000;54(1–3):241–57.
74. Paus T. Mapping brain maturation and cognitive development during adolescence. Trends Cogn Sci 2005;9(2):60–8.
75. Tsujimoto S. The prefrontal cortex: functional neural development during early childhood. Neuroscientist 2008;14(4):345–58.
76. Bunge SA, Wright SB. Neurodevelopmental changes in working memory and cognitive control. Curr Opin Neurobiol 2007;17(2):243–50.
77. Passarotti AM, Sweeney JA, Pavuluri MN. Neural correlates of incidental and directed facial emotion processing in adolescents and adults. Soc Cogn Affect Neurosci 2009;4(4):387–98.
78. Hooper CJ, Luciana M, Conklin HM, et al. Adolescents' performance on the Iowa gambling task: implications for the development of decision making and ventrome-dial prefrontal cortex. Dev Psychol 2004;40(6):1148–58.
79. Rubia K, Smith AB, Woolley J, et al. Progressive increase of frontostriatal brain activation from childhood to adulthood during event-related tasks of cognitive control. Hum Brain Mapp 2006;27(12):973–93.
80. Perlman SB, Pelphrey KA. Regulatory brain development: balancing emotion and cognition. Soc Neurosci 2010;5(5–6):533–42.
81. Yurgelun-Todd DA, Killgore WDS. Fear-related activity in the prefrontal cortex increases with age during adolescence: a preliminary fMRI study. Neurosci Lett 2006;406(3):194–9.
82. Kwon H, Reiss AL, Menon V. Neural basis of protracted developmental changes in visuo-spatial working memory. Proc Natl Acad Sci U S A 2002;99(20):13336–41.
83. Lau JY, Britton JC, Nelson EE, et al. Distinct neural signatures of threat learning in adolescents and adults. Proc Natl Acad Sci U S A 2011;108(11):4500–5.
84. Prencipe A, Kesek A, Cohen J, et al. Development of hot and cool executive function during the transition to adolescence. J Exp Child Psychol 2011;108(3):621–37.
85. Levin HS, Culhane KA, Hartmann J, et al. Developmental-changes in performance on tests of purported frontal-lobe functioning. Dev Neuropsychol 1991;7(3):377–95.
86. Brocki KC, Bohlin G. Executive functions in children aged 6 to 13: a dimensional and developmental study. Dev Neuropsychol 2004;26(2):571–93.
87. Welsh MC, Pennington BF, Groisser DB. A normative developmental-study of executive function—a window on prefrontal function in children. Dev Neuropsychol 1991;7(2):131–49.
88. Casey BJ. The storm and stress of adolescence: insights from human imaging and mouse genetics. Dev Psychobiol 2010;52(3):225–35.
89. Somerville LH, Jones RM, Casey B. A time of change: behavioral and neural correlates of adolescent sensitivity to appetitive and aversive environmental cues. Brain Cogn 2010;72(1):124–33.
90. Lange K, Williams LM, Young AW, et al. Task instructions modulate neural re-sponses to fearful facial expressions. Biol Psychiatry 2003;53(3):226–32.
91. Lieberman M, Inagaki T, Tabibnia G, et al. Subjective responses to emotional stimuli during labeling, reappraisal and distraction. Emotion 2011;11(3):468–80.
92. Pessoa L. On the relationship between emotion and cognition. Nat Rev Neurosci 2008;9:148–58.

93. Taylor SF, Phan KL, Decker LR, et al. Subjective rating of emotionally salient stimuli modulates neural activity. NeuroImage 2003;18(3):650–9.

94. Whalen PJ, Rauch SL, Etcoff NL, et al. Masked presentations of emotional facial expressions modulate amygdala activity without explicit knowledge. J Neurosci 1998;18(1):411–8.

95. Pessoa L, Adolphs R. Emotion processing and the amygdala: from a 'low road' to 'many roads' of evaluating biological significance. Nat Rev Neurosci 2010;11(11): 773–83.

96. Bar-Haim Y, Lamy D, Pergamin L, et al. Threat-related attentional bias in anxious and nonanxious individuals: a meta-analytic study. Psychol Bull 2007;133(1):1–24.

97. Fox NA, Pine DS. Temperament and the emergence of anxiety disorders [abstract]. J Am Acad Child Adolesc Psychiatry 2012;51(2):125–8.

98. Cisler JM, Koster EHW. Mechanisms of attentional biases towards threat in anxiety disorders: an integrative review. Clinical Psychology Review 2010;30:203–16.

99. Merikangas KR, Avenevoli S, Dierker L, et al. Vulnerability factors among children at risk for anxiety disorders. Biol Psychiatry 1999;46(11):1523–35.

100. Garcia-Coll C, Kagan J, Reznick JS. Behavioral inhibition in young children. Child Dev. 1984;55:1005–19.

101. Calkins SD, Fox NA, Marshall TR. Behavioral and physiological antecedents of inhibited and uninhibited behavior. Child Dev 1996;67(2):523–40.

102. Kagan J, Snidman N, Arcus D. Childhood derivatives of high and low reactivity in infancy. Child Dev 1998;69(6):1483–93.

103. Robinson JL, Reznick JS, Kagan J, et al. The heritability of inhibited and uninhibited behavior—a twin study. Dev Psychol 1992;28(6):1030–7.

104. Fox NA, Henderson HA, Marshall PJ, et al. Behavioral inhibition: linking biology and behavior within a developmental framework. Annu Rev Psychol 2005;56:235–62.

105. Hirshfeld-Becker DR, Biederman J, Rosenbaum JF. Behavioral inhibition. In: Morris TL, March JS, editors. Anxiety disorders in children and adolescents. 2nd ed. New York: Guilford Press; 2004. p. 27–58.

106. Kagan J, Reznick JS, Snidman N. The physiology and psychology of behavioral inhibition in children. Child Dev 1987;58(6):1459–73.

107. Kagan J, Reznick JS, Snidman N, et al. Childhood derivatives of inhibition and lack of inhibition to the unfamiliar. Child Dev 1988;59(6):1580–9.

108. Chronis-Tuscano A, Degnan KA, Pine DS, et al. Stable early maternal report of behavioral inhibition predicts lifetime social anxiety disorder in adolescence. J Am Acad Child Adolesc Psychiatry 2009;48(9):928–35.

109. Essex MJ, Klein MH, Slattery MJ, et al. Early risk factors and developmental pathways to chronic high inhibition and social anxiety disorder in adolescence. Am J Psychiatry 2010;167(1):40–6.

110. Schwartz CE, Snidman N, Kagan J. Adolescent social anxiety as an outcome of inhibited temperament in childhood. J Am Acad Child Adolesc Psychiatry 1999; 38(8):1008–15.

111. Blackford JU, Avery SN, Shelton RC, et al. Amygdala temporal dynamics: temperamental differences in the timing of amygdala response to familiar and novel faces. BMC Neurosci 2009;10:145.

112. Blackford JU, Avery SN, Cowan RL, et al. Sustained amygdala response to both novel and newly familiar faces characterizes inhibited temperament. Soc Cogn Affect Neurosc 2011;6(5):621–9.

113. Schwartz CE, Wright CI, Shin LM, et al. Inhibited and uninhibited infants "grown up": adult amygdalar response to novelty. Science 2003;300(5627):1952–3.

114. Schwartz CE, Kunwar PS, Greve DN, et al. A phenotype of early infancy predicts reactivity of the amygdala in male adults. Mol Psychiatry 2011; http://dx.doi.org/10.1038/mp.2011.96.
115. Blackford JU, Allen AH, Cowan RL, et al. Amygdala and hippocampus fail to habituate to faces in individuals with an inhibited temperament. Soc Cogn Affect Neurosci 2012; http://dx.doi.org/10.1093/scan/nsr078.
116. Schwartz CE, Kunwar PS, Greve DN, et al. Structural differences in adult orbital and ventromedial prefrontal cortex predicted by infant temperament at 4 months of age. Arch Gen Psychiatry 2010;67(1):78–84.
117. Clauss JA, Cowan RL, Blackford JU. Expectancy and temperament modulate amygdala and dorsal anterior cingulate responses to fear faces. Cogn Affect Behav Neurosci 2011;11(1):13–21.
118. American Psychiatric Association. Diagnostic and statistical manual of mental disorders (text revision). 4th edition. Washington, DC: American Psychiatric Association; 2000.
119. Thomas KM, Drevets WC, Dahl RE, et al. Amygdala response to fearful faces in anxious and depressed children. Arch Gen Psychiatry 2001;58(11):1057–63.
120. McClure EB, Monk CS, Nelson EE, et al. Abnormal attention modulation of fear circuit function in pediatric generalized anxiety disorder. Arch Gen Psychiatry 2007;64(1):97–106.
121. Beesdo K, Lau JYF, Guyer AE, et al. Common and distinct amygdala-function perturbations in depressed vs anxious adolescents. Arch Gen Psychiatry 2009;66(3):275–85.
122. Monk CS, Telzer EH, Mogg K, et al. Amygdala and ventrolateral prefrontal cortex activation to masked angry faces in children and adolescents with generalized anxiety disorder. Arch Gen Psychiatry 2008;65(5):568–76.
123. Roberson-Nay R, McClure EB, Monk CS, et al. Increased amygdala activity during successful memory encoding in adolescent major depressive disorder: an fMRI study. Biol Psychiatry 2006;60(9):966–73.
124. Monk CS, Nelson EE, McClure EB, et al. Ventrolateral prefrontal cortex activation and attentional bias in response to angry faces in adolescents with generalized anxiety disorder. Am J Psychiatry 2006;163(6):1091–7.
125. McClure E, Adler A, Monk C, et al. fMRI predictors of treatment outcome in pediatric anxiety disorders. Psychopharmacology (Berl) 2007;191(1):97–105.
126. Maslowsky J, Mogg K, Bradley BP, et al. A preliminary investigation of neural correlates of treatment in adolescents with generalized anxiety disorder. J Child Adolesc Psychopharmacol 2010;20(2):105–11.
127. De Bellis MD, Casey BJ, Dahl RE, et al. A pilot study of amygdala volumes in pediatric generalized anxiety disorder. Biol Psychiatry 2000;48(1):51–7.
128. Milham MP, Nugent AC, Drevets WC, et al. Selective reduction in amygdala volume in pediatric anxiety disorders: a voxel-based morphometry investigation. Biol Psychiatry 2005;57(9):961–6.
129. De Bellis MD, Keshavan MS, Shifflett H, et al. Superior temporal gyrus volumes in pediatric generalized anxiety disorder. Biol Psychiatry 2002;51(7):553–62.
130. Telzer EH, Mogg K, Bradley BP, et al. Relationship between trait anxiety, prefrontal cortex, and attention bias to angry faces in children and adolescents. Biol Psychol 2008;79(2):216–22.
131. Krain AL, Gotimer K, Hefton S, et al. A functional magnetic resonance imaging investigation of uncertainty in adolescents with anxiety disorders. Biol Psychiatry 2008;63(6):563–8.

132. Gentes EL, Ruscio AM. A meta-analysis of the relation of intolerance of uncertainty to symptoms of generalized anxiety disorder, major depressive disorder, and obsessive-compulsive disorder. Clin Psychol Rev 2011;31(6):923–33.

133. Dugas MJ, Marchand A, Ladouceur R. Further validation of a cognitive-behavioral model of generalized anxiety disorder: diagnostic and symptom specificity. J Anxiety Disord 2005;19(3):329–43.

134. Blair KS, Geraci M, Korelitz K, et al. The pathology of social phobia is independent of developmental changes in face processing. Am J Psychiatry 2011;168:1202–9.

135. Guyer AE, Lau JYF, Clure-Tone EB, et al. Amygdala and ventrolateral prefrontal cortex function during anticipated peer evaluation in pediatric social anxiety. Arch Gen Psychiatry 2008;65(11):1303–12.

136. Hirshfeld-Becker DR, Biederman J, Henin A, et al. Behavioral inhibition in preschool children at risk is a specific predictor of middle childhood social anxiety: a five-year follow-up. J Dev Behav Pediatr 2007;28(3):225–33.

137. Gest SD. Behavioral inhibition: stability and associations with adaptation from childhood to early adulthood. J Pers Soc Psychol 1997;72(2):467–75.

138. Bishop G, Spence SH, McDonald C. Can parents and teachers provide a reliable and valid report of behavioral inhibition? Child Dev 2003;74(6):1899–917.

139. Perez-Edgar K, Roberson-Nay R, Hardin MG, et al. Attention alters neural responses to evocative faces in behaviorally inhibited adolescents. NeuroImage 2007;35(4):1538–46.

140. Hardin MG, Perez-Edgar K, Guyer AE, et al. Reward and punishment sensitivity in shy and non-shy adults: relations between social and motivated behavior. Pers Indiv Differ 2006;40(4):699–711.

141. Guyer AE, Nelson EE, Perez-Edgar K, et al. Striatal functional alteration in adolescents characterized by early childhood behavioral inhibition. J Neurosci 2006;26(24):6399–405.

142. Bar-Haim Y, Fox NA, Benson B, et al. Neural correlates of reward processing in adolescents with a history of inhibited temperament. Psychol Sci 2009;20(8):1009–18.

143. Killgore WDS, Yurgelun-Todd DA. Social anxiety predicts amygdala activation in adolescents viewing fearful faces. NeuroReport 2005;16(15):1671–5.

144. March JS, Parker JDA, Sullivan K, et al. The multidimensional anxiety scale for children (MASC): factor structure, reliability, and validity. J Am Acad Child Adolesc Psychiatry 1997;36(4):554–65.

145. Mana S, Martinot MLP, Martinot JL. Brain imaging findings in children and adolescents with mental disorders: a cross-sectional review. Eur Psychiatry 2010;25(6):345–54.

146. Stein DJ, Fineberg NA, Bienvenu OJ, et al. Should OCD be classified as an anxiety disorder in DSM-V? Depress Anxiety 2010;27(6):495–506.

147. Kalra SK, Swedo SE. Children with obsessive-compulsive disorder: are they just "little adults"? J Clin Invest 2009;119(4):737–46.

148. Fireman B, Koran LM, Leventhal JL, et al. The prevalence of clinically recognized obsessive-compulsive disorder in a large health maintenance organization. Am J Psychiatry 2001;158(11):1904–10.

149. Lewinsohn PM, Hops H, Roberts RE, et al. Adolescent psychopathology .1. Prevalence and incidence of depression and other DSM-III-R disorders in high-school-students. J Abnorm Psychol 1993;102(1):133–44.

150. Rauch SL, Jenike MA. Neurobiological models of obsessive-compulsive disorder. Psychosomatics 1993;34(1):20–32.

151. Szeszko PR, Robinson D, Alvir JMJ, et al. Orbital frontal and amygdala volume reductions in obsessive-compulsive disorder. Arch Gen Psychiatry 1999;56(10): 913–9.

152. Rosenberg DR, Keshavan MS. Toward a neurodevelopmental model of obsessive-compulsive disorder. Biol Psychiatry 1998;43(9):623–40.

153. Saxena S, Rauch SL. Functional neuroimaging and the neuroanatomy of obsessive-compulsive disorder. Psychiatr Clin North Am 2000;23(3):563–86.

154. MacMaster FP, O'Neill J, Rosenberg DR. Brain imaging in pediatric obsessive-compulsive disorder. J Am Acad Child Adolesc Psychiatry 2008;47(11):1262–72.

155. Fitzgerald KD, MacMaster FP, Paulson LD, et al. Neurobiology of childhood obsessive-compulsive disorder. Child Adolesc.Psychiatr Clin N Am 1999;8(3):533–75.

156. Huyser C, Veltman DJ, de Haan E, et al. Paediatric obsessive-compulsive disorder, a neurodevelopmental disorder? Evidence from neuroimaging. Neurosci Biobehav Rev 2009;33(6):818–30.

157. Marsh R, Maia TV, Peterson BS. Functional disturbances within frontostriatal circuits across multiple childhood psychopathologies. Am J Psychiatry 2009;166(6):664–74.

158. Maia TV, Cooney RE, Peterson BS. The neural bases of obsessive-compulsive disorder in children and adults. Dev Psychopathol 2008;20(4):1251–83.

159. Gilbert AR, Akkal D, Almeida JR, et al. Neural correlates of symptom dimensions in pediatric obsessive-compulsive disorder: a functional magnetic resonance imaging study. J Am Acad Child Adolesc Psychiatry 2009;48(9):936–44.

160. Britton JC, Stewart SE, Killgore WD, et al. Amygdala activation in response to facial expressions in pediatric obsessive-compulsive disorder. Depress Anxiety 2010; 27(7):643–51.

161. Woolley J, Heyman I, Brammer M, et al. Brain activation in paediatric obsessive-compulsive disorder during tasks of inhibitory control. Br J Psychiatry 2008;192(1): 25–31.

162. Britton JC, Rauch SL, Rosso IM, et al. Cognitive inflexibility and frontal-cortical activation in pediatric obsessive-compulsive disorder. J Am Acad Child Adolesc Psychiatry 2010;49(9):944–53.

163. Diler RS, Kibar M, Avci A. Pharmacotherapy and regional cerebral blood flow in children with obsessive compulsive disorder. Yonsei Med J 2004;45(1):90–9.

164. Castillo ARGL, Buchpiguel CA, de Araujo LASB, et al. Brain SPECT imaging in children and adolescents with obsessive-compulsive disorder. J Neural Transm 2005;112(8):1115–29.

165. Lazaro L, Caldu X, Junque C, et al. Cerebral activation in children and adolescents with obsessive-compulsive disorder before and after treatment: a functional MRI study. J Psychiatr Res 2008;42(13):1051–9.

166. Szeszko PR, Christian C, MacMaster F, et al. Gray matter structural alterations in psychotropic drug-naive pediatric obsessive-compulsive disorder: an optimized voxel-based morphometry study. Am J Psychiatry 2008;165(10):1299–307.

167. Gilbert AR, Keshavan MS, Diwadkar V, et al. Gray matter differences between pediatric obsessive-compulsive disorder patients and high-risk siblings: a preliminary voxel-based morphometry study. Neurosci Lett 2008;435(1):45–50.

168. Zarei M, Mataix-Cols D, Heyman I, et al. Changes in gray matter volume and white matter microstructure in adolescents with obsessive-compulsive disorder. Biol Psychiatry 2011;70(11):1083–90.

169. Rosenberg DR, Keshavan MS, Ohearn KM, et al. Frontostriatal measurement in treatment-naive children with obsessive-compulsive disorder. Arch Gen Psychiatry 1997;54(9):824–30.

170. Szeszko PR, MacMillan S, McMeniman M, et al. Brain structural abnormalities in psychotropic drug-naive pediatric patients with obsessive-compulsive disorder. Am J Psychiatry 2004;161(6):1049–56.
171. Gilbert AR, Moore GJ, Keshavan MS, et al. Decrease in thalamic volumes of pediatric patients with obsessive-compulsive disorder who are taking paroxetine. Arch Gen Psychiatry 2000;57(5):449–56.
172. Tobe RH, Bansal R, Xu DR, et al. Cerebellar morphology in burette syndrome and obsessive-compulsive disorder. Ann Neurol 2010;67(4):479–87.
173. Rosenberg DR, Benazon NR, Gilbert A, et al. Thalamic volume in pediatric obsessive-compulsive disorder patients before and after cognitive behavioral therapy. Biol Psychiatry 2000;48(4):294–300.
174. Kendall PC, Compton SN, Walkup JT, et al. Clinical characteristics of anxiety disordered youth. J Anxiety Disord 2010;24(3):360–5.
175. Hakamata Y, Lissek S, Bar-Haim Y, et al. Attention bias modification treatment: a meta-analysis toward the establishment of novel treatment for anxiety. Biol Psychiatry 2010;68(11):982–90.

Psychopharmacologic Treatment of Children and Adolescents with Anxiety Disorders

Jeffrey R. Strawn, MD[a,b,]*, Dara J. Sakolsky, MD, PhD[c], Moira A. Rynn, MD[d]

KEYWORDS

- Benzodiazepine • Generalized anxiety disorder
- Selective serotonin norepinephrine reuptake inhibitor • Selective serotonin reuptake inhibitor
- Separation anxiety disorder • Social phobia

KEY POINTS

- Anxiety disorders often first emerge during childhood and adolescence and adversely affect social and family relationships and school performance.
- Children and adolescents with anxiety disorders are also more likely to report suicidal ideation or to attempt suicide than healthy subjects.
- Advances in pediatric psychopharmacology raise a number of opportunities to potentially decrease morbidity in youth with anxiety; emerging literature suggests that selective serotonin reuptake inhibitors and cognitive–behavioral therapy may modulate the activity of specific structures within central brain fear circuits.
- Neuroimaging markers of treatment response in pediatric anxiety will help to identify the specific neural circuits involved in successful treatment.
- Genetic markers of may enhance understanding of the molecular pathophysiology of treatment response in pediatric anxiety disorders.
- Biosignatures (eg, panel of genetic, neuroimaging, and/or physiologic biomarkers) in the future may be used to guide individualized treatment recommendations.

INTRODUCTION

Anxiety disorders often first emerge during childhood and adolescence,[1,2] and adversely affect social and family relationships as well as school performance.[3]

DISCLOSURES: Dr Strawn has received research support from Eli Lilly, Shire and from the American Academy of Child and Adolescent Psychiatry. Dr Sakolsky has received research support from NARSAD and NIMH. Dr Rynn has received research support from Eli Lilly, Shire, and Pfizer, and from the NIH and NICHD.

[a] Department of Psychiatry and Behavioral Neuroscience, University of Cincinnati, College of Medicine, Cincinnati, OH 45219, USA; [b] Department of Psychiatry, Cincinnati Children's Hospital Medical Center, Cincinnati, OH 45267, USA; [c] Department of Psychiatry, University of Pittsburgh, Western Psychiatric Institute and Clinic, University of Pittsburgh Medical Center, Bellefield Towers, Room 515, 100 North Bellefield Avenue, Pittsburgh, PA 15213, USA; [d] Department of Psychiatry and New York State Psychiatric Institute (NYSPI), Columbia University, New York, NY, USA
* Corresponding author. Department of Psychiatry, University of Cincinnati, Box 670559, Cincinnati, OH 45267-0559.
E-mail address: strawnjr@uc.edu

Child Adolesc Psychiatric Clin N Am 21 (2012) 527–539
http://dx.doi.org/10.1016/j.chc.2012.05.003
1056-4993/12/$ – see front matter © 2012 Elsevier Inc. All rights reserved.

childpsych.theclinics.com

Children and adolescents with anxiety disorders are also more likely to report suicidal ideation or to attempt suicide than healthy subjects, and are more likely to report or attempt suicide than those with depression alone. These findings suggest that anxiety disorders heighten the risk of suicidal ideation or suicide attempts in children and adolescents.[4,5] However, despite the prevalence of these conditions and their associated morbidity, children and adolescents suffering from anxiety disorders are often not identified and frequently do not receive treatment with psychotherapy or psychopharmacologic interventions.[6,7]

Psychopharmacologic trials in youth with anxiety disorders (other than obsessive–compulsive disorder [OCD] and posttraumatic stress disorder) have largely focused on studying the "anxiety triad" of symptoms and disorders (eg, the combination of separation anxiety disorder [SAD], generalized anxiety disorder [GAD], and social phobia [SoP]).[8] The tendency to evaluate the treatment of these three anxiety disorders (specifically GAD, SAD, and SoP) together has generally been the result of several clinical and theoretical issues. For example, these anxiety disorders are (1) highly comorbid, (2) are considered physiologically distinct from other child onset anxiety disorders (eg, OCD or posttraumatic stress disorder), and (3) they have shown similar responses to treatment with pharmacotherapy (eg, selective serotonin re-uptake inhibitors [SSRIs] and cognitive behavioral therapy [CBT]).[9–11] However, several studies have recently focused on specific anxiety disorders (eg, GAD or SoP) in these populations. In this review, we have summarized all randomized, controlled trials of SSRIs, serotonin norepinephrine reuptake inhibitors (SNRIs), benzodiazepines, and other agents (eg, buspirone and tricyclic antidepressants) that have included pediatric patients with non-OCD, non-posttraumatic stress disorder anxiety disorders.

GENERALIZED ANXIETY DISORDER
Sertraline

In the first placebo-controlled trial of the SSRI sertraline to be conducted in youth with GAD, children and adolescents, aged 5–17 years (n = 22), were treated with fixed-dose sertraline (50 mg/d) for 9 weeks. Compared with placebo-treated youth, significant improvement was noted in the sertraline-treated patients on the Hamilton Anxiety Rating Scale,[12] Clinical Global Impression—Severity (CGI-S; from 1 [not mentally ill] to 7 [severely ill]) and CGI—Improvement (CGI-I; from 1 [very much improved] to 7 [very much worse]) scores. Additionally, the authors of this study controlled for the severity of co-occurring depressive symptoms and observed a highly significant "main treatment effect for anxiety," but not for depression.[13] No differences in side effects were observed between the sertraline-treated patients and those who received placebo. In addition, sertraline was recently compared with placebo, CBT, and their combination (sertraline plus CBT) in the Child/Adolescent Anxiety Multimodal Study (CAMS) in which GAD was present in 78% of the 488 patients.[8] In CAMS, sertraline was found to be superior to placebo and equally as effective as CBT.

Fluoxetine

A small study of 14 youth with GAD revealed that treatment with flexibly dosed fluoxetine (5–40 mg/d) or CBT was associated symptomatic improvement in youth with GAD[14] and revealed increased activation of the right ventrolateral prefrontal cortex in response to pictures of angry faces after treatment with both fluoxetine and CBT, suggesting that increased activity within the ventrolateral prefrontal cortex may have compensatory function in youth with GAD.[14] In addition, several studies have evaluated the efficacy of fluoxetine in patients with GAD or overanxious disorder (*DSM-III-R* forerunner for GAD) in studies of mixed anxiety disorders in youth,[15–17] and these are discussed later in the section on mixed anxiety disorders.

Venlafaxine

The SNRI venlafaxine has been evaluated in 2 randomized, 8-week, placebo-controlled trials in youth diagnosed with GAD, aged 6–17 years (n = 323).[18] Extended-release (ER) venlafaxine was initiated at 37.5 mg/d in all participants. For youth weighing between 25 and 39 kg, the highest dose allowed was 112.5 mg/d; for patients weighing 40 kg and greater it was 225 mg/d. In this report, which includes data from 2 identically designed studies (Study 1 and Study 2), venlafaxine ER was superior to placebo in producing improvements in scores on the GAD section of the Columbia K-SADS as well as the Pediatric Anxiety Rating Scale (PARS),[19] Hamilton Anxiety Rating Scale,[12] and Screen for Anxiety Related Emotional Disorders (parent and child)[20] scores only in Study 1 ($P<.001$), but failed to reach significance in Study 2 ($P<.06$). In the pooled analysis of Study 1 and Study 2, venlafaxine ER, compared with placebo, demonstrated significant differences for improving anxiety symptoms ($P<.001$) and had a higher response rate (69% vs 48%; $P<.04$).[18] Children and adolescents who received venlafaxine were more likely to experience asthenia, pain, anorexia, and somnolence as well as weight loss compared with those receiving placebo.[18]

Buspirone

To date, 2 open-label studies have evaluated the efficacy and tolerability of the 5-HT$_{1A}$ agonist buspirone in pediatric patients with overanxious disorder (now defined as *DSM-IV-TR* GAD). Kutcher and colleagues[21] reported that over 6 weeks of treatment with flexibly-dosed buspirone (15–30 mg/d), anxiety significantly improved in youth with overanxious disorder. Subsequently, Simeon[22] reported that in a sample of 13 children and adolescents (9 of whom had primary or secondary diagnoses of overanxious disorder), anxiety symptoms significantly improved over 4 weeks of treatment. In addition, buspirone was generally noted to be well tolerated, although some patients experienced sedation, nausea, stomach aches, and headaches.[22] Two randomized, placebo-controlled trials of buspirone have examined the efficacy and tolerability of this agent in pediatric patients (age range, 6–17 years; n = 559). In these studies, which utilized 15–60 mg of buspirone per day, no significant differences between buspirone and placebo were noted for GAD symptoms,[23] despite pharmacokinetic studies of this agent which have revealed plasma exposure to buspirone [and its active metabolite, 1-(2-pyrimidinyl)-piperazine] are equivalent or greater in pediatric patients compared with adults.[24]

Benzodiazepines

Despite the common use of benzodiazepines for the treatment of anxiety disorders in adults,[25–27] there are few studies completed with anxious youth and the results have been mixed. In 1 open-label trial, 12 adolescents with overanxious disorder (*DSM-III-R* criteria) were treated with open-label alprazolam (0.5–1.5 mg/d) for 4 weeks and significant improvements were noted in terms of anxiety and insomnia.[22] Of note, alprazolam was generally well tolerated, despite some sedation, agitation, headaches, and nausea.[28] A double-blind, placebo-controlled trial of alprazolam in youth aged 8 to 16 years (n = 30) with overanxious disorder (*DSM-III-R* criteria) found no difference between alprazolam and placebo on a clinical global rating of improvement. However, this study may have failed to find a difference between groups because it was underpowered. Alprazolam was well-tolerated, with some reports of fatigue and dry mouth; there were no reports of withdrawal symptoms.[28]

SOCIAL PHOBIA
Paroxetine

In a multicenter, double-blind, placebo-controlled trial of paroxetine, Wagner and colleagues[29] randomized 322 youth with SoP to paroxetine or placebo. In this 16-week study, the last-observation carried forward analyses revealed a greater response (by CGI-I score) for paroxetine (78% response) as compared with placebo (38.3% response). Insomnia, decreased appetite, and vomiting were among the most common side effects (experienced at least twice as often in the medication group than the placebo group), although the medication was generally well tolerated. In addition, 4 paroxetine-treated patients expressed suicidal ideation or had threatened suicide (versus none in the placebo group). Finally, and of clinical importance, upon discontinuation, SSRI withdrawal symptoms including nausea, dizziness, and vomiting were experienced twice as frequently by the paroxetine-treated patients than those who received placebo.[29]

Venlafaxine ER

The efficacy of venlafaxine ER has been evaluated in a randomized, double-blind, placebo controlled trial of 293 outpatient children and adolescents (age 8–17 years; mean, 13.6) with SoP.[30] Venlafaxine ER was initiated at 37.5 mg/d and titrated to a maximum dose over 16 weeks. Specifically, in youth weighing between 25 and 33 kg, the maximum dose was 112.5 mg/d, whereas in patients weighing between 34 and 49 kg, venlafaxine ER was titrated to a maximum dose of 150 mg/d and in youth weighing more than 50 kg, venlafaxine ER could be increased to 225 mg/d. March and colleagues[30] noted that youth receiving venlafaxine ER had a greater reduction in their social anxiety symptoms compared with placebo (response rates in the 2 groups were 56 vs 37%, respectively; **Table 1**). Although both groups reported mild-to-moderate adverse events, events that occurred at least twice as often as in placebo included asthenia, pain, anorexia, and somnolence. Significant weight loss was noted in patients treated with venlafaxine ER. Also, 3 patients treated with venlafaxine ER developed suicidal ideation, whereas no patients in the placebo group reported suicidal ideation.[30]

Fluoxetine

In a double-blind, randomized trial, Beidel and colleagues[31] compared Social Effectiveness Therapy for Children (SET-C), fluoxetine (forced titration 10–40 mg/d), and a pill placebo in children and adolescents (aged 7–17 years) with SoP.[31] Patients were randomized to 1 of 3 treatment groups: SET-C, fluoxetine, or pill placebo. Of the SET-C group, 53% no longer met diagnostic criteria (compared with 21.2% of patients treated with fluoxetine and 3.1% of those treated with placebo). There were no severe adverse events reported, although some fluoxetine-treated participants experienced side effects (eg, diarrhea).[31]

Sertraline

An open-label study of sertraline (mean dose 123 ± 37 mg/d) in children and adolescents (age 10–17 years; 8 boys and 6 girls) with SoP, evaluated 14 youth during 8 weeks of treatment with sertraline.[32] Analysis of CGI-I scores revealed that 36% (5/14) of subjects were responders and 29% (4/14) as partial responders by the end

Table 1
Randomized, controlled trials of SSRIs and SNRIs and atypical anxiolytics in pediatric anxiety disorders

Reference	Diagnosis	Duration (wks)	Treatment	n	Dose Range (mg/d)	Average Dose	NNT*	Outcome
Walkup et al[8]	GAD SoP SAD	12	Sertraline CBT Combination Placebo	133 139 140 76	25–200 25–200	146.0 ± 60.8 to 133.7 ± 59.8 mg	3 (3.2–3.5)	CBT, SSRIs, or CBT + SSRIs > placebo
Rynn et al[13]	GAD	9	Sertraline Placebo	11 11	50	Fixed dose	2 (1–2)	Sertraline >placebo
Beidel et al[31]	SoP	12	Fluoxetine SET Placebo	33 57 32	10–40	Not specified		SET = fluoxetine >placebo
Wagner et al[29]	SoP	16	Paroxetine Placebo	163 156	10–50	24.8 mg for all patients, 21.7 mg for children, and 26.1 mg for adolescents	3 (3–4)	Paroxetine >placebo
March et al[30]	SoP	16	Venlafaxine ER Placebo	137 148	37.5–225	2.6–3.0 mg/kg	6 (4–14)	Venlafaxine ER >placebo
Rynn et al[18]	GAD	8	Study 1: Venlafaxine ER Placebo Study 2: Venlafaxine ER Placebo	76 77 78 82	37.5–225 37.5–225		5 (4–11)	Study 1: Venlafaxine ER Placebo Study 2: Venlafaxine ER = Placebo
Birmaher et al[17]	GAD SoP SAD	12	Fluoxetine Placebo	37 37	20	Fixed dose	4 (3–27)	Fluoxetine >placebo
RUPP[40]	GAD SoP SAD	8	Fluvoxamine Placebo	61 63		2.9 ± 1.3 mg/kg	3 (2–4)	Fluvoxamine >placebo
BMS, 2010	GAD	8	Buspirone Placebo		15–60 mg	Not specified	N/A	Buspirone = placebo

Abbreviation: SET, Social Effectiveness Therapy for Children.
* Number needed to treat (NNT) for medication versus placebo.

of the 8-week trial. Response occurred by week 6 and sertraline was generally well tolerated with no subject developing significant behavioral disinhibition, mania, or suicidal ideation. Nausea, diarrhea, and headaches were the most frequently reported adverse events and were generally mild.[32] In addition, patients with SoP (82% of sample) were included CAMS, which compared placebo, sertraline, CBT, their combination (sertraline plus CBT) in youth with multiple anxiety disorders[8] and is discussed in the mixed anxiety disorders section.

Citalopram

No randomized, controlled trials have evaluated the efficacy of citalopram in the treatment of pediatric SoP. One open-label study of citalopram evaluated the efficacy of flexibly dosed citalopram (10–40 mg/d, mean dose 35 ± 7 mg/d) in 12 children and adolescents (aged 8–17 years; mean, 13.4 ± 3) with social anxiety disorder over 12 weeks.[33] In this study, 83% of youth reported improvement (as measured by CGI-I); significant improvement was also observed on self-report and parental reports of social anxiety symptoms.[33] In general, citalopram was well-tolerated.

SEPARATION ANXIETY DISORDER
Tricyclic Antidepressants

Several studies have evaluated youth with school refusal in whom SAD and or SoP are often present. In the first, 35 children (aged 6–14 years) were treated with flexibly dosed imipramine (100–200 mg/d) and imipramine-treated patients treated with imipramine improved more so than those who received placebo. However, subsequent trials of tricyclic antidepressants in youth with school refusal, overanxious disorder, and SAD have failed to find differences between imipramine[34,35] or clomipramine[36] and placebo. Finally, Bernstein and colleagues[37] compared CBT plus imipramine with CBT plus placebo in 63 adolescents with major depressive disorder and an anxiety disorder, and found clinician and self-report measures of anxiety showed no significant difference between groups.

Benzodiazepines

One study has evaluated the efficacy of clonazepam (up to 2 mg/d) in 15 children (aged 7–13 years; 8 males and 7 females) with SAD (SAD, n = 14; GAD, n = 5; total, n = 15). This study was unique in that it utilized a crossover design, which should have been powered to detect a "clearly beneficial effect."[38] No difference in the clinical global improvement scale was observed between the clonazepam-treated and placebo groups. In general, patients experienced frequent side effects (83% clonazepam vs 58% placebo). Drowsiness, irritability, and "oppositional behavior" were the most frequent side effects seen the clonazepam group.[38]

Of note, most psychopharmacologic trials of youth with "mixed anxiety disorders" have included children and adolescents with SAD in addition to GAD and SoP because of their high comorbidity. For example, in CAMS, more than half of patients met *DSM-IV-TR* criteria for SAD, thus the results of this placebo-controlled trial of sertraline and CBT,[8] which are described in the mixed anxiety disorders would likely be applicable to youth with SAD.

PANIC DISORDER

Studies of pharmacologic interventions in youth with panic disorder are rare and many recent studies of pediatric anxiety disorders have excluded patients with panic disorder. In fact, we are only able identify 2 open-label studies of SSRIs in pediatric patients with panic disorder. In the first study, several SSRIs (fluoxetine, sertraline, and paroxetine) were evaluated in 12 children and adolescents with panic disorder (mean age, 14.5 ± 3.4 years; 7 girls) over the course of 6 months, and the authors observed that 75% of patients were "much" to "very much improved," and that SSRIs were generally well-tolerated in this population. Importantly, at the conclusion of the trial, 67% of patients no longer fulfilled criteria for panic disorder, although 4 youth continued to experience "significant residual symptoms." In this study, a benzodiazepine adjunct (clonazepam and lorazepam) was used in 67% of patients and the authors suggest that "treatment [with a benzodiazepine] might be helpful for patients with severe panic disorder" while awaiting the clinical response to the SSRI.[39]

Additionally, in a study which is described in greater detail in the mixed anxiety disorders section, Fairbanks and colleagues[15] treated 16 children and adolescents with flexibly dosed fluoxetine and noted that only 3 of 5 patients with panic disorder exhibited clinical response.[15] To date, we are unable to locate any placebo-controlled trials of any psychopharmacologic treatment in youth with panic disorder.

MIXED ANXIETY DISORDERS
Fluvoxamine

Fluvoxamine has been evaluated in a double-blind, placebo-controlled trial in youth with anxiety disorders including SAD, SoP, and GAD.[40] In this study, 128 children with anxiety disorders were treated with fluvoxamine titrated to 300 mg/d (mean dose, 2.9 + 1.3 mg/kg) and significant differences were found in CGI-I and endpoint PARS scores ($P<.001$). In addition, fluvoxamine was well tolerated with only abdominal discomfort and increased motor activity occurring more frequently in the fluvoxamine-treated youth than in those who received placebo.[40] In addition, a 6-month, open-label extension of this study revealed that 94% of fluovoxamine responders maintained response and 71% (10/14) of the fluvoxamine-treated patients who had not responded to fluvoxamine responded to fluoxetine.[41]

Fluoxetine

Two open-label studies have evaluated the SSRI fluoxetine in youth with mixed anxiety disorders.[15,16] In the first study, youth with mixed anxiety disorders (overanxious disorders, SoP, or SAD) who were not depressed and whom had failed to respond to psychotherapy were treated for 6 months with flexibly dosed fluoxetine for up to 10 months. Birmaher and colleagues[17] observed moderate to marked improvement in 81% of patients and noted fluoxetine to be very well tolerated. Later, Fairbanks and colleagues[15] evaluated 16 outpatients (aged 9–18) who had failed psychotherapy and treated them with flexibly dosed fluoxetine (5 mg/d, flexibly titrated to a maximum of 40 mg in children and 80 mg/d in adolescents [mean dose, 0.7 mg/kg] in both groups). Clinical improvement occurred in all patients with current SAD (n = 10), whereas clinical improvement occurred in 8 of 10 with SoP, 4 of 6 with specific phobia, 3 of 5 with panic disorder, and 1 of 7 with GAD. Fluoxetine was well tolerated and the most frequently reported side effects included drowsiness, sleep problems, decreased appetite, nausea, and abdominal pain. No treatment-emergent suicidality was noted in this trial and the authors concluded that fluoxetine may be effective in "SAD and SoP." Also of interest, the authors observed that patients with only 1 anxiety disorder tended to respond to lower doses of fluoxetine than patients with multiple anxiety disorders (0.49 ± 0.14 vs 0.80 ± 0.28 mg/kg).[15]

Birmaher and colleagues[17] evaluated the efficacy and tolerability of fluoxetine in a randomized, placebo-controlled trial of youth with GAD, SAD, and SoP (mean age, 11.6 ± 3 years; range, 7–17). In this 12-week trial, fluoxetine was initiated at 10 mg/d and was titrated to 20 mg/d at the end of the first week and was generally well tolerated; 76% of the fluoxetine-treated patients completing the trial (versus 84% placebo completion; $P = .39$). Compared with placebo, significant improvements were noted in the fluoxetine-treated patients on the Screen for Anxiety Related Emotional Disorders (both child and parent versions) scores, PARS score, CGI-I, CGI-S, and CGAS. Rates of CGI-I scale response were significantly higher in the fluoxetine group than in the placebo group and treatment effects. In addition, a follow-up study suggested that fluoxetine may be effective as a maintenance treatment in children and adolescents with anxiety disorders.[42]

Sertraline Plus Cognitive Behavioral Therapy

Recently, CAMS evaluated the comparative efficacy of sertraline, CBT, or the combination of sertraline plus CBT (COMB) in patients aged 7 to 17 years (mean, 11.8) with SoP, SAD, GAD, or any combination of these anxiety disorders.[8] Sertraline was initiated at 25 mg/d and was titrated to 200 mg/d (mean, 146 ± 61; 25–200). Improvement (CGI-I) scores for the children treated with COMB were greater (80.7%) than for those youth who received CBT (59.7%) or sertraline alone (54.9%). All treatments were superior to placebo in this 12-week study.[8] With regard to remission rates after 12 weeks of treatment were 46% to 68% for COMB, 34% to 46% for sertraline, 20% to 46% for CBT, and 15% to 27% for placebo.[43] Sertraline was well tolerated and rates of adverse events were similar to placebo. However, those children who received CBT were less likely to report insomnia, fatigue, sedation, restlessness, or fidgeting than those who received sertraline.[8] Finally, a recent analysis of remission in this study revealed that predictors of posttreatment remission included younger age, nonminority status, lower baseline anxiety severity, absence of other internalizing disorders (eg, depression), and absence of SoP.[43]

Atomoxetine

The SNRI atomoxetine has been evaluated in a placebo-controlled trial of children and adolescents (age 8–17 years) with ADHD and comorbid anxiety (defined as SAD, GAD, SoP, or a combination of these conditions). Atomoxetine was initiated at 0.8 mg/kg per day for 3 days and increased to the target dose of 1.2 mg/kg per day with a maximum dose of 1.8 mg/kg per day; treatment was continued for 12 weeks. Last observation carried forward analysis of PARS scores revealed improvement with atomoxetine versus placebo (effect size = 0.5) and significant improvements were also noted for ADHD symptoms. In general, atomoxetine was well tolerated.[44]

TREATMENT GUIDELINES

Over the last 2 decades, substantial advances have been made in both psychotherapeutic and psychopharmacologic treatment of youth with anxiety disorders. Of the available studies of psychotherapy, most have evaluated the efficacy of CBT,[45–47] although several alternate forms of psychotherapy that are efficacious in other types of psychopathology in youth remain understudied in youth with anxiety disorders (eg, interpersonal psychotherapy for adolescents and mentalization-based therapy).

As these studies suggest, the SSRIs are considered to be first-line medication treatments for childhood anxiety disorders. Additionally, there are some preliminary data for the use of SNRIs (eg, venlafaxine ER) for GAD and SoP. Because of the lack of positive results and their side effect profile, TCAs are generally not recommended for the treatment of the triad anxiety disorders. The research data are limited in terms of the use of benzodiazepine; however, with careful dosing and monitoring, this class of medication may be helpful as adjunctive treatment to the SSRI during the acute phase of treatment. Unfortunately, there are very few medication trials that provide information on the efficacy, tolerability, and safety for long-term medication treatment. Of those that are available, they seem to suggest with continued treatment response is maintained and adverse events are tolerable.

However, when considering prescribing medication for a pediatric patient, the clinician needs to consider the risks versus the benefits for this treatment and to convey this information to the parent and child. As reviewed herein, antidepressants can lead to adverse events in 2 main categories: Physical (eg, headaches, gastric distress, and sleep difficulties) and psychiatric (eg, disinhibition, agitation, increased anxiety symptoms, and suicidal ideation and behaviors). Of particular concern is the "black-box" warning placed by the US Food and Drug Administration in 2004 on antidepressant medications, including SSRIs and SNRIs, publicizing a 2-fold increased risk for suicidal thinking or behavior in children and adolescents taking these medications. Bridge and colleagues[48] conducted a meta-analysis based on pediatric medication trials including all indications (n = 39, of which 6 were OCD trials).[48] The results showed a small, increased risk of suicidal ideation and attempts for youth treated with antidepressant medications as compared with placebo (0.7%; 95% confidence interval, 0.1%–1.3%) in all studies for both anxiety and depression trials. It was found the number needed to harm was 143 (95% confidence interval, 77–1000) and there were no completed suicides. **Table 1** shows the NNT for each of the studies discussed herein.

Finally, the field has shown significant, positive, synergistic effects of the combination of psychotherapy and psychopharmacologic interventions,[8,43] and current practice guidelines from the American Academy of Child and Adolescent Psychiatry recommend a multimodal treatment approach.[49]

IMPLICATIONS FOR RESEARCH AND CLINICAL PRACTICE

The exciting advances in pediatric psychopharmacology described herein raise a number of opportunities to potentially decrease morbidity in youth with anxiety. First, distinct lines of research have begun to converge as studies have integrated the clinical effects of successful treatment with SSRIs and psychotherapy with the accompanying changes in the underlying neurophysiology of pediatric anxiety disorders.[14,50] In short, this emerging literature suggests that SSRIs and CBT may modulate the activity of specific structures within these central brain fear circuits (those involving the anterior limbic network; see Strawn and colleagues[50] for a recent review) and lays the groundwork for studies which may predict treatment outcome based on neural responses obtained in specific functional magnetic resonance imaging tasks.[51]

Although neuroimaging markers of treatment response in pediatric anxiety will help to identify the specific neural circuits involved in successful treatment, genetic markers may enhance our understanding of the molecular pathophysiology of treatment response in pediatric anxiety disorders. Preliminary data analyses from the CAMS study suggest that genetic variation in *GRIK4*, the gene that codes for the KA1 subunit of the kainate-preferring glutamate receptor, and *SLC6A4*, the gene that codes for serotonin transporter, may help to predict treatment response in pediatric anxiety disorders.[52,53] In the future, biosignatures (eg, a panel of genetic, neuroimaging, and/or physiologic biomarkers) may be used to guide individualized treatment recommendations.

Given that 20% to 35% of youth treated with SRIs and CBT may not receive significant benefit from available current treatment interventions,[8] it will be important to identify medications with novel mechanisms of action to our psychopharmacologic armamentarium. In this regard, studies of adults with anxiety spectrum disorders have observed increased central glutamate concentrations[54,55] and glutamatergic hyperactivity is hypothesized to be implicated in the pathophysiology of anxiety disorders and is an emerging target of novel therapeutics being developed for the treatment of anxiety disorders.[56,57] Thus, it will be important to evaluate glutamatergic modulators in youth with anxiety disorders such as D-cycloserine, memantine, and minocycline.[58] Finally, some data implicate other neurochemical systems in youth with anxiety disorders, including clonidine-challenge studies, which suggest enhanced central adrenergic sensitivity in pediatric patients with anxiety disorders,[59] raising the possibility that anti-adrenergics (eg, guanfacine, clonidine) may hold promise as treatments for anxious youth. However, despite some evidence, which suggests that these agents may be effective in treating anxiety disorders in adults,[60] only single-dose studies exist in anxious children and adolescents.[61]

REFERENCES

1. Beesdo K, Pine DS, Lieb R, et al. Incidence and risk patterns of anxiety and depressive disorders and categorization of generalized anxiety disorder. Arch Gen Psychiatry 2010;67:47–57.
2. Beesdo K, Knappe S, Pine DS. Anxiety and anxiety disorders in children and adolescents: developmental issues and implications for DSM-V. Psychiatr Clin North Am 2009;32:483–524.
3. Birmaher B, Yelovich AK, Renaud J. Pharmacologic treatment for children and adolescents with anxiety disorders. Pediatr Clin North Am 1998;45:1187–204.
4. Foley DL, Goldston DB, Costello EJ, et al. Proximal psychiatric risk factors for suicidality in youth: the Great Smoky Mountains Study. Arch Gen Psychiatry 2006; 63:1017–24.
5. Jacobson CM, Muehlenkamp JJ, Miller AL, et al. Psychiatric impairment among adolescents engaging in different types of deliberate self-harm. J Clin Child Adolesc Psychol 2008;37:363–75.
6. Costello EJ, Janiszewski S. Who gets treated? Factors associated with referral in children with psychiatric disorders. Acta Psychiatr Scand 1990;81:523–9.
7. Chavira DA, Stein MB, Bailey K, et al. Child anxiety in primary care: prevalent but untreated. Depress Anxiety 2004;20:155–64.
8. Walkup JT, Albano AM, Piacentini J, et al. Cognitive behavioral therapy, sertraline, or a combination in childhood anxiety. N Engl J Med 2008;359:2753–66.
9. Compton SN, Walkup JT, Albano AM, et al. Child/Adolescent Anxiety Multimodal Study (CAMS): rationale, design, and methods. Child Adolesc Psychiatry Ment Health 2010;4:1.
10. Kendall PC, Compton SN, Walkup JT, et al. Clinical characteristics of anxiety disordered youth. J Anxiety Disord 2010;24:360–5.
11. Verduin TL, Kendall PC. Differential occurrence of comorbidity within childhood anxiety disorders. J Clin Child Adolesc Psychol 2003;32:290–5.
12. Hamilton M. The assessment of anxiety states by rating. Br J Med Psychol 1959;32: 50–5.
13. Rynn MA, Siqueland L, Rikels K. Placebo-controlled trial of sertraline in the treatment of children with generalized anxiety disorder. Am J Psychiatry 2001;158:2008–14.
14. Maskowsky J, Mogg K, Bradley BP, et al. A preliminary investigation of the neural correlates of treatment in adolescents with generalized anxiety disorder. J Child Adolesc Psychopharmacol 2010;20:105–11.

15. Fairbanks JM, Pine DS, Tancer NK, et al. Open fluoxetine treatment of mixed anxiety disorders in children and adolescents. J Child Adolesc Psychopharmacol 1997;7:17–29.
16. Birmaher B, Waterman GS, Ryan N, et al. Fluoxetine for childhood anxiety disorders. J Am Acad Child Adolesc Psychiatry 1994;33:993–9.
17. Birmaher B, Axelson DA, Monk K, et al. Fluoxetine for the treatment of childhood anxiety disorders. J Am Acad Child Adolesc Psychiatry 2003;42:415–23.
18. Rynn MA, Riddle MA, Yeung PP, et al. Efficacy and safety of extended-release venlafaxine in the treatment of generalized anxiety disorder in children and adolescents: two placebo-controlled trials. Am J Psychiatry 2007;164:290–300.
19. The Pediatric Anxiety Rating Scale (PARS): development and psychometric properties. J Am Acad Child Adolesc Psychiatry 2002;41:1061–9.
20. Birmaher B, Khetarpal S, Brent D, et al. The Screen for Child Anxiety Related Emotional Disorders (SCARED): scale construction and psychometric characteristics. J Am Acad Child Adolesc Psychiatry 1997;36:545–53.
21. Kutcher SP, Reiter S, Gardner DM, et al. The pharmacotherapy of anxiety disorders in children and adolescents. Psychiatr Clin North Am 1992;15:41–67.
22. Simeon JG, Ferguson HB. Alprazolam effects in children with anxiety disorders. Can J Psychiatry 1987;32:570–4.
23. Bristol-Meyers Squibb Company. Buspirone package insert. Princeton, NJ; 2010.
24. Salazar DE, Frackiewicz EJ, Dockens R, et al. Pharmacokinetics and tolerability of buspirone during oral administration to children and adolescents with anxiety disorder and normal healthy adults. J Clin Pharmacol 2001;41:1351–8.
25. Ballenger JC, Burrows GD, DuPont RL, et al. Alprazolam in panic disorder and agoraphobia: results from a multicenter trial. Arch Gen Psychiatry 1988;45:413–22.
26. Rickels K, Case G, Downing RW. Long-term diazepam therapy and clinical outcome JAMA 1983;250;767–71.
27. Tesar G, Rosenbaum J, Pollack M, et al. Clonazepam versus alprazolam in the treatment of panic disorder: interim analysis of data from a prospective, double-blind, placebo-controlled trial. J Clin Psychiatry 1987;15:16–21.
28. Simeon JG, Ferguson HB, Knott V, et al. Clinical, cognitive, and neurophysiological effects of alprazolam in children and adolescents with overanxious and avoidant disorders. J Am Acad Child Adolesc Psychiatry 1992;31:29–33.
29. Wagner KD, Berard R, Stein MB, et al. A multicenter, randomized, double-blind, placebo-controlled trial of paroxetine in children and adolescents with social anxiety disorder. Arch Gen Psychiatry 2004;61:1153–62.
30. March JS, Entusah AR, Rynn M, et al. A randomized controlled trial of venlafaxine ER versus placebo in pediatric social anxiety disorder. Biol Psychiatry 2007;62:1149–54.
31. Beidel DC, Turner SM, Sallee FR, et al. SET-C versus fluoxetine in the treatment of childhood social phobia. J Am Acad Child Adolesc Psychiatry 2007;46:1622–32.
32. Compton SN, Grant PJ, Chrisman AK, et al. Sertraline in children and adolescents with social anxiety disorder: an open trial. J Am Acad Child Adolesc Psychiatry 2001;40:564–71.
33. Chavira DA, Stein MB. Combined psychoeducation and treatment with selective serotonin reuptake inhibitors for youth with generalized social anxiety disorder. J Child Adolesc Psychopharmacol 2002;12:47–54
34. Klein RG, Koplewicz HS, Kanner A. Imipramine treatment of children with separation anxiety disorder. J Am Acad Child Adolesc Psychiatry 1992;31:21–8.
35. Bernstein GA, Garfinkel BD, Borchardt CM. Comparative studies of pharmacotherapy for school refusal. J Am Acad Child Adolesc Psychiatry 1990;29:773–81.

36. Berney T, Kolvin I, Bhate SR, et al. School phobia: a therapeutic trail with clomipramine and short-term outcome. Br J Psychiatry 1981;138:110–8.

37. Bernstein GA, Borchardt CM, Perwien AR, et al. Imipramine plus cognitive-behavioral therapy in the treatment of school refusal. J Am Acad Child Adolesc Psychiatry 2000;39:276–83.

38. Graae F, Milner J, Rizzotto L, et al. Clonazepam in childhood anxiety disorders. J Am Acad Child Adolesc Psychiatry 1994;33:372–6.

39. Renaud J, Birmaher B, Wassick SC, et al. Use of selective serotonin reuptake inhibitors for the treatment of childhood panic disorder: a pilot study. J Child Adolesc Psychopharmacol 1999;9:73–83.

40. Fluvoxamine for the treatment of anxiety disorders in children and adolescents. N Engl J Med 2001;344:1279–85.

41. Walkup J, Labellarte M, Riddle MA, et al. Treatment of pediatric anxiety disorders: an open-label extension of the research units on pediatric psychopharmacology anxiety study. J Child Adolesc Psychopharmacol 2002;12:175–88.

42. Clark DB, Birmaher B, Axelson D, et al. Fluoxetine for the treatment of childhood anxiety disorders: open-label, long-term extension to a controlled trial. J Am Acad Child Adolesc Psychiatry 2005;44:1263–70.

43. Ginsburg GS, Kendall PC, Sakolsky D, et al. Remission after acute treatment in children and adolescents with anxiety disorders: findings from the CAMS. J Consult Clin Psychol 2011;79:806–13.

44. Geller D, Donnelly C, Lopez F, et al. Atomoxetine treatment for pediatric patients with attention-deficit/hyperactivity disorder with comorbid anxiety disorder. J Am Acad Child Adolesc Psychiatry 2007;46:1119–27.

45. Kendall PC. Treating anxiety disorders in children: results of a randomized clinical trial. J Consult Clin Psychol 1994;62:100–10.

46. Kendall PC, Flannery-Schroeder E, Panichelli-Mindel SM, et al. Therapy for youths with anxiety disorders: a second randomized clinical trial. J Consult Clin Psychol 1997;65:366–80.

47. James A, Soler A, Weatherall R. Cognitive behavioural therapy for anxiety disorders in children and adolescents. Cochrane Database Syst Rev 2005:19:CD004690.

48. Bridge JA, Iyengar S, Salary CB, et al. Clinical response and risk for reported suicidal ideation and suicide attempts in pediatric antidepressant treatment: a meta-analysis of randomized controlled trials. JAMA 2007;297:1683–96.

49. Connolly SD, Bernstein GA; Work Group on Quality Issues. Practice parameter for the assessment and treatment of children and adolescents with anxiety disorders. J Am Acad Child Adolesc Psychiatry 2007;46:267–83.

50. Strawn JR, Wehry AM, DelBello MP, et al. Establishing the neurobiologic basis of treatment for children and adolescents with generalized anxiety disorder. Depress Anxiety 2012;29:328–39.

51. McClure EB, Adler A, Monk CS, et al. fMRI predictors of treatment outcome in pediatric anxiety disorders. Psychopharmacology (Berl) 2007;191:97–105.

52. Sakolsky D, Nurmi E, Birmaher B, et al. Association of GRIK4 with treatment response in the Child/Adolescent Anxiety Multimodal Study (CAMS). Annual Meeting of the American Academy of Child and Adolescent Psychiatry (AACAP), New York, October 26–31, 2010.

53. Sakolsky D, Nurmi E, Birmaher B, et al. Academy of Child and Adolescent Psychiatry in the Child/Adolescent Anxiety Multimodal Study (CAMS). American Academy of Child and Adolescent Psychiatry (AACAP) and Canadian Academy of Child and Adolescent Psychiatry (CACAP) Joint Annual Meeting, Toronto, Canada, October 18–23, 2011.

54. Pollack MH, Jensen JE, Simon NM, et al. High-field MRS study of GABA, glutamate and glutamine in social anxiety disorder: response to treatment with levetiracetam. Progr Neuropsychopharmacol Biol Psychiatry 2008;32:739–43.
55. Yücel M, Harrison BJ, Wood SJ, et al. Functional and biochemical alterations of the medial frontal cortex in obsessive-compulsive disorder. Arch Gen Psychiatry 2007; 64:946–55.
56. Kugaya A, Sanacora G. Beyond monoamines: glutamatergic function in mood disorders. CNS Spectr 2005;10:808–19.
57. Palucha A, Pilc A. Metabotropic glutamate receptor ligands as possible anxiolytic and antidepressant drugs. Pharmacol Ther 2007;115:116–47.
58. Rynn M, Puliafico A, Heleniak C, et al. Advances in pharmacotherapy for pediatric anxiety disorders. Depress Anxiety 2011;28:76–87.
59. Sallee FR, Sethuraman G, Sine L, et al. Yohimbine challenge in children with anxiety disorders. Am J Psychiatry 2000;157:1236–42.
60. Hoehn-Saric R, Merchant AF, Keyser ML, et al. Effects of clonidine on anxiety disorders. Arch Gen Psychiatry 1981;38:1278–82.
61. Sallee FR, Richman H, Sethuraman G, et al. Clonidine challenge in childhood anxiety disorder. J Am Acad Child Adolesc Psychiatry 1998;37:655–62.

Cognitive Behavior Therapy for the Anxiety Triad

Olga Jablonka, BA[a], Alix Sarubbi, PsyD[b], Amy M. Rapp, BA[a],
Anne Marie Albano, PhD, ABPP[b,c],*

KEYWORDS

- Cognitive behavior therapy • Anxiety triad • Children and adolescent anxiety
- Separation anxiety • Generalized anxiety • Social phobia
- Treatment for pediatric anxiety

KEY POINTS

- Cognitive behavior therapy (CBT) should be strongly considered by any provider for a child or adolescent who experiences anxiety.
- The three most common anxiety disorders among youth—separation anxiety disorder (SAD), generalized anxiety disorder (GAD), and social phobia (SoP)—known as the child and adolescent anxiety triad, are frequently comorbid.
- Children with SAD primarily worry about being away from their caregiver for fear that something bad will happen to either of them.
- Children with GAD typically focus their worry on realistic concerns or self-directed worries regarding performance, perfectionism, or other unrealistic expectations.
- Children with SoP fear embarrassment or humiliation in front of others.
- CBT addresses physiologic, cognitive, and behavioral aspects of anxiety through various treatment components including psychoeducation, affective identification, somatic management, cognitive restructuring, behavioral exposure, family involvement, and relapse prevention.

INTRODUCTION

When childhood anxiety is treated through empirically supported psychosocial treatments (eg, The Coping Cat Program[1]), the likelihood of improvement is high.

Disclosures: Olga Jablonka, none; Alix Sarubbi, none; Amy Rapp, none; Anne Marie Albano, National Institute of Mental Health, Bracket Global, Oxford University Press.
[a] Children's Day Unit, Department of Child and Adolescent Psychiatry, Columbia University/New York State Psychiatric Institute, 1051 Riverside Drive, Unit 74, New York, NY 10032, USA;
[b] Columbia University Clinic for Anxiety and Related Disorders, 3 Columbus Circle, New York, NY 10019, USA; [c] Columbia University/New York State Psychiatric Institute, 1051 Riverside Drive, Unit 74, New York, NY, USA
* Corresponding author. Columbia University Clinic for Anxiety and Related Disorders, Columbia University/NYSPI, 1051 Riverside Drive, Unit 74, New York, NY 10032.
E-mail address: AlbanoA@nyspi.columbia.edu

Research has shown that approximately 60% to 70% of children over age 7 years no longer met criteria for an anxiety disorder[2–5] after receiving cognitive behavior therapy (CBT) based on the Coping Cat Program.[1] Although medication performs well in clinical trials in treating anxious youth as a monotherapy, and when combined with CBT,[4] CBT is rated as more acceptable, believable, and effective in the short- and long-term by parents.[6] CBT should be strongly considered by any provider for a child or adolescent who experiences anxiety.

The current article discusses the existing as well as the newly developed CBT methods for the three most common anxiety disorders among youth:

1. Separation anxiety disorder (SAD)
2. Generalized anxiety disorder (GAD)
3. Social phobia (SoP).

These three disorders, otherwise known as the child and adolescent anxiety triad, are frequently comorbid and have been studied together in several clinical trials examining the efficacy of CBT for anxiety.[2,5,7,8] These three anxiety disorders are hypothesized to share similar causes and have demonstrated similar response profiles to CBT and medication treatment. It is for these reasons that the current article focuses on the childhood anxiety triad.

OVERVIEW OF THE EXISTING CBT METHODS FOR THE CHILD ANXIETY TRIAD

The past two decades have witnessed a surge of clinical trials examining the efficacy of CBT for childhood anxiety disorders with good effect.[9,10] Consequently, the Coping Cat Program[1] has been deemed as "probably efficacious" in the treatment of childhood anxiety.[10,11] Of note, this designation came prior to the comparison of the Coping Cat with medication in the National Institute of Mental Health–sponsored Child/Adolescent Anxiety Multimodal Study,[5] which added strong support for a new Coping Cat classification of efficacious. CBT protocols, including the Coping Cat Program,[1] have been adapted to group formats that have also demonstrated efficacy in treating anxious youth with the triad.[12,13]

In the Coping Cat Program, anxiety is conceptualized through a tripartite model[9,14] involving physiologic, cognitive, and behavioral components. CBT addresses these three aspects of anxiety through various treatment components including psychoeducation, affective identification, somatic management, cognitive restructuring, behavioral exposure, family involvement, and relapse prevention.[15] Psychoeducation helps the child and family understand the nature of anxiety and how CBT specifically works in reducing anxiety, whereas affective identification and somatic management skills training address the physiologic and emotional aspects of anxiety. Cognitive restructuring targets the cognitive component of anxiety by assisting the child in recognizing anxious thoughts and then teaching age-appropriate ways for the child to engage in more rational, balanced, and coping-focused thinking. Behavioral exposure, long understood as the cornerstone of CBT treatments for anxiety, enables the child to make small steps toward approaching feared situations. The goal of exposure is to provide a personally salient experience in coping as the child learns that feared ideas about a situation were either untrue or, if a negative experience, something they can cope with and handle. Exposure directly reverses the avoidance behavior that accompanies and maintains anxiety. The use of family involvement is essential, because parents can provide valuable information regarding their child's specific fears. Parents also learn how to effectively manage their child's anxiety and how to coach him or her through behavioral exposures. Relapse prevention strategies then help the child maximize treatment gains through the design of coping plans for future obstacles.

The Coping Cat Program[1] has strongly influenced CBT programs in treating childhood anxiety. The remainder of this review discusses the clinical presentations of the anxiety triad as well as the recent innovations in CBT for each disorder.

SEPARATION ANXIETY DISORDER
Definition and Diagnostics

As defined in the current edition of the *Diagnostic and Statistical Manual of Mental Disorders, Fourth Edition, Text Revision* (DSM-IV-TR),[16] SAD is excessive anxiety regarding separation from home or from major attachment figures. In young children, some level of separation anxiety is developmentally appropriate.[17] In order to meet diagnostic criteria for SAD, the separation anxiety must lead to significant interference in social and academic functioning and must have occurred continuously for at least 1 month. Clinical features of SAD include repeated and excessive distress when separation from home or from attachment figures occurs, worry about harm befalling major attachment figures, worry that an untoward event will happen to oneself or attachment figures when separation occurs, extreme reluctance to leave attachment figures to attend school or social events, a fear of being alone, a refusal to go to sleep without being close to attachment figures, nightmares including a separation theme, and physical symptoms. It is important to note that SAD is the only anxiety disorder based on specific child criteria as well as the only anxiety disorder to specifically have a childhood onset.[18] Adults can be diagnosed with SAD as long as the disorder onset is before the age of 18. Indeed, SAD is the most common childhood anxiety disorder and the age of onset is typically 7 to 12 years of age.[19,20]

Clinical Presentations

Children who present for treatment for SAD specifically report fears of being alone, being abandoned, getting kidnapped, becoming ill, or some other harmful, catastrophic event occurring when separation occurs.[18]

Children with SAD engage in extreme avoidance behaviors, such as refusing to attend school, sleep alone at night, or go to a friend's house/birthday party because of their fear of separation. Often, even when at home with the attachment figure, children with SAD require that the person remain in sight (eg, in the same room as the child) and will become distressed if they cannot physically see their attachment figure.

Through a process of negative reinforcement, parents of separation-anxious children inadvertently reinforce the child's anxiety by giving in and allowing the child access to their presence. For example, when a separation situation is approaching, such as the child needing to leave for school, the child may increase yelling, screaming, or crying and other expressions of extreme distress. Parents are often upset by this expression, and some believe that this distress "damages" their child. Hence, a parent may then give in and allow the child to remain at home (eg, "You can take a break today, but you must go tomorrow"). The child feels an immediate sense of relief from anxiety (negative reinforcement), and this approach deprives the child of calming one's self, coping with the separation, and gaining positive reinforcement for engaging in the school day (through the attention of peers and teachers, and praise for coping/attending from the parents).

Recently, Eisen and colleagues[21–24] proposed a schematic of four SAD subtypes to facilitate individualized case conceptualization and prescriptive treatment:

FOLLOWER

Eisen and colleagues[18] identify that among the subtypes, children may fall under the "follower" subtype, in which the child's primary fear is of being alone.

Children within this subtype may also worry that if alone, they will develop a medical illness.

VISITOR

Another subtype includes fear of a "visitor," in which children worry that when alone, someone will break into the child's house.

MISFORTUNE TELLER

A third subtype, named by Eisen and colleagues as the "misfortune teller," suggests that some children are worried that when separation occurs they will be abandoned, and that personal harm/illness will occur to the child if abandoned.

TIME KEEPER

In the "time keeper" subtype, the child's fear of abandonment emerges as a result of worry about parental safety/harm befalling the parent.

These subtypes, if explored more vigorously in research, may hold important implications for applying specific types of cognitive restructuring and behavioral exposure exercises within CBT procedures in treating SAD.

CBT for Separation Anxiety Disorder in Youth

The focus of treatment with CBT for children suffering from SAD typically is on teaching children fundamental skills in recognizing their anxious feelings and thoughts in regard to separation, identifying their physical responses to anxiety, and developing appropriate coping strategies, such as engaging in balanced, rational thinking about separation or using relaxation strategies to better manage anxious, physiologic responses to separation. This approach has shown efficacy in individualized treatment,[2] as well as in CBT treatments targeting family involvement.[25,26] A group treatment approach for anxious youth has been found to be efficacious in treating childhood anxiety disorders, including SAD.[13]

Researchers have recently examined the modification of parent-child interaction therapy (PCIT) in the treatment of separation anxiety in young children.[27] In essence, PCIT focuses on reshaping the development of problematic behavior by modifying interactions between the parent and child. Treatment sessions, which combine elements of play therapy and behavioral training and feature real-time, in-session training for parents, emphasize the important of positive attention, problem-solving, and effective communication between the parent and child. This method has been proved to be effective in many studies examining the treatment of disruptive behavior disorders.[28–30] Choate and colleagues[31] and Pincus and colleagues[27] first speculated that there may be clinical utility in modifying PCIT in the treatment of childhood anxiety disorders, by targeting the overinvolved, intrusive, and controlling parenting that is often associated with anxiety disorders.[32–37] Please see the article by Puliafico and colleagues elsewhere in this issue on adapting parent-child interaction therapy to treat anxiety disorders in young children to learn more about the fundamental principles underlying PCIT and the rationale for adapting this treatment to target anxiety symptoms in young children.

Implications for Research

Further research may allow clinicians to pinpoint the "central active ingredients"[2] that are effective in targeting SAD symptoms. Identifying such aspects (eg, child engagement through treatment materials, therapist-child relationship, parental factors) would serve to elucidate the active elements of effective treatment. Parental involvement, specifically, is a promising area of further examination and treatment development.

GENERALIZED ANXIETY DISORDER
Definition and Diagnostics

As defined in the current edition of the DSM-IV-TR,[16] GAD is excessive and uncontrollable anxiety and worry about a number of topics for more days than not for at least 6 months, where the worry is accompanied by at least one physiologic symptom, such as stomachaches, headaches, muscle tension, sleep disturbance, or restlessness, and the anxiety results in impairment in functioning. The one-physiologic-symptom criterion for children is in contrast to adults, who need three or more physiologic symptoms to meet diagnostic criteria. Although many children worry about school, their friends, and their classmates,[38] children or adolescents who meet criteria for GAD typically perceive their worry as more intense compared with nonanxious children.[38–41] In clinical populations, children typically report worry in various areas, but they also report an inability or difficulty controlling their worry.[14] In other words, even with reassurance or when attempting to distract themselves from their worry, children who meet diagnostic criteria for GAD have difficulty refraining from engaging in their worry, thus leading to greater experience of anxiety, physiologic distress, and impairment in functioning.

Clinical Presentations

Children and adolescents with GAD report worrying about various issues. Weems and colleagues[41] found that their clinic-referred population of youth who met criteria for GAD reported worries predominantly in areas of health, school, disasters, and personal harm. Wagner[42] found that youth with GAD worried most about school performance, natural phenomena, social situations, and punctuality. Children with GAD may also worry about events that have a low probability of occurring but may overestimate (without recognizing that they are doing so) the likelihood that a problematic situation may occur.[38] They engage in future-oriented worry, asking themselves and others "what if" questions, such as, "What if I fail my test," "What if you get sick," "What if the car crashes."[14]

In addition to worry, youth with GAD typically present with frequent need for reassurance, experience tension in their bodies, have a negative self-image, and report physical complaints.[43–45] Children and adolescents with GAD may also struggle with striving for perfectionism, experience frequent self-doubt, and have a fear of failure.[14]

CBT for Generalized Anxiety Disorder in Youth
Imaginal exposures

The CBT program most frequently used when treating childhood GAD is Kendall's Coping Cat program, which Kendall developed for youth ages 8 to 13.[46] One aspect of conducting the Coping Cat program that is particularly helpful in treating GAD is the use of imaginal exposures. For instance, several children with GAD worry about their parents becoming ill, or about death and dying. In these situations it is helpful to conduct role-plays or imaginal exposures with the child about what would happen if their parents died or became ill.[47] Having the child role-play this scenario with the therapist, or imagining it, helps the child confront irrational fears around the experience. However, it is cautioned that experienced CBT therapists conduct exposures to upsetting ideas such as death and dying with children, within the context of a solid therapeutic relationship and overall treatment plan. Other exposures that are helpful for children with GAD are having them make mistakes on purpose, such as writing something out with spelling or grammatical errors and then showing it to the therapist, a friend, or parent, because many children with GAD worry about perfectionism and have a fear of making mistakes.

Emotion regulation

In addition to the Coping Cat Program, innovative areas of CBT that have recently been researched to target GAD include emotion regulation and mindfulness techniques. In terms of emotion regulation, recent research on anxiety in youth suggests that children who meet criteria for an anxiety disorder have difficulty regulating their emotional experiences.[48,49] Additionally, whereas CBT targets worry and anxiety, it may not adequately target a child's overall ability to regulate other emotional experiences, such as sadness and anger.[50]

Based on emotion regulation theory, Suveg and colleagues[51] developed emotion-focused cognitive behavior therapy (ECBT) for youth with anxiety disorders. They posited that adding an emotion regulation component to standard CBT for childhood anxiety may be associated with improved treatment outcomes, given that research has demonstrated that anxious children self-reported higher levels of emotion and decreased ability to regulate their emotions compared with their nonanxious counterparts.[49,51] Although CBT has proved itself as effective in treating childhood anxiety, Suveg and colleagues[51] highlighted that over one-third of children who receive CBT do not respond to treatment; therefore, improvements in CBT for childhood anxiety may be beneficial for treatment nonresponders.

Suveg and colleagues'[51] ECBT program consists of standard CBT procedures consistent with the Coping Cat Program,[1] however it adds emotion-focused content to several treatment sessions. In ECBT, not only are anxiety and worry targeted, but children are also taught how to identify and describe situations, emotions, and cognitive content related to several different emotional experiences, such as sadness and anger. Exposures consist of anxiety-provoking situations but also anger-provoking situations, or exposure to any emotionally salient trigger for the child. Results of this new program are promising[50,51] in that children report decreases in anxiety and improvement in emotion regulation skills.

Mindfulness

Mindfulness has been described as being nonjudgmentally aware of the present moment, on purpose, with a specific quality of attention.[52] Mindfulness-based strategies, although researched and implemented mostly with adult populations dealing with anxiety,[53,54] depression,[55] difficulties with emotion regulation,[56] and chronic pain[57] are currently being investigated with youth as well.[58,59] Mechanisms of mindfulness that may garner positive changes have been hypothesized to be improving attentional control.[59] These improvements may be particularly helpful for anxious youth, who frequently allow their worries to become excessive or repetitive. Initial studies examining mindfulness-based programs in schools have found that in nonclinically referred children, mindfulness programs have improved children's selective attention, reduced test anxiety, increased their ability to pay attention, and improved their social skills.[60] These initial data, combined with the success of implementing mindfulness strategies in clinically referred adult populations, warrant further investigation of mindfulness-based programs for anxious youth.

Studies examining mindfulness in youth are few,[58,59,61] however research is promising in that (a) youth seem capable of learning and understanding mindfulness techniques, and (b) they seem to benefit from mindfulness training in areas such as executive functioning,[58] stress reduction,[61] and anxiety management.[59] Specific to anxiety, in Semple and colleagues'[59] pilot study, they examined five children (ages 7 to 8) who were identified by teachers and a school psychologist in an inner-city school as being anxious. The purpose of the study was to examine the feasibility and acceptability of conducting mindfulness-based interventions with young children. Study participants were taught various mindfulness techniques for a 6-week treatment program. During the program, children were taught how to observe and describe their experiences without judgment, as well as focus their attention on one object, such as the breath or other sensory experiences. Children were also taught how to identify their worries and distance themselves from their worries by writing their worries down and then placing them in a "worry wastebasket." Results from this pilot study suggested that children improved in managing their anxiety, because teachers rated a decrease in participant anxiety posttreatment via the Achenbach Children Behavior Check List, Teacher Report Form.[62] However, results should be interpreted with caution, because the study included a small sample size and was exploratory in nature.

Implications for Research

Taken together, key techniques in treating GAD in youth seem to be using standard CBT procedures, such as behavioral exposures, whereas more innovative methods include incorporating emotion-regulation procedures with CBT, as Suveg and colleagues[50,51] have demonstrated through their ECBT program. Although Suveg and colleagues'[51] work demonstrates promising initial results, more research is necessary to confirm the additive benefit of including emotion regulation procedures in CBT for childhood anxiety. Mindfulness-based methods may be beneficial when working with children with GAD as well, because these methods may teach children to notice their worries without judgment and how to distance themselves from their worry. However, randomized controlled trials examining the effectiveness of implementing mindfulness-based methods with children in clinically referred samples are warranted to confirm that mindfulness is effective when working with anxious youth.

SOCIAL PHOBIA
Definition and Diagnostics

Per the DSM-IV-TR,[16] SoP is defined as a chronic fear of social or performance situations, in which the individual worries about embarrassing himself or herself, or about being judged by others. When faced with such anxiety-producing situations, the person almost invariably feels an immediate increase in anxiety symptoms, which are often coupled with physical symptoms such as palpitations, sweating, or nausea, and may even experience a panic attack. This extreme fear often leads to avoidance behaviors, which may cause significant declines in the individual's academic, social, and occupational functioning, and negatively impact the person's quality of life.

As commonly seen in other pediatric anxiety disorders, children, as compared with adolescents and adults, may not recognize their fear and avoidance of social situations as irrational or excessive. Younger children in particular may exhibit disproportionate crying or tantrums, or shying away from social situations with people they do not know well. DSM-IV-TR criteria also require that children have the capacity for age-appropriate social relationships with familiar people and that the anxiety must occur in peer settings, not just in interactions with adults. Last, children and adolescents must experience impairment for at least 6 months to meet diagnostic criteria.

Clinical Presentations

Children and adolescents with SoP are typically described as "shy" or "loners."[63] Although they would like to develop friendships, many have poor social skills and lack confidence. In addition, ordinary situations, such as speaking to a store clerk or participating in a sports or dance team, can cause significant distress for these children, creating further isolation and feelings of loneliness.[64] Furthermore, Beidel and colleagues[63] found that children with SoP have a higher level of general emotional overresponsiveness and general fearfulness than children without SoP.

CBT for SoP in Youth

Psychosocial treatments for SoP are limited, but overall studies maintain the efficacy of CBT treatment.[65,66] Studies have shown treatment gains from both individual and group approaches,[67,68] which, similar to the treatment approach for SAD and GAD, target irrational thoughts related to social settings and emphasize exposures that challenge the child to approach social situations that they would typically avoid. Tracey and colleagues[69] conducted a randomized, controlled trial for group CBT treatment for adolescents with or without family involvement and found both treatment conditions to be superior to waitlist, with 70% of the sample no longer meeting criteria at posttreatment. This protocol was adapted by Albano and colleagues and based on Heimberg's empirically supported adult Cognitive Behavioral Group Treatment program. Similar results were duplicated in research findings by Spence and colleagues,[65] who examined a comprehensive CBT program that included social skills training, relaxation, social problem-solving, and cognitive interventions and exposures, as well as in a study by Gallagher and colleagues,[68] which focused on education, identification and replacement of negative self-talk, and exposure in group CBT.

Behavioral therapy has also received a great deal of support in the treatment of SoP in children and adolescents. Beidel and colleagues[70] examined a behavioral approach called social effectiveness therapy for children (SET-C), which incorporates social skills training, peer generalization sessions, and personalized in-vivo exposures, in a randomized trial of 67 children and found promising results. Please refer to the article on SoP and selective mutism by Keeton and Budinger elsewhere in this issue for further information about SET-C.

Implications for Research

Future research may examine gains over time for both SET-C and fluoxetine, in addition to combination therapy. Furthermore, as noted in the article by Keeton and Budinger on SoP and selective mutism, existing interventions should be examined, particularly to develop options for treatment-resistant conditions.

ATTENTIONAL RETRAINING FOR ANXIETY TREATMENT

Despite the established efficacy of CBT, there are children and adolescents who do not respond to this treatment. Thus, novel interventions are necessary for treatment-resistant conditions. One such intervention is attention bias modification treatment (ABMT). The basic tenet of ABMT is one shared with models of CBT—that cognitive biases cause clinically significant anxiety.[71] MacLeod[72] was first to suggest the utility of ABMT as an augment to currently available treatments for anxious populations. The rationale for this assumption came from a study that used a modified dot-probe to produce attentional bias in healthy adults.[73] Participants were trained to focus on either negative or neutral stimuli. Those participants who were trained to focus on threat cues reported increases in negative mood and anxiety after completing an experimental stressor. Results suggest that emotional vulnerability may be mediated by attentional bias.[73] Several pediatric studies using a modified dot-probe task have shown that anxious children demonstrate attentional bias toward emotional stimuli.[74-76] ABMT strives to reduce cognitive bias toward threat thought to cause and perpetuate patterns of elevated anxiety reactions to the environment, thus normalizing how emotional information is processed and reducing vulnerability to anxiety.

Given the small body of work investigating attentional bias toward threat cues in the pediatric GAD population, and the inconsistencies within these studies, more research needs to be conducted to test for validity and reliability. For example, functional magnetic resonance imaging studies using visual probes in pediatric populations demonstrated attentional avoidance of threat,[77] whereas other studies using word probes demonstrated attention toward threat.[75] This disparity, among others, suggests the necessity of exploring various methods of ABMT before it can be established as an effective intervention for CBT nonresponders. Furthermore, these treatments are designed to be brief, which may not be beneficial for patients with severe anxiety who need longer and more frequent interventions. Last, ABMT lacks the involvement of a professional, who plays a critical role in anxiety treatment. Future research should examine the use of ABMT as an adjunctive treatment, perhaps as homework or extra practice, in the context of CBT treatment.

Implications for Assessment in Clinical Practice

There may be some difficulty in assessing and differentiating these three anxiety disorders from each other, because many symptoms may overlap. It is important to remember that children with SAD primarily worry about being away from their caregiver, for fear that something bad will happen to either of them; in children with GAD, the worry is typically focused on realistic concerns or self-directed worries regarding performance, perfectionism, or other unrealistic expectations; and children with SoP fear embarrassment or humiliation in front of others. Clinicians should also remember that comorbidity is high among anxiety disorders, with most children meeting criteria for more than one of these anxiety disorders.

Another assessment issue in diagnosing the anxiety triad is that some children and adolescents struggle to report their cognitive experience. Although youth are generally able to report physiologic symptoms as well as irritability, sleep disturbance, or difficulty concentrating, it seems more difficult for them to be aware of their thought processes. It is important to extensively interview both child and parent for this reason, because the parent may have more insight into the child's worries or cognitions. To this end, teacher and guidance counselor data may be helpful as well.

SUMMARY

It is clear that CBT has been validated as the gold standard treatment for the anxiety triad. The fundamental principles of CBT have established the foundation on which newer models of therapy can be created. This article did a preliminary review and identified a few innovative strategies for modifying components of CBT in the treatment of SAD, GAD, and SoP. Additional research will be needed in discerning the value and efficacy of these novel treatment modalities.

REFERENCES

1. Kendall PC, Hedtke KA. Cognitive-behavioral therapy for anxious children: therapist manual. 3rd edition. Ardmore (PA): Workbook Publishing; 2006.
2. Kendall PC, Flannery-Schroeder E, Panichelli-Mindel SM, et al. Therapy for youths with anxiety disorders: a second randomized clinical trial. J Consult Clin Psychol 1997;65(3):366–80.
3. Kendall PC, Hudson JL, Gosch E, et al. Cognitive-behavioral therapy for anxiety disordered youth: a randomized clinical trial evaluating child and family modalities. J Consult Clin Psychol 2008;76(2):282–97.
4. Silverman WK, Kurtines WM, Ginsburg GS, et al. Treating anxiety disorders in children with group cognitive-behavioral therapy: a randomized clinical trial. J Consult Clin Psychol 1999;67(6):995–1003.
5. Walkup JT, Albano AM, Piacentini J, et al. Cognitive behavioral therapy, sertraline, or a combination in childhood anxiety. N Engl J Med 2008;359(26):2753–66.
6. Brown AM, Deacon BJ, Abramowitz JS, et al. Parents' perceptions of pharmacological and cognitive-behavioral treatments for childhood anxiety disorders. Behav Res Ther 2007;45(4):819–28.
7. Kendall PC. Treating anxiety disorders in children: results of a randomized clinical trial. J Consult Clin Psychol 1994;62(1):100–10.
8. Kendall PC, Southam-Gerow MA. Long-term follow-up of a cognitive–behavioral therapy for anxiety-disordered youth. J Consult Clin Psychol 1996;64(4):724–30.
9. Kendall PC, Furr JM, Podell JL. Child-focused treatment of anxiety. In: Kazdin AE, Weisz JK, editors. Evidence-based psychotherapies for children and adolescents. 2nd edition. New York: Guilford Press; 2010. p. 243–94. Chapter 4.
10. Silverman WK, Pina AA, Viswesvaran C. Evidence-based psychosocial treatments for phobic and anxiety disorders in children and adolescents. J Clin Child Adolesc Psychol 2008;37(1):105–30.
11. Ollendick TH, King NJ, Chorpita BF. Empirically supported treatments for children and adolescents. Child and adolescent therapy: cognitive-behavioral procedures. 3rd edition. New York: Guilford Press; 2006:492–520.
12. Barrett PM. Evaluation of cognitive-behavioral group treatments for childhood anxiety disorders. J Clin Child Psychol 1998;27(4):459–68.
13. Flannery-Schroeder EC, Kendall PC. Group and individual cognitive-behavioral treatments for youth with anxiety disorders: A randomized clinical trial. Cognit Ther Res 2000;24(3):251–78.
14. Albano AM, Hack S. Children and adolescents. New York: The Guilford Press; 2004.
15. Albano AM, Kendall PC. Cognitive behavioural therapy for children and adolescents with anxiety disorders: clinical research advances. Int Rev Psychiatry 2002;14(2):128–33.
16. American Psychiatric Association. Diagnostic and statistical manual of mental disorders. 4th edition, text revision. Washington (DC): American Psychiatric Association; 2000.
17. Hanna GL, Fischer DJ, Fluent TE. Separation anxiety disorder and school refusal in children and adolescents. Pediatr Rev 2006;27(2):56–63.
18. Eisen AR, Sussman JM, Schmidt T, et al. Separation anxiety disorder. In: McKay D, Storch EA, editors. Handbook of child and adolescent anxiety disorders. New York: Springer; 2011. p. 245–59.
19. Allen J, Rapee R, Sandberg S. Severe life events and chronic adversities as antecedents to anxiety in children: a matched control study. J Abnorm Child Psychol 2008;36(7):1047–56.

20. Compton SN, Nelson AH, March JS. Social phobia and separation anxiety symptoms in community and clinical samples of children and adolescents. J Am Acad Child Adolesc Psychiatry 2000;39(8):1040–6.
21. Eisen AR, Engler LB. Helping your child overcome separation anxiety or school refusal: a step-by-step guide for parents. Oakland (CA): New Harbinger Publications; 2006.
22. Eisen AR, Pincus DB, Hashim R, et al. Seeking safety. In: Eisen AR, editor. Treating childhood behavioral and emotional problems: a step-by-step evidence-based approach. New York: Guilford; 2008. Chapter 1.
23. Eisen AR, Raleigh H, Neuhoff CC. The unique impact of parent training for separation anxiety disorder in children. Behav Ther 2008;39(2):195–206.
24. Eisen AR, Schaefer CE. Separation anxiety in children and adolescents: an individualized approach to assessment and treatment. New York: Guilford Press; 2005.
25. Barrett PM, Dadds MR, Rapee RM. Family treatment of childhood anxiety: a controlled trial. J Consult Clin Psychol 1996;64(2):333–42.
26. Mendlowitz SL, Manassis K, Bradley S, et al. Cognitive-behavioral group treatments in childhood anxiety disorders: the role of parental involvement. J Am Acad Child Adolesc Psychiatry 1999;38(10):1223–9.
27. Pincus DB, Eyberg SM, Choate ML. Adapting parent-child interaction therapy for young children with separation anxiety disorder. Educ Treat Children 2005;28(2): 163–81.
28. Eyberg SM, Funderburk BW, Hembree-Kigin TL, et al. Parent-child interaction therapy with behavior problem children: one and two year maintenance of treatment effects in the family. Child Fam Behav Ther 2001;23(4):1–20.
29. Hood KK, Eyberg SM. Outcomes of parent-child interaction therapy: mothers' reports of maintenance three to six years after treatment. J Clin Child Adolesc Psychol 2003;32(3):419–29.
30. Nixon RD, Sweeney L, Erickson DB, et al. Parent-child interaction therapy: a comparison of standard and abbreviated treatments for oppositional defiant preschoolers. J Consult Clin Psychol 2003;71(2):251–60.
31. Choate ML, Pincus DB, Eyberg SM. Parent-child interaction therapy for treatment of separation anxiety disorder in young children: a pilot study. Cognitive Behavioral Therapy 2005(12):136–45.
32. Hudson JL, Comer JS, Kendall PC. Parental responses to positive and negative emotions in anxious and nonanxious children. J Clin Child Adolesc Psychol 2008; 37(2):303–13.
33. McLeod BD, Wood JJ, Weisz JR. Examining the association between parenting and childhood anxiety: a meta-analysis. Clin Psychol Rev 2007;27(2):155–72.
34. Moore PS, Whaley SE, Sigman M. Interactions between mothers and children: impacts of maternal and child anxiety. J Abnorm Psychol 2004;113(3):471–6.
35. Siqueland L, Kendall PC, Steinberg L. Anxiety in children: perceived family environments and observed family interaction. J Clin Child Psychol 1996;25(2):225–37.
36. Wood JJ, McLeod BD, Sigman M, et al. Parenting and childhood anxiety: theory, empirical findings, and future directions. J Child Psychol Psychiatry 2003;44(1): 134–51.
37. Rapee RM. Potential role of childrearing practices in the development of anxiety and depression. Clin Psychol Rev 1997;17(1):47–67.
38. Silverman WK, La Greca AM, Wasserstein S. What do children worry about? Worries and their relation to anxiety. Child Dev 1995;66(3):671–86.
39. Muris P, Meesters CO, Merckelbach H, et al. Worry in normal children. J Am Acad Child Adolesc Psychiatry 1998;37(7):703–10.

40. Perrin S, Last CG. Worrisome thoughts in children clinically referred for anxiety disorder. J Clin Child Psychol 1997;26(2):181–9.
41. Weems CF, Silverman WK, La Greca AM. What do youth referred for anxiety problems worry about? Worry and its relation to anxiety and anxiety disorders in children and adolescents. J Abnorm Child Psychol 2000;28(1):63–72.
42. Wagner KD. Generalized anxiety disorder in children and adolescents. Psychiatr Clin North Am 2001;24(1):139–53.
43. Masi G, Mucci M, Favilla L, et al. Symptomatology and comorbidity of generalized anxiety disorder in children and adolescents. Compr Psychiatry 1999;40(3):210–5.
44. Masi G, Favilla L, Millepiedi S, et al. Somatic symptoms in children and adolescents referred for emotional and behavioral disorders. Psychiatry 2000;63(2):140–9.
45. Masi G, Millepiedi S, Mucci M, et al. Generalized anxiety disorder in referred children and adolescents. J Am Acad Child Adolesc Psychiatry 2004;43(6):752–60.
46. Kendall PC, Kane M, Howard B, et al. Cognitive-behavioral therapy for anxious children: treatment manual. [Available from: Philip C. Kendall, Department of Psychology, Temple University, Philadelphia] 1990.
47. Kendall PC, Robin JA, Hedtke KA, et al. Considering CBT with anxious youth? Think exposures. Cogn Behav Pract 2005;12(1):136–48.
48. Carthy T, Horesh N, Apter A, et al. Patterns of emotional reactivity and regulation in children with anxiety disorders. J Psychopathol Behav Assess 2010;32(1):23–36.
49. Suveg C, Zeman J. Emotion regulation in children with anxiety disorders. J Clin Child Adolesc Psychol 2004;33(4):750–9.
50. Suveg C, Sood E, Comer JS, et al. Changes in emotion regulation following cognitive-behavioral therapy for anxious youth. J Clin Child Adolesc Psychol 2009;38(3):390–401.
51. Suveg C, Kendall P, Comer J, et al. Emotion-focused cognitive-behavioral therapy for anxious youth: a multiple-baseline evaluation. J Contemp Psychother 2006;36(2):77–85.
52. Kabat-Zinn J. Wherever you go, there you are: mindfulness meditation in everyday life. New York: Hyperion; 1994.
53. Kabat-Zinn J, Massion AO, Kristeller J, et al. Effectiveness of a meditation-based stress reduction program in the treatment of anxiety disorders. Am J Psychiatry 1992;149(7):936–43.
54. Roemer L, Orsillo SM. Expanding our conceptualization of and treatment for generalized anxiety disorder: integrating mindfulness/acceptance-based approaches with existing cognitive-behavioral models. Clin Psychol (New York) 2002;9(1):54–68.
55. Segal ZV, Williams JM, Teasdale JD. Mindfulness-based cognitive therapy for depression: a new approach to preventing relapse. New York: Guilford Press; 2002.
56. Linehan MM. Cognitive behavioral treatment of borderline personality disorder. New York: Guilford Press; 1993.
57. Kabat-Zinn J, Lipworth L, Burncy R, et al. Four-year follow-up of a meditation-based program for the self-regulation of chronic pain: treatment outcomes and compliance. Clin J Pain 1986;2(3):159–774.
58. Flook L, Smalley SL, Kitil MJ, et al. Effects of mindful awareness practices on executive functions in elementary school children. Journal of Applied School Psychology 2010;26(1):70–95.
59. Semple RJ, Reid EF, Miller L. Treating anxiety with mindfulness: an open trial of mindfulness training for anxious children. J Cogn Psychother 2005;19(4):379–92.
60. Napoli M, Krech PR, Holley LC. Mindfulness training for elementary school students. Journal of Applied School Psychology 2005;21(1):99–125.
61. Biegel GM, Brown KW, Shapiro SL, et al. Mindfulness-based stress reduction for the treatment of adolescent psychiatric outpatients: a randomized clinical trial. J Consult Clin Psychol 2009;77(5):855–66.

62. Achenbach TM. Child behavior checklist; youth self-report; teacher's report form. Burlington (VT): Dept. of Psychiatry, University of Vermont; 1991.

63. Beidel DC, Turner SM, Morris TL. Psychopathology of childhood social phobia. J Am Acad Child Adolesc Psychiatry 1999;38(6):643–50.

64. Spence SH, Donovan C, Brechman-Toussaint M. Social skills, social outcomes, and cognitive features of childhood social phobia. J Abnorm Psychol 1999;108(2):211–21.

65. Spence SH, Donovan C, Brechman-Toussaint M. The treatment of childhood social phobia: the effectiveness of a social skills training-based, cognitive-behavioral intervention, with and without parental involvement. J Child Psychol Psychiatry 2000; 41(6):713–26.

66. Tracey SA, Chorpita BF, Albano AM, et al. Cognitive-behavioral group treatment of social phobia in adolescents: preliminary examination of parental involvement. Presented at the Annual Meeting of the Association for Advancement of Behavior Therapy. Washington (DC), November 1998.

67. Albano AM, Marten PA, Holt CS, et al. Cognitive-behavioral group treatment for social phobia in adolescents. A preliminary study. J Nerv Ment Dis 1995;183(10):649–56.

68. Gallagher HM, Rabian BA, McCloskey MS. A brief group cognitive-behavioral intervention for social phobia in childhood. J Anxiety Disord 2004;18(4):459–79.

69. Tracey SA, Mattis SG, Chorpita BF, et al. Cognitive-behavioral group treatment of social phobia in adolescents: preliminary examination of the contribution of parental involvement. Presented at the Association for Advancement of Behavior Therapy Annual Convention. Washington, DC, 1998.

70. Beidel DC, Turner SM, Sallee FR, et al. SET-C versus fluoxetine in the treatment of childhood social phobia. J Am Acad Child Adolesc Psychiatry 2007;46(12):1622–32.

71. Hakamata Y, Lissek S, Bar-Haim Y, et al. Attention bias modification treatment: a meta-analysis toward the establishment of novel treatment for anxiety. Biol Psychiatry 2010;68(11):982–90.

72. MacLeod C. Training selective attention: a cognitive-experimental technique for reducing anxiety vulnerability? World Congress of Behavioral and Cognitive Therapies Abstracts 1995;118.

73. MacLeod CR, Campbell L, Ebsworthy G, et al. Selective attention and emotional vulnerability: assessing the causal basis of their association through the experimental manipulation of attentional bias. J Abnorm Psychol 2002;111:107–23.

74. Vasey MW, Daleiden EL, Williams LL, et al. Biased attention in childhood anxiety disorders: a preliminary study. J Abnorm Child Psychol 1995;23(2):267–79.

75. Taghavi MR, Neshat-Doost HT, Moradi AR, et al. Biases in visual attention in children and adolescents with clinical anxiety and mixed anxiety-depression. J Abnorm Child Psychol 1999;27:215–23.

76. Waters AM, Mogg K, Bradley BP, et al. Attentional bias for emotional faces in children with generalized anxiety disorder. J Am Acad Child Adolesc Psychiatry 2008;47(4): 435–42.

77. Monk CS, Nelson EE, McClure EB, et al. Ventrolateral prefrontal cortex activation and attentional bias in response to angry faces in adolescents with generalized anxiety disorder. Am J Psychiatry 2006;163(6):1091–7.

Obsessive-Compulsive and Tic-Related Disorders

Martin E. Franklin, PhD*, Julie P. Harrison, BA, Kristin L. Benavides, BA

KEYWORDS

- Obsessive-compulsive disorder • Tic disorders • Tourette syndrome
- Exposure response prevention • Cognitive behavior therapy
- Habit reversal training

KEY POINTS

- Significant distress, functional impairment, and psychiatric comorbidity, collectively, compromise quality of life and achievement of developmental milestones for youth affected by obsessive compulsive disorder (OCD) and chronic tic disorders.
- The *Diagnostic and Statistical Manual of Mental Disorders, Fourth Edition, Text Revision*, characterizes OCD as the presence of recurrent obsessions and/or compulsions that interfere substantially with daily functioning.
- A diagnosis of a tic disorder is given only when either a motor or a vocal tic is present; when both motor and vocal tics are present, the diagnosis of Tourette syndrome is assigned.
- A version of cognitive behavior therapy, known as exposure plus response prevention, is considered as a first line intervention for OCD, either alone or in combination with pharmacotherapy.
- Habit reversal training has been shown to be a promising treatment option for adults and youth with tic disorders, including Tourette syndrome.

INTRODUCTION

Obsessive-compulsive disorder (OCD) and tic disorders (TDs) affect many children and adolescents worldwide and are associated with substantial functional impairment in afflicted youth. Fortunately, in the last decade both conditions have been the focus of clinical research that has clarified key phenomenologic issues and provided empirical support for treatments including disorder-specific cognitive-behavioral interventions (eg, Refs[1–6]). The co-occurrence of these disorders, which seems to be common, poses a particular challenge to clinicians with respect to making treatment recommendations to families and to implementing the chosen interventions.

Department of Psychiatry, University of Pennsylvania School of Medicine, 3535 Market Street, 6th Floor, Philadelphia, PA 19104, USA
* Corresponding author.
E-mail address: marty@upenn.edu

Child Adolesc Psychiatric Clin N Am 21 (2012) 555–571
http://dx.doi.org/10.1016/j.chc.2012.05.008
1056-4993/12/$ – see front matter Published by Elsevier Inc.

childpsych.theclinics.com

This review provides information regarding the psychopathology of each of these conditions separately and when comorbid, as well as an outline of the empirically grounded and clinically informed approach to treatment of OCD and TDs. Moderator analyses of treatment response in the Pediatric OCD Treatment Study (POTS) I[7] indicated that secondary, comorbid tic symptoms predicted poorer response to pharmacotherapy alone but not to cognitive behavior therapy (CBT) alone or to combined treatment in a trial in which OCD was classified as the primary disorder.[8] However, the mediating variable that produced this result has yet to be fully uncovered. As yet, the converse (moderator analyses of the effect of OCD on treatment response in primary TDs) has not been explored in the context of a randomized treatment trial, and thus clinicians need to exercise their empirically informed judgment when considering treatment of primary TD when OCD is also present.

First the authors provide a focused review of psychopathology for each of these conditions, describe the core CBT protocols for treating each condition separately, and then take into consideration what is known about psychopathology and treatment when they are both present (see **Table 1** for a comparison of OCD, tics, and OCD with comorbid tics). The authors' view is that there is much reason for optimism that children who have comorbid OCD and TDs can be successfully treated, but that treating clinicians have several factors to keep in mind as they attempt to do so. Reduction of core symptoms in both OCD and TDs is important in improving the quality of life for affected youth and their families, but the judgment of which of the two conditions is driving current functional impairment and which disorder influences the symptoms of the other one directly must guide the initial treatment plan.

OBSESSIVE-COMPULSIVE DISORDER
Prevalence

OCD's prevalence rate in youth has been estimated at 1% to 3% (eg, Refs[9,10]) with variability occurring perhaps as a result of research method variance.[11] OCD is evident across development[12] and is associated with substantial dysfunction and psychiatric comorbidity.[13,14] The National Comorbidity Survey Replication Study involving over 9000 adult participants in the United States estimated that the 12-month prevalence rate of OCD was 1.0%[15]; epidemiologic studies with children and adolescents suggest similar lifetime prevalence rates in these samples (eg, Refs[9,10]). Data concerning younger children suggest that approximately 1 in 200 young people has OCD, which in many cases severely disrupts academic, social, and vocational functioning.[9]

Phenomenology

According to the *Diagnostic and Statistical Manual of Mental Disorders, Fourth Edition, Text Revision* (DSM-IV-TR),[16] OCD is characterized as the presence of recurrent obsessions and/or compulsions that interfere substantially with daily functioning. Obsessions are "persistent ideas, thoughts, impulses, or images that are experienced as intrusive and inappropriate and cause marked anxiety or distress."[16(p457)] Compulsions are "repetitive behaviors or mental acts, the goal of which is to prevent or reduce anxiety or distress."[16(p457)]

There is typically a functional link between obsessions and compulsions in OCD, such that obsessions cause marked anxiety and distress and compulsions are performed in an attempt to reduce the distress or, in the case of patients with specific feared consequences, reducing the likelihood of a feared outcome (eg, catching a deadly disease, injuring someone as a result of an act of omission or commission).

Table 1
Features of OCD and tics and their comorbidity

	OCD	Tics	OCD with Comorbid Tics
Prevalence	1%–3% of youth in the general population	1% of youth in the general population	• No prevalence rates have been empirically determined for the general population • 20%–30% of individuals with OCD have tics • 22%–44% of individuals with tics have OCD
Onset	• Childhood onset	• Childhood onset	• Childhood onset, typically at earlier age than OCD or tics alone
Phenomenology	• Persistent, intrusive, and inappropriate ideas, thoughts, impulses, or images that cause anxiety or distress • Repetitive behaviors or mental acts that serve to prevent or reduce anxiety or distress	• Sudden, rapid, recurrent, nonrhythmic, stereotyped motor movements or vocalizations • Classifications include simple versus complex tics and vocal versus motor tics • Performed to relieve aversive physical sensation • Presence of premonitory urge	• Chronic waxing and waning course of symptoms • Repetitive behaviors • Intrusive sensations • Impairment in behavioral inhibition • Higher rates of the physical sensations typically only seen in Tourette syndrome preceding or accompanying the cognitive processes surrounding OCD compulsions • Increased mental sensations such as "just-right" feelings and energy release • Higher frequencies of repetitive behaviors preceded by both cognitive and sensory phenomena • Higher rates of compulsions that look like complex motor tics • Higher frequencies of hoarding, counting rituals, intrusive violent and sexual thoughts or images, somatic obsessions, and repetitive movement compulsions
Treatment	• Exposure and response prevention • Psychoeducation • Hierarchy development • Exposure • Relapse prevention • Pharmacotherapy may augment treatment response	• Habit reversal training • Psychoeducation • Awareness training • Hierarchy development • Competing response strategies • Relapse prevention • Pharmacotherapy may augment treatment response	• Little empirical evidence for standardized treatment protocol • Psychoeducation • Awareness training • Hierarchy development • Exposure • Competing response strategies • Relapse prevention • Pharmacotherapy may augment treatment response

In the DSM-IV field trial on OCD, over 90% of participants reported that their compulsions aim to either prevent harm associated with their obsessions or to reduce obsessional distress.[17] If the patient cannot describe a clear relationship between the obsession and the compulsion (obsessions are distressing and compulsions aim at reducing this distress), another diagnosis (eg, stereotypic movement disorder) should be considered. Furthermore, in order to distinguish diagnosable OCD from the occasional phenomena of unwanted thoughts and repetitive behaviors reported by the vast majority of individuals without OCD,[18,19] obsessions and/or compulsions must be found to be of sufficient severity to cause marked distress, be time consuming, and interfere with daily functioning. Youth and their parents do not always agree on the degree of impairment, thus it is important to gather information about functioning from multiple sources to determine if this criterion has been met and, by extension, if treatment is indeed warranted.

There are a number of typical symptoms found in the presentation of OCD. The Children's Yale-Brown Obsessive Compulsive Scale (CY-BOCS)[20] checklist assesses for a wide variety of obsessions and compulsions, including obsessions characterized as pertaining to contamination, aggressive, sexual, hoarding/saving, magical thoughts/superstitious, somatic, and religious scrupulosity.

The categories of compulsions on the CY-BOCS checklist include washing/cleaning, checking, repeating, counting, ordering, arranging, hoarding/saving, excessive games/superstitious behavior, and rituals involving others. The compulsions are often performed according to rigid rules that need to be followed in order to provide relief from the intrusive thought or feeling.[21] Compulsions can be both cognitive (eg, mental reviewing, praying) or behavioral (eg, physical checking, hand washing) and can include content that might be considered unusual or illogical (eg, repeatedly tapping on desk at school in order to prevent a parent from dying in a motor vehicle accident).

Onset of OCD often occurs in childhood or during adolescence, although adult onset is also seen.[22,23] Among adults with OCD, one-third to one-half developed the disorder during childhood or adolescence.[24] Development of OCD is typically gradual, but more rapid onset has been reported in some cases. The course of OCD is most often chronic with some waxing and waning of symptoms, with patients reporting some responsiveness to external stressors as well.[25] In rare pediatric cases, however, onset is very sudden (eg, overnight) and associated with strep infection; treatment of the infection is then associated with substantial reduction of symptoms, but recurrence of infection is associated with symptom exacerbation (pediatric autoimmune neuropsychiatric disorders associated with strep).[26]

Treatment

Among adults, OCD is ranked 10th among the leading causes of disability worldwide including heart disease, diabetes, and cancer.[27] Because it has been established that OCD symptoms tend to persist over time (eg, Ref[28]), it is prudent for clinicians who evaluate OCD in their practices to share this information with families and to be prepared to provide the CBT protocols of established efficacy for this condition (eg, Ref[1]). Pharmacotherapy with selective serotonin reuptake inhibitors (SSRIs) has been consistently found efficacious compared with pill placebo. Cognitive behavior therapy, known as exposure plus response prevention, may be considered as a first line intervention for OCD, either alone or in combination with pharmacotherapy, specifically, selective serotonin reuptake inhibitors.

A version of cognitive behavior therapy, known as exposure plus response prevention (ERP) (Ref[1]), is considered as a first line intervention for OCD, either alone or in combination with pharmacotherapy. Pharmacotherapy with selective serotonin reuptake inhibitors (SSRIs) has been consistently found efficacious compared with pill placebo. Notably, however, medication trials in pediatric and adult OCD indicate that residual impairment is the norm even after adequate treatment (eg, Ref[3]), and thus, ERP either alone or in combination with SSRIs should also be considered whenever ERP is available.

ERP has been studied around the world for the last 40 years and has proved to be both effective and durable for patients with OCD across the developmental spectrum from childhood to adulthood (eg, Refs[1,3,7,29-37]). The course of ERP for youth typically includes 12 to 20 sessions delivered weekly, although more intensive formats have also proved effective and efficient (eg, Refs[38-41]). The main components of ERP include[42]:

- Psychoeducation
- Externalization of OCD
- Mapping a hierarchy for necessary exposures
- Graded exposure and response prevention
- Relapse prevention.

Exposures are often done in real-life settings and involve prolonged contact with the feared external (eg, contaminated surfaces) or internal (eg, images of harming a family member) stimuli that the patient reports as distressing.

For patients who fear specific consequences if they refrain from performing rituals, these fears can be addressed through "imaginal exposure": creating very detailed scripts of the feared consequence and listening to or reading these scripts repeatedly until they are perceived as less anxiety-provoking. According to Foa and Kozak's[43] information processing theory, in vivo and imaginal exposures are designed specifically to prompt obsessional distress. It is believed that repeated, prolonged exposure to feared thoughts and situations serves to disconfirm mistaken associations and evaluations held by the patient, thereby promoting habituation.[43]

Exposures are typically done gradually, with situations provoking moderate distress confronted before more upsetting ones. Exposure "homework" is routinely assigned between sessions, and patients are asked to refrain from rituals during exposures but also, to the extent possible, throughout the day more generally speaking. The stated goal is complete abstinence from rituals, yet therapists must be cognizant of the need to encourage patients to achieve this goal over time rather than simply insisting upon it immediately. Patients are reminded throughout treatment that ritualizing maintains fear or "feeds the beast," whereas refraining from rituals promotes its dissipation; accordingly, they are given recommendations as to how best to refrain from rituals, such as externalizing the obsessive thoughts and "bossing back" OCD.

TIC DISORDERS AND TOURETTE SYNDROME
Prevalence

In a large community sample of 4475 youth, it was determined that .8% had chronic motor tics, .5% had chronic vocal tics, and .6% had Tourette syndrome (TS).[44] Worldwide, TDs and TS are reported to affect 1% of youth.[45] Notably, after the age of 20, fewer than 20% of individuals with TS continue to bear moderate to severe impairment,[46] and 20% to 90% of individuals with TS reported experiencing at least slight to moderate impairment into their adult years.[46-48] Unfortunately, efforts to predict which children with tic disorders including TS will continue to exhibit tic symptoms and experience significant functional impairment into adulthood have not yielded consistent findings. Accordingly, the decision about whether to treat or not to treat current symptoms in youth must be based exclusively on current symptom levels, associated impairment, and ability and willingness to engage in treatment rather than by an empirically informed decision tree that takes likely future course into account.

Phenomenology

TDs and TS are neuropsychiatric disorders whose symptoms tend to mimic fragments of typical behavior (eg, eye blinking, throat clearing). According to the American Psychiatric Association, tics are defined as "sudden, rapid, recurrent, non-rhythmic, stereotyped motor movements or vocalizations."[16] Diagnostic criteria for a chronic motor or vocal TD state that tics must occur numerous times each day, either most days or intermittently for at least 1 year and surface before the age of 18. Depending on the presentation of the tics, chronic TDs are classified as either motor or phonic, and the tics themselves can be simple or complex in nature. The classification of simple motor tic is assigned when muscle spasms are brief and only affect one muscle group, as seen in eye blinking or head jerking. The classification of complex tic would be assigned to longer or sequenced movements, as seen in squatting, jumping, or touching motions. Vocal tics can also be classified as simple or complex with simple phonic tics occurring as short, meaningless utterances, such as grunting, sniffing, humming, or throat clearing. In contrast, complex vocal tics tend to be longer and more meaningful and seem more purposeful. Complex vocal tics might present as echoing the words or phrases of others or repeating one's own utterances.[16] An important clarification to note is that a diagnosis of a tic disorder is given only when either a motor or a vocal tic is present; when an individual exhibits both motor and vocal tics, the diagnosis of TS is assigned. Individuals with TS tend to present with numerous motor tics and at least one vocal tic, whereas the motor and vocal tics occur simultaneously or at separate times throughout the course of illness.[16]

Those naïve to TDs and TS might assume the impairment that arises from these disorders is due to the outward expression of the tics. However, for individuals with tic disorders, the enacting of tics themselves causes only a portion of the distress; much of the suffering associated with tics is actually due to the unpleasant urges that precede, and induce, the tic. The comparison of tics and hyperkinetic movement disorders (eg, Parkinson disease and Huntington chorea) helps to elucidate this concept. On the surface, TDs can be difficult to distinguish from symptoms of hyperkinetic movement disorders because both disorder types display convulsive, sporadic motions. The core distinguishing feature resides in the fact that in TDs, the nature of the tics is volitional, whereas the movements produced by hyperkinetic movement disorders are involuntary.[49]

Accordingly, tics have been described as semivolitional in the literature because most individuals, if they extend much effort and concentration, do have the ability to suppress the outward expression of tics. Typically, tics are produced voluntarily in response to unpleasant, involuntary sensations or phenomenologic experiences that have come to be referred to as premonitory urges. These premonitory urges are frequently described as a building up of tension that is relieved by the performance of a tic; something similar to the uncomfortable sensation that precedes the scratching of an itch.[50,51] Clinical investigations have shown that a variety of premonitory sensory phenomena exist in patients with TS and TDs. These phenomena consist of uncomfortable physical and cognitive sensations such as warmth, coldness, pressure, tension, tickling, or as a generalized inner tension or anxiety that is relieved through motor discharge.[50] For many, the struggle to control these urges can be very distressing: for example, in a study performed by Cohen and Leckman,[52] 57% of their sample revealed the premonitory urges to be more bothersome than the tics themselves.

Prevalence rates for these premonitory urges are apparently quite high. One study reported that 93% of their 135 participants reported the existence of these premonitory urges.[53] Another study revealed that 82% of the 28 child and adult participants reported the presence of premonitory urges immediately preceding their tics.[52] Researchers who have examined this facet of TDs have noted that awareness of these urges and their functional relationship to tics occurs mostly in older children and adults, but not young children. Perception of these premonitory sensations is more reliably reported by children who are at least 10 years old.[53] Children under the age of 10, who often display simple tics, may be insufficiently aware of the premonitory urges, or at least unable to link the presence of the urge with the tic itself.[54]

Interestingly, not only does the awareness of the entire cycle of tics increase around the age of 10, but this is also typically the age at which the symptoms of TDs are at their most severe.[47,55,56] The typical pattern of TDs is that onset will occur between the range of 5.6 to 7.6 years,[47,57-60] will peak in severity around age 10,[47] and will likely decline in severity around the age of 20.

Not only do the symptoms of TDs appear and disappear at intermittent times throughout the illness, but the severity and frequency of the tics themselves also exhibit a waxing and waning pattern. Reasoning for why tic severity and frequency display such a cyclic pattern is that the pattern is due in part to the heightened sensitivity of tics to factors that are common and often unavoidable.[61] Triggering situations could range from an array of daily environmental occurrences (eg, watching television, fatigue, heightened emotions, social settings, or isolation) to anxiety-provoking situations.[62-64] Given how sensitive tics are to an array of common triggers, impairment caused by TDs and TS can be severe and far-reaching. The negative effects of these disorders can impede numerous facets of a child's or adolescent's life including social, family, academic, and occupational domains.

In terms of associated impairment, one study reported that, in a sample of 59 youth, those with tics indicated an overall lower quality of life than their healthy counterparts.[65] Because motor and vocal tics frequently occur at inappropriate times, where utterances or sporadic movements would be deemed strange or distracting, a main negative effect of these disorders is extreme social discomfort. Individuals with TDs commonly report heightened feelings of sadness, shame, and self-consciousness.[16] In addition, individuals with TDs have reported social difficulties with creating and maintaining friendships, hardships in dating, rejection from peers, social withdrawal, teasing, aggression, low popularity, negative social perceptions, and lower social acceptability.[35,66-72]

Impairment in the academic realm also seems to be common in individuals with TS. Research indicates that tics contribute to declines in academic functioning, with one survey reporting that 50% of their sample (71 guardians of children with TS) insisted tics produced moderate interference in their children's reading and writing abilities.[69] Another study reported that of 59 children with TS, 36% claimed that their tics hampered their class preparedness, ability to write, ability to complete homework, and concentration levels.[35]

Mental health disorders rarely only affect the afflicted individual, and TS is no exception. Studies report that families with at least one member with TS incur a heightened burden on caregivers, a diminished family cohesion, trouble with solving family issues, and increased interference in the daily functioning of family members.[35,73-75] These effects should be evaluated and acknowledged in the evaluation context and may well become targets for clinical intervention in and of themselves.

Treatment

Habit reversal training (HRT) has been shown to be a promising treatment option for adults and youth with TDs including TS. Although the neurologic basis of tics is explicitly acknowledged in HRT protocols (eg, Ref[5]), HRT is implemented under the assumption that situational and environmental factors, including the perception of premonitory urges, contribute to the performance or suppression of tics. A detailed review of pharmacotherapy strategies for TDs and TS is beyond the scope of this review, but HRT has been found efficacious in both youth and adults (eg, Refs[4,76,77]), and seems to yield effect sizes that are comparable with those reported in pharmacotherapy trials but with many fewer untoward side effects.[4] Unfortunately, head-to-head comparisons of HRT versus monotherapy with medications known to be effective for TS or randomized, controlled comparisons of those monotherapies against combined treatment approaches have yet to be conducted.

According to Piacentini and colleagues,[4] the two core components of HRT are training in tic awareness and competing response. When planning the course of treatment, the patient's developmental level should be a main factor of consideration. Clinical observations have indicated younger children exhibit greater success with tic reduction when treatment has placed greater emphasis on implementing competing responses and focused less on awareness training.[78] Because the awareness of premonitory urges and their functional relationship to tics tend to increase with age, adolescents and adults can typically implement both awareness training and competing response training with little difficulty. Therefore, depending on the base awareness level the patient has of premonitory urges, HRT either develops or simply increases the perception of these urges in order to prevent the performance of tics. To foster greater awareness, patients are typically taught how to self-monitor the premonitory urges and other warning signs (eg, situations that consistently predict tic onset) that frequently accompany tic occurrences. Competing response training is geared around disrupting the negative reinforcement cycle that is produced by the performance of tics; in other words, the performance of the tic reduces the unwanted premonitory urge sensations and provides temporary relief. One of the goals of the intervention, therefore, is achieved by training patients to complete a physical behavior that is incompatible with the expression of the tic. Ideally, this competing response is exercised when the patient feels the presence of a premonitory urge or notices the warning signs of a tic. Optimally, the competing responses are designed to be more socially acceptable than the tic expression, and it is hoped that they allow the patient to continue to function unobtrusively while tolerating the uncomfortable sensation of the premonitory urge.

Typically, during the first few sessions of treatment, the therapist and patient create a tic hierarchy based on level of distress each tic causes. With this hierarchy as a guide, the therapist and patient collaborate to structure the awareness and competing response training to first tackle the most distressing tics before gearing treatment toward eliminating the more residual ones. This model differs from traditional OCD and anxiety hierarchy-building in that it is more typical in treating OCD to begin with less distressing and impairing exposures and gradually work up toward more and more distress-evoking situations. HRT sessions typically occur once a week for about an hour and include features of psychoeducation, awareness training, competing response training, and problem-solving around treatment barriers. Additionally, depending on the situation, sessions might also include family education and training, including efforts to create a "tic-neutral" environment at home in order to reduce any reinforcement provided for tics that may serve to maintain the cycle, such as receiving additional attention from parents or being allowed to discontinue difficult tasks (eg, schoolwork) whenever tics occur.

OCD AND TIC DISORDERS: PHENOMENOLOGIC OVERLAP, DISTINCTIONS, AND COMORBIDITY

Although classified as separate disorders, the overlap between the symptoms of complex motor tic disorders and the compulsions associated with OCD is considerable, which makes the task of distinguishing the two phenomena challenging. Common clinical correlates that characterize these two disorders include typical childhood onset, a chronic waxing and waning course, and familial occurrence.[79] TDs and OCD can also share similar clinical presentations including repetitive behaviors, intrusive sensations, and impairment in behavioral inhibition.[80]

Phenomenologic differences between these two disorders do exist, however, and the key to their division resides in the distinguishing feature of the functional relationship between the repetitive movements and any preceding thoughts. These differences can be categorized into cognitive processes and physical sensations. Although the end goal of both compulsions and complex motor tics is the same—to produce relief—compulsions carry a cognitive component to the behavior that tics typically do not.[81] For accurate diagnosis, it is critical to understand the function of the repetitive behavior. Although some complex tics seem to be purposeful, such as certain grooming movements (ie, brushing hair behind one's ear), there is no specific fear that precedes tics that demands the stereotyped movement to be performed (eg, "My mom will get hurt if I don't fix my hair repeatedly"). However, if an individual repeatedly brushed hair behind his or her ear to neutralize some superstitious fear, then the behavior would fall into the classification of a compulsion because its function in such a case would be to reduce the likelihood of a feared outcome. When assessing an individual with comorbidity, the diagnostician must be adept at making and then teaching the patient these kinds of fine-tuned distinctions, because different treatment strategies could be implemented at different times in treatment depending on whether the behavior was conceptualized as a compulsion or a tic.

In short, our current nosology labels the same repetitive behavior differently based on the nature of the subjective experience that precedes it. To elaborate, specific cognitions are associated with OCD, and these cognitive phenomena, known as obsessions, give rise to urges to perform compulsions that serve to alleviate the associated obsessional distress; elaborated thoughts and fears do not typically precede the performance of tics, because they function as the physical response to reduce sensory urges and somatic tension.[82–86] Although no conventional techniques exist to differentiate "pure" compulsions from tics, the incisive diagnostician should know that OCD with pure compulsions is exceptionally rare.[17]

To further complicate the task of differentiating these conditions, high comorbidity rates of OCD and tics exist, with studies indicating that 22% to 44% of individuals with TS also have OCD.[87–89] Studies measuring the inverse have found that 20% to 30% of individuals with OCD also carry a current or past history of tics.[90] Additionally, in the recently completed POTS II OCD study, the comorbidity rate for TDs was approximately 22%.[3]

When comorbidity does occur, the clinical presentation may be somewhat different from either OCD or TS symptoms alone, with symptoms often seeming to fall right in the middle of a theoretical continuum between the two. Individuals exhibiting the comorbidity pattern of OCD plus TDs tend to report higher rates of the physical sensations typically only seen in TS preceding or accompanying the cognitive processes surrounding OCD compulsions.[84,91] Mental sensations, such as "just-right" feelings, and energy release (described as mental energy that builds up and calls for release) are sensory phenomena that tend to be more frequent in OCD and TS patients than in patients with OCD alone.[21] Individuals with OCD plus tics have shown higher frequencies of repetitive behaviors that are preceded by both cognitive and sensory phenomena. This population has higher rates of compulsions that look like complex motor tics, such as tapping, rubbing, and touching.[92,93] Higher frequencies of certain OCD symptoms, such as hoarding, counting rituals, intrusive violent and sexual thoughts or images, somatic obsessions, and repetitive movement compulsions are seen in the comorbidity between TS and OCD.[92,94–96] Additionally, research has shown that patients with tics and OCD incur symptom onset at an earlier age[83,93,97] and are more likely to be male.[92]

Impairment caused by the comorbidity of TDs and OCD depends on the presentation, severity, and frequency of the symptoms. Results obtained from studies that focus on this topic are mixed. Thibert and colleagues[98] revealed that individuals with TS and obsessive-compulsive symptoms had higher levels of anxiety and lower self-concepts than individuals with TS alone. Lewin and colleagues[80] reported that having a diagnosis of both TDs and OCD did not increase the level of impairment caused by either disorder in children when examining severity levels, comorbidity burden, emotional and behavioral problems, or global functioning. However, research in adults with both TDs and OCD indicates that having comorbid TDs and OCD is associated with higher levels of symptom severity when compared with individuals with only TDs or OCD.[79] These varied outcomes could be reflective of the developmental differences in the study populations, but more research is needed to examine whether sampling strategies and method variance are responsible for the inconsistent findings. Clinically it is important to examine patterns of onset (eg, OCD first vs tics first), patient and family evaluation of which condition is currently more impairing, patient interest and confidence to tackle the symptoms of one disorder first as opposed to the other, and the degree to which symptoms of one condition exacerbate those of the other (eg, increased tic urges when triggered by OCD stimuli).

IMPLICATIONS FOR CLINICAL PRACTICE WITH COMORBID OCD AND TDS

Unfortunately, little has been done empirically to examine the treatment for comorbid OCD and TDs in children and adolescents. In their review of the literature, Ferrao and colleagues[21] suggest that ERP alone is probably not as effective in treating TDs as it is for treating OCD, but that more research is needed; however, an adult study indicated that ERP was quite effective in treating TS and was actually more effective on some outcome measures than HRT.[99] Other research concerning the influence of tics on OCD treatment has suggested similar treatment outcomes for adolescents with OCD with or without tics.[100] However, when both OCD and TDs are present in a child or adolescent, there is some support for the possibility that exposure treatment, which has been found efficacious for OCD across the developmental spectrum, may also have positive effects on tics and tic urges.[99] However, it is important to note that the methods and perhaps even the function of exposure may differ when being used to combat urges to do compulsions as opposed to tics. For example, an emphasis on imaginal exposure to obsessional content would be prominent in treating an individual who engages in repetitive tapping behavior to prevent a specific dreaded outcome (eg, death of a parent in an accident), whereas an individual who reports engaging in a nearly identical tapping behavior in order to reduce discomfort associated with premonitory urges would be unlikely to benefit from imaginal exposure.[5] Thus, the degree to which the OCD and tic symptoms are formally similar may well assist the clinician in devising approaches that can be used for both phenomena.

There are several potentially reasonable options to consider when treating a child or adolescent with both conditions. Several options may be weighed in this clinical circumstance[101]:

1. Continue the focus on the disorder classified as primary regardless of the presence of other symptoms.
2. Attempt to incorporate some clinical procedures and session time to manage the symptoms of the co-occurring disorder but continue to focus most session time and effort on the primary disorder.
3. Shift the focus of treatment to address the symptoms of the secondary disorder because their presence makes it difficult to treat the primary disorder successfully, but move back to the primary disorder as soon as possible.
4. Treat the primary disorder only after the symptoms of the secondary disorder are under better control.

Considering the high likelihood that OCD drives the functional impairment when both disorders are present, option 1 is usually the authors' default decision unless the OCD symptoms are very mild and are not of particular relevance to the child. The conceptual overlap between the disorders and the procedural similarity between some of the core interventions for OCD and TDs also probably renders option 4 perhaps the least preferable choice for this particular comorbidity pattern, because differentiating so clearly between the two phenomena is difficult and in some cases may not even be necessary.

Thus, when the authors proceed with treatment of children and adolescents with OCD plus a comorbid tic disorder, they are most likely to either incorporate procedures for both conditions into one treatment or, given the likelihood that OCD will drive the majority of the functional impairment, address the OCD first while carefully examining the effects of the OCD treatment procedures on tic symptoms. It may be optimal to blend both treatment approaches and have the patient engage in exposures but incorporate habit reversal techniques to help the patient remain focused on the exposure tasks at hand without being distracted by tic urges. What is important clinically is that patients are taught to use the proper techniques to address those symptoms that are clearly emanating from one disorder or the other and that they become comfortable experimenting with different techniques for those symptoms that could be classified as either one.

IMPLICATIONS FOR RESEARCH

There is much still to be determined regarding the optimal strategy or sequence of strategies for addressing comorbid OCD and TDs. The lack of empirical evidence on this topic currently hampers clinical decision-making with respect to providing empirically informed treatment recommendations for OCD and TDs in youth. Data from multiple clinical trials already support the efficacy of ERP and HRT, respectively, for these conditions, but more work is needed to determine whether a sequenced or a transdiagnostic approach would be best in handling disorder-specific symptoms that, although certainly sharing overlap, also have distinguishing features that could be more or less responsive to particular interventions available in the ERP or HRT protocols. Ultimately, it is important to determine whether and how best to modify and combine these approaches for patients who have both diagnoses.

CLINICAL CONTROVERSIES

Perhaps the most interesting development in the field with implications for the treatment of OCD and disorders involving impulse control has to do with underlying assumptions related to the centrality of habituation. ERP and HRT theorists have consistently acknowledged the neurobiological nature of obsessions and premonitory urges that give rise to compulsions and tics, respectively. However, each treatment is predicated on the notion that, if the individual can refrain from acting on the urge, the result will be a temporary increase in discomfort that will be followed by habituation of the urge, at least to some extent.[102] The degree of emphasis on habituation has varied within treatment protocols—some have suggested that the frequency and intensity of the associated emotion will substantially diminish with repeated practice,[8] whereas others have emphasized that using behavioral methods to deal with these phenomena will provide the patient a way to manage urges more successfully in situations in which it matters to them.[5] The emergence of acceptance and commitment therapy as an efficacious treatment for OCD[103] raises questions about whether a habituation model needs to be emphasized, and the authors' clinical observations across patients with OCD and tic disorders actually suggests a range of responses in that some patients do report great reduction of urge strength, whereas others report that the use of ERP or HRT simply allows them to manage urges more effectively even when the urge intensity does not diminish substantially. These observations need to be followed up in laboratory work as we seek to better elucidate the mechanisms by which these treatments' effects are realized.

REFERENCES

1. Abramowitz JS, Whiteside SP, Deacon RJ. The effectiveness of treatment for pediatric obsessive-compulsive disorder: A meta-analysis. Behav Ther 2005;36: 55–63.
2. Cook CR, Blacher J. Evidence-based psychosocial treatments for tic disorders. Clin Psychol (New York) 2007;14:252–67.
3. Franklin ME, Sapyta J, Freeman JB, et al. Cognitive behavior therapy augmentation of pharmacotherapy in pediatric obsessive compulsive disorder: The pediatric OCD treatment study II randomized controlled trial. JAMA 2011;306:1224–32.
4. Piacentini J, Woods DW, Scahill L, et al. Behavior therapy for children with Tourette disorder: a randomized controlled trial. JAMA 2010;303:1929–37.
5. Woods DW, Piacentini J, Chang S, et al. Managing Tourette syndrome: a behavioral intervention for children and adults. New York: Oxford University Press; 2008.
6. Woods D, Himle M, Miltenberger R, et al. Durability, negative impact, and neuropsychological predictors of tic suppression in children with chronic tic disorder. J Abnorm Child Psychol 2008;36(2):237–45.
7. Pediatric OCD Treatment Study (POTS) Team. Cognitive-behavior therapy, sertraline, and their combination for children and adolescents with obsessive-compulsive disorder: the pediatric OCD treatment study (POTS) randomized controlled trial. JAMA 2004;292:1969–76.
8. March JS, Mulle K. OCD in children and adolescents: a cognitive-behavioral treatment manual. New York: The Guilford Press; 1998.
9. Flament MF, Whitaker A, Rapoport JL, et al. Obsessive compulsive disorder in adolescence: an epidemiological study. J Am Acad Child Adolesc Psychiatry 1988; 27:764–71.

10. Valleni-Basille LA, Garrison CZ, Jackson KL. Frequency of obsessive compulsive disorder in a community sample of young adolescents. J Am Acad Child Adolesc Psychiatry 1994;33:782–91.

11. Ruscio AM, Stein DJ, Chiu WT, et al. The epidemiology of obsessive-compulsive disorder in the National Comorbidity Survey Replication. Mol Psychiatry 2010;15: 53–63.

12. Piacentini J, Bergman RL. Obsessive-compulsive disorder in children. Psychiatr Clin North Am 2000;23:519–33.

13. Piacentini J, Bergman RL, Keller M. et al. Functional impairment in children and adolescents with obsessive-compulsive disorder. J Child Adolesc Psychopharmacol 2003;13:S61–9.

14. Swedo SE, Rapoport JL, Leonard HL, et al. Obsessive-compulsive disorder and children and adolescents: clinical phenomenology of 70 consecutive cases. Arch Gen Psychiatry 1989;46:335–41.

15. Kessler RC, Chiu WT, Demler O, et al. Prevalence, severity, and comorbidity of 12 month DSM-IV disorders in the national comorbidity survey replication. Arch Gen Psychiatry 2005;62:617–27.

16. American Psychiatric Association. Diagnostic and statistical manual of mental disorders. 4th edition, text revision. Washington (DC): American Psychiatric Association; 2000.

17. Foa EB, Kozak MJ, Goodman WK, et al. DSM-IV field trial: obsessive compulsive disorder. Am J Psychiatry 1995;152:90–6.

18. Crye J, Laskey B, Cartwright-Hatton S. Non-clinical obsessions in a young adolescent population: frequency and association with metacognitive variables. Psychol Psychother 2010;83:15–26.

19. Rachman S, de Silva P. Abnormal and normal obsessions. Behav Res Ther 1978; 16:233–48.

20. Scahill LD, Riddle MA, McSwiggin-Hardin M, et al. Children's Yale-Brown Obsessive Compulsive Scale: reliability and validity. J Am Acad Child Adolesc Psychiatry 1997;36:844–52.

21. Ferrao YA, Miguel E, Stein DJ. Tourette's syndrome, trichotillomania, and obsessive compulsive disorder: how closely are they related? Psychiatry Research 2009;170: 32–42.

22. Rasmussen SA, Eisen JL. Epidemiology of obsessive compulsive disorder. J Clin Psychiatry 1990;51:10–3.

23. Spitzer M, Sigmund D. The phenomenology of obsessive compulsive disorder. Int Rev Psychiatry 1997;9:7–14.

24. DeVeaugh-Geiss J, Moroz G, Biederman J, et al. Clomipramine hydrochloride in childhood and adolescent obsessive-compulsive disorder—a multicenter trial. J Am Acad Child Adolesc Psychiatry 1992;31:45–9.

25. Franklin ME, Foa EB. Treatment of obsessive compulsive disorder. Annu Rev Clin Psychol 2011;7:229–43.

26. Swedo SE, Leonard HL, Garvey M, et al. Pediatric autoimmune neuropsychiatric disorders associated with streptococcal infections: clinical description of the first 50 cases. Am J Psychiatry 1998;155;264–71.

27. Murray CJ, Lopez AD. Global health statistics. Cambridge (MA): Harvard University Press; 1996.

28. Skoog G, Skoog I. A 40 year follow up of patients with obsessive compulsive disorder. Arch Gen Psychiatry 1999;56:121–7.

29. Abramowitz JS. Variants of exposure and response prevention in the treatment of obsessive-compulsive disorder: a meta-analysis. Behav Ther 1996;27:583–600.

30. National Institute for Health and Clinical Excellence (NICE). Obsessive compulsive disorder: core interventions in the treatment of obsessive-compulsive disorder and body dysmorphic disorder. Available at: www.nice.org.uk/CG031. Accessed June 6, 2012.

31. Rosa-Alcazar AI, Sanchez-Meca J, Gomez-Conesa A, et al. Psychological treatment of obsessive-compulsive disorder: a meta-analysis. Clin Psychol Rev 2008;28: 1310–25.

32. Barret P, Healey-Farrell A, March JS. Cognitive-behavioral family treatment of childhood obsessive-compulsive disorder: a controlled trial. JAMA 2004;43:46–62.

33. Bolton D, Perin S. Evaluation of exposure with response-prevention for obsessive compulsive disorder in children and adolescence. J Behav Ther Exp Psychiatry 2008;39:11–22.

34. Freeman JB, Garcia AM, Coyne L, et al. Early childhood OCD: preliminary findings from a family-based cognitive-behavioral approach. JAMA 2008;47:593–602.

35. Storch EA, Lack CW, Simons LE, et al. A measure of functional impairment in youth with Tourette's syndrome. J Pediatr Psychol 2007;32:950–9.

36. Watson HJ, Rees CS. Meta-analysis of randomized, controlled treatment trials for pediatric obsessive-compulsive disorder. J Child Psychol Psychiatry 2008;49: 489–98.

37. Williams TI, Salkovskis PM, Forrester L, et al. A randomised controlled trial of cognitive behavioural treatment for obsessive-compulsive disorder in children and adolescents. Eur Child Adolesc Psychiatry 2010;19:449–56.

38. Piacentini J, Bergman RL, Chang S, et al. Controlled comparison of family cognitive behavioral therapy and psychoeducation/relaxation training for child obsessive-compulsive disorder. J Am Acad Child Adolesc Psychiatry 2011;50:1149–61.

39. Franklin ME, Kozak MJ, Cashman LA, et al. Cognitive-behavioral treatment of pediatric obsessive-compulsive disorder: an open clinical trial. J Am Acad Child Adolesc Psychiatry 1998;37:412–9.

40. Storch EA, Geffken GR, Merlo LJ, et al. Family-based cognitive-behavioral therapy for pediatric obsessive-compulsive disorder: comparison of intensive and weekly approaches. J Am Acad Child Adolesc Psychiatry 2007;46:469–78.

41. Whiteside SP, Brown AM, Abramowitz JS. Five-day intensive treatment for adolescent OCD: a case series. J Anxiety Disord 2008;22:495–504.

42. Sapyta JJ, Freeman J, Franklin ME, et al. Obsessive compulsive disorder. In: Szigethy E, Weisz JR, Findling RL, editors. Cognitive-behavior therapy for children and adolescents. Washington (DC): American Psychiatric Publishing; 2012. p. 299–330.

43. Foa EB, Kozac MJ. Emotional processing of fear: exposure to corrective information. Psychol Bull 1986;99:20–35.

44. Khalifa N, von Knorring AL. Prevalence of tic disorders and Tourette syndrome in a Swedish school population. Dev Med Child Neurol 2003;45:31531–9.

45. Robertson MM. The prevalence and epidemiology of Gilles de la Tourette syndrome part 1: the epidemiological and prevalence studies. J Psychosom Med 2008;65: 461–72.

46. Bloch MH, Peterson BS, Scahill L, et al. Adulthood outcome of tic and obsessive-compulsive symptom severity In children with Tourette syndrome. Arch Pediatr Adolesc Med 2006;160:65–9.

47. Leckman JF, Zhang H, Vitale A, et al. Course of tic severity in Tourette syndrome: the first two decades. Pediatrics 1998;102:14–9.

48. Pappert EJ, Goetz CG, Louis ED, et al. Objective assessments of longitudinal outcome in Gilles de la Tourette's syndrome. Neurology 2003;61:936–40.

49. Kompoliti K, Goetz CG. Hyperkinetic movement disorders misdiagnosed tics in Gilles de la Tourette syndrome. Mov Disord 2008;13:477–80.
50. Banaschewski T, Woerner W, Rothenberger A. Premonitory sensory phenomena and suppressibility of tics in Tourette syndrome: developmental aspects in children and adolescents. Dev Med Child Neurol 2003:45:700–3.
51. Kwak C, Vuong KD, Jankovic J. Premonitory sensory phenomenon in Tourette's syndrome. Mov Disord 2003;18:1530–3.
52. Cohen AJ, Leckman JF. Sensory phenomena associated with Gilles de la Tourette's syndrome. J Clin Psychiatry 1992;53:319–23.
53. Leckman JF, Walker DE, Cohen DJ. Premonitory urges in Tourette's syndrome. Am J Psychiatry 1993:150:98–102.
54. Woods DW, Piacentini J, Himle MB, et al. Premonitory Urge for Tics Scale (PUTS): initial psychometric results and examination of the premonitory urge phenomenon in youths with tic disorders. J Dev Behav Pediatr. 2005;26:397–403.
55. Lin H, Yeh C, Peterson BS, et al. Assessment of symptom exacerbations in a longitudinal study of children with Tourette's syndrome or obsessive compulsive disorder. J Am Acad Child Adolesc Psychiatry 2002;41:1070–7.
56. Robertson MM, Banerjee S, Kurlan RR, et al. The Tourette syndrome diagnostic confidence index: developmental and clinical associations. Neurology 1999;53; 2108–12.
57. Comings DE, Comings BG. Tourette syndrome: clinical and psychological aspects of 250 cases. Am J Hum Genet 1985;37:435–45.
58. Freeman RD, Fast DK, Burd L, et al. An international perspective on Tourette syndrome: selected findings from 3500 individuals in 22 countries. Dev Med Child Neurol 2000;42:436–47.
59. Janik P, Kalbarczyk, Sitek M. Clinical analysis of Gilles de la Tourette syndrome based on 126 cases. Neurol Neurochir Pol 2007;41:381–7.
60. Lees AJ, Robertson M, Trimble MR, et al. A clinical study of Gilles de la Tourette syndrome in the United Kingdom. J Neurol Neurosurg Psychiatry 1984;47:1–8.
61. Conelea CA, Woods DW. The influence of contextual factors on tic expression in Tourette's syndrome: a review. J Psychosom Res 2008;65:487–96.
62. Findley DB, Leckman JF, Katsovich L, et al. Development of the Yale Children's Global Stress Index (YCGSI) and its application in children and adolescents with Tourette's syndrome and obsessive-compulsive disorder. J Am Acad Child Adolesc Psychiatry 2003;42:450–7.
63. Hoekstra PJ, Anderson GM, Limburg PC, et al. Neurobiology and neuroimmunology of Tourette's syndrome: an update. Cell Mol Life Sci 2004;61:886–98.
64. Silva RR, Munoz DM, Barickman J, et al. Environmental factors and related fluctuation of symptoms in children and adolescents with Tourette's disorder. J Child Psychiatry 1995;36:305–12.
65. Storch EA, Merlo LJ, Lack C, et al. Quality of life in youth with Tourette's syndrome and chronic tic disorder. J Clin Child Adolesc Psychol 2007;36:216–27.
66. Champion LM, Fulton WA, Shady GA. Tourette syndrome and social functioning in a Canadian population. Neurosci Biobehav Rev 1988;12:255–7.
67. Elstner KK, Selai CE, Trimble MR, et al. Quality of life (QOL) of patients with Gilles de la Tourette's syndrome. Acta Psychiatr Scand 2001;103:52–9.
68. Lin H, Katsovich L, Ghebremichael M, et al. Psychosocial stress predicts future symptom severities in children and adolescents with Tourette syndrome and/or obsessive-compulsive disorder. J Child Psychol Psychiatry 2007;48:157–66.
69. Packer LE. Tic-related school problems: Impact on functional accommodations and interventions. Behav Modif 2005;29:876–99.

70. Stokes A, Bawden HN, Camfield PR, et al. Peer problem in Tourette's disorder. Pediatrics 1991;87:936–42.
71. Marcks BA, Woods DW, Ridosko JL. The effects of trichotillomania disclosure on peer perceptions and social acceptability. Body Image 2005;2:299–306.
72. Woods DW, Fuqua R, Outman RC. Evaluating the social acceptability of persons with habit disorders: the effects of topography frequency and gender manipulation. J Psychopathol Behav Assess 1999;21:1–18.
73. Bawden HN, Stokes A, Camfield CS, et al. Peer relationship problems in children with Tourette's disorder or diabetes mellitus. J Child Psychol Psychiatry, 1998;39:663–8.
74. Cooper C, Robertson MM, Livingston G. Psychological morbidity and caregiver burden in parents of children with Tourette's disorder and psychiatric comorbidity. J Am Acad Child Adolesc Psychiatry 2003;42:1370–5.
75. Hubka GB, Fulton WA, Shady GA, et al. Tourette syndrome: impact on Canadian family functioning. Neurosci Biobehav Rev 1988;12:259–61.
76. Deckersbach T, Rauch S, Buhlmann U, et al. Habit reversal versus supportive psychotherapy in Tourette's disorder: a randomized controlled trial and predictors of treatment response. Behav Res Ther 2006;44:1079–99.
77. Wilhelm S, Deckersbach T, Coffey BJ, et al. Habit reversal versus supportive psychotherapy for Tourette's disorder: a randomized controlled trial. Am J Psychiatry 2003;160:1175–7.
78. Piacentini J, Chang S. Behavioral treatments for Tourette syndrome and tic disorders.In: Cohen DJ, Jankcovicz J, Goetz CG. Advances in neurology,vol. 85, Tourette syndrome. Philadelphia: Lippincott, Williams & Wilkins; 2001. p. 319–32.
79. Coffey BJ, Miguel EC, Biederman J, et al. Tourette's disorder with and without obsessive-compulsive disorder in adults: are they different? J Nerv Ment Dis 1998;186:201–6.
80. Lewin AB, Chang S, McCracken J, et al. Comparison of clinical features among youth with tic disorders, obsessive-compulsive disorder (OCD), and both conditions. Psychiatry Res 2010;178:317–22.
81. Mansueto CS, Keuler DJ. Tic or compulsion?: it's Tourettic OCD. Behav Modif 2005;29:784–99.
82. Miguel EC, Coffey BJ, Baer L, et al. Phenomenology of intentional repetitive behaviors in obsessive-compulsive disorder and Tourette's disorder. J Clin Psychiatry 1995;56:246–55.
83. Miguel EC, Baer L, Coffey BJ, et al. Phenomenological differences appearing with repetitive behaviours in obsessive-compulsive disorder and Gilles de la Tourette's syndrome. Br J Psychiatry 1997;170:140–5.
84. Miguel EC, do Rosario-Campos MC, Prado HS, et al. Sensory phenomena in obsessive-compulsive disorder and Tourette's disorder. J Clin Psychiatry 2000;61:150–6.
85. Scahill LD, Leckman JF, Marek KL. Sensory phenomena in Tourette's syndrome. Adv Neurology 1995;65:273–80.
86. Shapiro AK, Shapiro E. Evaluation of the reported association of obsessive compulsive symptoms or disorder with Tourette's disorder. Compr Psychiatry 1992;33:152–65.
87. Freeman RD. Tourette Syndrome International Database Consortium. Tic disorders and ADHD: answers from a world-wide clinical dataset on Tourette syndrome. Eur Child Adolesc Psychiatry 2007;16:536.
88. King RA, Leckman JF, Scahill LD, et al. Obsessive-compulsive disorder, anxiety, and depression. In: Leckman JF, Cohen DJ. Tourette's syndrome tics,obsessions, compulsions: developmental psychopathology and clinical care. New York: John Wiley & Sons; 1998. p. 43–62.

89. Termine C, Balottin U, Rossi G, et al. Psychopathology in children and adolescents with Tourette's syndrome: a controlled study. Brain Dev 2006;28:69–75.
90. Pauls DL, Towbin KD, Leckman JF, et al. Gilles de la Tourette's syndrome and obsessive-compulsive disorder. Arch Gen Psychiatry 1986;43:1180–2.
91. Leckman JF, Walker DE, Goodman WK, et al. "Just-right" perceptions associated with compulsive behavior in Tourette's syndrome. Am J Psychiatry 1994;151: 675–80.
92. Holzer JC, Goodman WK, McDougle CJ, et al. Obsessive-compulsive disorder with and without a chronic tic disorder: a comparison of symptoms in 70 patients. Br J Psychiatry 1994;164:469–73.
93. Leckman JF, Goodman WK, Anderson GM, et al. Cerebrospinal fluid biogenic amines in obsessive compulsive disorder, Tourette's syndrome, and healthy controls. Neuropsychopharmacology 1995;12:73–86.
94. Swerdlow NR, Zinner S, Farber RH, et al. Symptoms in obsessive-compulsive disorder and Tourette syndrome: a spectrum? SNS Spectrum, 1999;4:21–33.
95. Zohar AH, Pauls DL, Ratzoni G, et al. Obsessive-compulsive disorder with and without tics in an epidemiological sample of adolescents. Am J Psychiatry 1997;154: 274–6.
96. Cath DC, Spinhovern P, van de Wetering BJ, et al. The relationship between types and severity of repetitive behaviors in Gilles de la Tourette's disorder and obsessive-compulsive disorder. J Clin Psychiatry 2000;61:505–13.
97. Rosario-Campos MC, Leckman JF, Mercadante MT, et al. Adults with early-onset obsessive-compulsive disorder. Am J Psychiatry 2001;158:1899–903.
98. Thibert AL, Day HI, Sandor P. Self-concept and self-consciousness in adults with Tourette's syndrome. Can J Psychiatry 1995;40:35–9.
99. Verdellen CW, Keijsers GP, Cath DC, et al. Exposure with response prevention versus habit reversal in Tourette's syndrome: a controlled study. Behav Res Ther 2004;42:501–11.
100. Himle JA, Fischer DJ, Van Etten ML, et al. Group behavioral therapy for adolescents with tic-related and non tic-related obsessive-compulsive disorder. Depress Anxiety 2003;17:73–7.
101. Franklin ME, Tolin DF, editors. Treating trichotillomania: cognitive behavioral therapy for hair pulling and related problems. New York: Springer Science and Business Media; 2007.
102. Himle MB, Franklin ME. The more you do it, the easier it gets: exposure and response prevention for OCD. Cogn Behav Pract 2008;16:29–39.
103. Twohig MP, Hayes SC, Plumb JC, et al. A randomized clinical trial of acceptance and commitment therapy vs. progressive relaxation training for obsessive compulsive disorder. J Consult Clin Psychol 2010;78:705–16.

Posttraumatic Stress Disorder
Shifting Toward a Developmental Framework

Victor G. Carrion, MD*, Hilit Kletter, PhD

KEYWORDS

- Pediatric posttraumatic stress disorder • Childhood trauma
- Childhood development • Neurobiology • Interventions

KEY POINTS

- It has been proposed that posttraumatic stress disorder (PTSD) should be conceptualized as a dimensional and continuous, rather than a categorical, clinical entity in youth.
- As a result of young children's limitations in their verbal capacity, they may use other means to express themselves such as being fussy or having temper tantrums, types of behavior often overlooked as symptoms of PTSD.
- Chronic periods of stress may impair the hypothalamic–pituitary–adrenal (HPA) axis resulting in dysregulation of cortisol secretion, which has been suggested as a marker for PTSD; though neuroendocrine studies have yielded mixed results regarding the relationship of cortisol and pediatric PTSD, the majority of studies report high levels of cortisol to be indicative of PTSD.
- Psychotherapeutic interventions have the potential to modulate negative effects of PTSD by providing new experiences that repair brain function and promote the growth of neural connections.

INTRODUCTION

Childhood exposure to trauma is a common phenomenon, with 25% of young people experiencing a traumatic event such as physical abuse; sexual abuse; witnessing violence, war, and terrorism; natural disasters; illness; or injury by the time they reach age 16 years.[1] Internal (eg, genetics and individual traits) and environmental (eg, home, school, community) factors interact to determine the outcome that trauma will have on a child. Many young people demonstrate resilience, the ability to adapt and cope despite adversity, and continue to develop normally.[2] Some will be susceptible to develop mood and/or anxiety disorders.[3] Yet others are at risk to develop posttraumatic stress disorder (PTSD), which can

The authors have nothing to disclose.
Department of Psychiatry and Behavioral Sciences, Division of Child and Adolescent Psychiatry, Stanford School of Medicine, Stanford University, 401 Quarry Road, Stanford, CA 94305, USA
* Corresponding author.
E-mail address: vcarrion@stanford.edu

Child Adolesc Psychiatric Clin N Am 21 (2012) 573–591
http://dx.doi.org/10.1016/j.chc.2012.05.004
1056-4993/12/$ – see front matter © 2012 Elsevier Inc. All rights reserved.

childpsych.theclinics.com

have a negative impact on biological, cognitive, emotional, behavioral, and social domains of the child.[4] Although trauma exposure is associated with the development of different conditions, this article focuses specifically on PTSD because it is the disorder (or injury) with the most widely studied outcome across populations and trauma types.

CLASSIFICATION OF PTSD

It has long been established that PTSD occurs in adults; however, it was not until the publication of the DSM-III-R that it was recognized that young people experience similar symptoms.[5] The diagnosis of PTSD is based on six major criteria, two of which define the trauma (criterion A). The DSM-IV-TR provides the following description:

1. The person experienced, witnessed, or was confronted with an event or events that involved actual or threatened death or serious injury, or a threat to the physical integrity of self or others.
2. The person's response involved intense fear, helplessness, or horror.[6]

In children, the latter may be expressed as disorganized or agitated behavior. Symptoms of PTSD are divided into three clusters:

1. **Reexperiencing of the traumatic event** (criterion B), which includes flashbacks, nightmares, exaggerated startle response, and intrusive recollections.
2. **Avoidance of trauma** with regard to relevant stimuli and numbing of general responsiveness (criterion C), which includes feeling detached or estranged from others and deriving markedly less pleasure from activities that previously were enjoyed.
3. **Hyperarousal** (criterion D), which includes irritability, hypervigilance, and difficulties in sleep and concentration.

Symptoms must persist for at least 1 month (criterion E) and cause significant distress or impairment in functioning (criterion F).

Proposed changes to the PTSD diagnosis for DSM-V take into account developmental variations in symptom manifestation, including a separate subtype for children younger than age 6 years.[7] Additional changes include clarification of what constitutes a traumatic event, elimination of criterion A2, division of cluster C avoidance and numbing into two separate criteria, and elimination of the acute versus chronic designation. In addition, cluster D (numbing) has new symptoms emphasizing the role of self or other blaming and persistently negative emotional states and cluster E (hyperarousal) has an added symptom of reckless or self-destructive behavior. **Table 1** shows the current DSM-IV criteria and highlights the proposed DSM-V changes.

There are instances in which PTSD symptoms may differ in young people. For example, children may engage in repetitive play and experience frightening dreams without specific content.[8] Many children develop fears associated with certain aspects of a trauma that may develop into phobias.[9] Increased irritability and anger may lead to aggressive behavior in such cases.[9] Children with PTSD often experience guilt over what they should or could have done in a particular situation.[10] A number of cognitive problems have also been observed in traumatized youth. Children with PTSD frequently report difficulties in concentration, especially with regard to schoolwork.[11] They may develop memory problems, both in learning new material and in remembering previously acquired skills.[11]

Table 1
Proposed changes in the diagnostic criteria of PTSD in the DSM-V

DSM-IV Criteria	DSM-V Proposed Changes
A. The person has been exposed to a traumatic event in which both of the following were present: 1. The person experienced, witnessed, or was confronted with an event or events that involved actual or threatened death or serious injury, or a threat to the physical integrity of self or others. 2. The person's response involved intense fear, helplessness, or horror. Note: In children, this may be expressed instead by disorganized or agitated behavior.	A. The person was exposed to one or more of the following event(s): death or threatened death, actual or threatened serious injury, or actual or threatened sexual violation, in one or more of the following ways: 1. Experiencing the event(s) him/herself 2. Witnessing, in person, the event(s) as they occurred to others 3. Learning that the event(s) occurred to a close relative or close friend; in such cases, the actual or threatened death must have been violent or accidental 4. Experiencing repeated or extreme exposure to aversive details of the event(s) (eg, first responders collecting body parts; police officers repeatedly exposed to details of child abuse); this does not apply to exposure through electronic media, television, movies, or pictures, unless this exposure is work related. Criterion A2 eliminated.
B. The traumatic event is persistently reexperienced in one (or more) of the following ways: 1. Recurrent and intrusive distressing recollections of the event, including images, thoughts, or perceptions. Note: In young children, repetitive play may occur in which themes or aspects of the trauma are expressed. 2. Recurrent distressing dreams of the event. Note: In children, there may be frightening dreams without recognizable content. 3. Acting or feeling as if the traumatic event were recurring (includes a sense of reliving the experience, illusions, hallucinations, and dissociative flashback episodes, including those that occur on awakening or when intoxicated). Note: In young children, trauma-specific reenactment may occur. 4. Intense psychological distress at exposure to internal or external cues that symbolize or resemble an aspect of the traumatic event. 5. Physiological reactivity on exposure to internal or external cues that symbolize or resemble an aspect of the traumatic event.	B. Intrusion symptoms that are associated with the traumatic event(s) (that began after the traumatic event[s]), as evidenced by one or more of the following: 1. Spontaneous or cued recurrent, involuntary, and intrusive distressing memories of the traumatic event(s). Note: In children, repetitive play may occur in which themes or aspects of the traumatic event(s) are expressed. 2. Recurrent distressing dreams in which the content and/or affect of the dream is related to the event(s). Note: In children, there may be frightening dreams without recognizable content. 3. Dissociative reactions (eg, flashbacks) in which the individual feels or acts as if the traumatic event(s) were recurring (Such reactions may occur on a continuum, with the most extreme expression being a complete loss of awareness of present surroundings.) Note: In children, trauma-specific reenactment may occur in play. 4. Intense or prolonged psychological distress at exposure to internal or external cues that symbolize or resemble an aspect of the traumatic event(s). 5. Marked physiological reactions to reminders of the traumatic event(s).

(continued on next page)

Table 1 (continued)	
DSM-IV Criteria	**DSM-V Proposed Changes**
C. Persistent avoidance of stimuli associated with the trauma and numbing of general responsiveness (not present before the trauma), as indicated by three (or more) of the following: 1. Efforts to avoid thoughts, feelings, or conversations associated with the trauma. 2. Efforts to avoid activities, places, or people that arouse recollections of the trauma. 3. Inability to recall an important aspect of the trauma. 4. Markedly diminished interest or participation in significant activities 5. Feeling of detachment or estrangement from others. 6. Restricted range of affect (eg, unable to have loving feelings). 7. Sense of a foreshortened future (eg, does not expect to have a career, marriage, children, or a normal life span).	Avoidance and numbing as two separate clusters. C. Persistent avoidance of stimuli associated with the traumatic event(s) (that began after the traumatic event(s)), as evidenced by efforts to avoid one or more of the following: 1. Avoids internal reminders (thoughts, feelings, or physical sensations) that arouse recollections of the traumatic event(s). 2. Avoids external reminders (people, places, conversations, activities, objects, situations) that arouse recollections of the traumatic event(s). D. Negative alterations in cognitions and mood that are associated with the traumatic event(s) (that began or worsened after the traumatic event(s)), as evidenced by three or more of the following: Note: In children, as evidenced by two or more of the following: 1. Inability to remember an important aspect of the traumatic event(s) (typically dissociative amnesia; not due to head injury, alcohol, or drugs). 2. **Persistent and exaggerated negative expectations about one's self, others, or the world (eg, "I am bad," "no one can be trusted," "I've lost my soul forever," "my whole nervous system is permanently ruined," "the world is completely dangerous").** 3. **Persistent distorted blame of self or others about the cause or consequences of the traumatic event(s).** 4. **Pervasive negative emotional state, eg, fear, horror, anger, guilt, or shame** 5. Markedly diminished interest or participation in significant activities. 6. Feeling of detachment or estrangement from others. 7. Persistent inability to experience positive emotions (eg, unable to have loving feelings, psychic numbing).
D. Persistent symptoms of increased arousal (not present before the trauma), as indicated by two (or more) of the following: 1. Difficulty falling or staying asleep 2. Irritability or outbursts of anger 3. Difficulty concentrating 4. Hypervigilance 5. Exaggerated startle response.	E. Alterations in arousal and reactivity that are associated with the traumatic event(s) (that began or worsened after the traumatic event(s)), as evidenced by three or more of the following: Note: In children, as evidenced by two or more of the following: 1. Irritable or aggressive behavior 2. **Reckless or self-destructive behavior** 3. Hypervigilance 4. Exaggerated startle response 5. Problems with concentration 6. Sleep disturbance, eg, difficulty falling or staying asleep, or restless sleep.

From American Psychiatric Association. DSM-V Development. www.dsm5.org.

Table 2	
Single-event versus multiple-event trauma	
Single-Event Trauma	**Multiple-Event Trauma**
Acute, one-time event.	Chronic and/or many events.
Classic symptoms of PTSD.	Symptoms are more intrinsic (eg, numbing, denial, personality changes).
Normal development is resumed.	Normal development is inhibited.

SINGLE-EVENT VERSUS MULTIPLE-EVENT TRAUMA

The distinction between single-event and multiple-event trauma (**Table 2**) has been referred to by various designations such as *acute versus chronic trauma, type I versus type II trauma*, and *simple versus complex trauma*.[12,13]

Type I Trauma

Type I trauma has been defined as a single-event trauma that usually meets the DSM criteria for PTSD and is characterized by the classic symptom clusters of repetition, avoidance, and increased arousal.[12] In addition, young people with single-event trauma may experience symptoms of trauma including specific fears; regressive behavior; loss and grief reactions; cognitive–perceptual distortions; changed attitudes about the self, others, or the future; and reexperiencing of perceptual, affective, ideational, or somatic components of the trauma. This type of trauma generally occurs along with a background of normal development. Although impairments are expected in such areas as academic performance, maintenance of peer and family relationships and, at times, in daily living activities, individuals are expected to make a full recovery in functioning.[14]

Type II Trauma

Type II trauma refers to multiple-event trauma and often presents with the classic symptoms of PTSD. Repeated exposure can also lead to the development of more severe symptoms such as massive denial, psychic numbing, self-anesthesia, and personality problems.[12] In this type of trauma, the deviation from the normal trajectory of development occurs earlier and the chronic nature inhibits the trajectory from returning to its normal course. Herman (1992) coined the term "complex trauma" to describe the chronic effects of type II trauma and maintains that the much more diverse consequences of this type of trauma require a more comprehensive diagnosis than the PTSD normally observed in single-incident trauma.[13] In line with this, a new provisional diagnosis of Developmental Trauma Disorder has been proposed to better capture the experiences of youth with complex trauma such as community violence that is characterized by multiple events and/or prolonged exposure.[15] The premise of this proposed diagnosis is that multiple trauma exposures have consistent and predictable outcomes that impact on many domains of functioning. Specifically, impairment occurs in seven domains: attachment, biology, affect regulation, dissociation, behavioral regulation, cognition, and self-concept.[16] The diagnosis centers on triggered dysregulation in response to traumatic reminders, stimulus generalization, and behavioral attempts to avoid the reexperiencing of traumatic effects. Thus it is suggested that treatment should target three key areas: establishing safety and competence, dealing with traumatic reenactments, and integrating body and mind.[15]

Studies Comparing Single-Event and Multiple-Event Trauma

Several studies have compared single-event and multiple-event traumas in youth. In a sample of sexually abused children, common type I trauma symptoms included reexperiencing events such as nightmares, avoidant behaviors (ie, fear of certain places and situations, withdrawal), and increased hyperarousal (ie, difficulties with sleep and concentration, irritability).[17] Furthermore, it was found that those with type II trauma experienced more anxiety and depression, and had deficits in coping strategies related to daily and extreme stresses. They tended to have an enduring maladaptive attributional style (ie, learned helplessness); often experienced dissociative states (ie, massive denial and numbing); and frequently had excessive, poorly regulated responses to anger-provoking stimuli. In a sample of South African adolescents, those exposed to multiple-event traumas experienced more PTSD symptoms and depression than those exposed to single-event traumas.[18] Hagenaars and colleagues found that individuals with multiple-event trauma experienced more dissociation and shame compared to those with single-event trauma.[19]

LIMITATIONS OF THE CURRENT CLASSIFICATION OF PTSD

There has been much debate regarding whether the current diagnostic criteria, which rely on behavioral descriptions, adequately capture the presentation of PTSD in youth.[20,21] It has been proposed that PTSD should be conceptualized as a dimensional and continuous, rather than a categorical, clinical entity in youth.[22] Developmental variations may affect children's expression of PTSD symptoms and there has been much criticism that the current DSM criteria do not account for the developmental nature of the disorder.[23,24] For example, young children are limited in their verbal capacity and thus they may use other means to express themselves such as being fussy or having temper tantrums.[25,26] These types of behavior are often overlooked as symptoms of PTSD. Furthermore, relying on the current categorical model for diagnosis of PTSD may result in neglect of individuals who fall short of meeting the full criteria but may still be experiencing significant impairment. Several studies have found that subthreshold PTSD is similar to full-criteria PTSD in terms of its adverse effects.[27–29] This suggests that the diagnosis of PTSD in youth might be more accurate based on the intensity of symptoms related to functional impairment rather than number of symptoms met.

Another major limitation of behavioral descriptions is the lack of recognition that fear networks underlying the mechanism of PTSD may perpetuate other forms of anxiety. Young people with PTSD are at greater risk of the future development of anxiety disorders such as obsessive–compulsive disorder, generalized anxiety disorder, and phobias.[30] Thus, the diagnostic criteria ought to consider that PTSD may precede the development of other anxiety disorders and that there is potential for symptom overlap. Comorbidity rates for mood and anxiety disorders are as high as 80% in posttraumatic populations,[31] which suggests that these comorbidities may need to be included in the classification of PTSD.

ASSESSMENT OF PTSD

Numerous instruments exist for screening and diagnosis of childhood PTSD, as well as evaluation of trauma exposure and associated symptoms. Although a full review of all available measures is beyond the scope of this discussion, some of the most widely used instruments are described.

Clinician-Administered PTSD Scale for Children and Adolescents

The Clinician-Administered PTSD Scale for Children and Adolescents (CAPS-CA) is considered the gold standard in childhood PTSD assessment.[32] The CAPS-CA is used to assess PTSD and associated symptoms in youth ages 8 to 18. It consists of 36 questions based on a specific event that the child identifies as most distressing. The CAPS-CA evaluates current and lifetime diagnosis; frequency and intensity of symptoms; and functioning in social, developmental, and academic domains.

UCLA PTSD Reaction Index for DSM-IV

The UCLA PTSD Reaction Index for DSM-IV (PTSD-RI) is a self-report measure with child (ages 7–12), adolescent (ages 13–18), and parent versions.[33] The PTSD-RI contains 48 items that assess exposure to 26 types of traumatic events and evaluates DSM-IV PTSD criteria for the event that the child identifies as the most distressing. Youth rate symptoms on a 5-point Likert scale (0 = "none of the time" to 4 = "most of the time") and the parent version has an option of responding "don't know" to account for symptoms that the parent may not have observed. It also evaluates associated symptoms of guilt and fear of recurrence of the event.

Child PTSD Interview

This is a 95-item semistructured interview that assesses DSM-IV PTSD criteria and associated symptoms.[34] Questions are written at a third-grade level, though the measure has been used with younger children.[34] Each symptom item is rated as either being present or absent. There is also a parent form that assesses the same dimensions as the child form.

Children's PTSD Inventory

The Children's PTSD Inventory (CPTSDI) is a clinician-administered measure for children ages 6 to 18 based on the DSM-IV criteria for PTSD.[35] The child is first screened for exposure to various traumatic events by being asked if he or she ever experienced it or felt upset for not being able to stop it from happening. If an event meets the screening criteria, then symptoms are assessed in reference to the event. In addition to a PTSD total score, the CPTSDI also yields scores on five subscales: Situational Reactivity, Reexperiencing, Avoidance and Numbing, Increased Arousal, and Significant Impairment.

Child PTSD Symptom Scale

The Child PTSD Symptom Scale (CPSS) is a 26-item self-report that assesses PTSD and symptom severity in youth ages 8 to 18.[36] Items are rated on a 4-point Likert scale (0 = "not at all" to 3 = "5 or more times a week"). Functional impairment is also assessed (0 = "absent" and 1 = "present") but is not based on DSM-IV criteria. The measure provides total scores for symptom severity and severity of impairment, as well as scores for PTSD symptom clusters.

Trauma Symptom Checklist for Children

The Trauma Symptom Checklist for Children (TSCC) is a brief self-report for children ages 8 to 16 that screens for trauma exposure and posttraumatic stress but is not intended to be diagnostic.[37] It consists of two validity scales (over- and under-reporting) and six clinical scales (anxiety, depression, posttraumatic stress, sexual concerns, dissociation, and anger). Children are presented with thoughts, feelings, and behaviors related to traumatic events and are asked to mark how often they happened on a 4-point Likert scale (0 = "never" to 3 = "almost all the time").

Childhood Trauma Questionnaire

The Childhood Trauma Questionnaire (CTQ) is a 28-item, self-report that screens for a history of abuse and neglect in children over the age of 12.[38] It assesses exposure to five types of trauma: emotional, physical, and sexual abuse, and emotional and physical neglect. In addition, it contains a three-item minimization/denial scale for detecting under-reporting.

THE ROLE OF NEUROBIOLOGY IN UNDERSTANDING PTSD
The Role of Cortisol

The endocrine system, crucial to growth and development, is influenced by the hypothalamic–pituitary–adrenal (HPA) axis that secretes the hormone cortisol during times of stress to mobilize an individual into action.[39] Chronic periods of stress, however, may impair the HPA axis, resulting in dysregulation of cortisol secretion, which has been suggested as a marker for PTSD.[39] Neuroendocrine studies have yielded mixed results regarding the relationship of cortisol and pediatric PTSD. The majority of studies report high levels of cortisol to be indicative of PTSD.[40–46] On the other hand, lower cortisol levels have been associated with PTSD in youth exposed to an earthquake, sexually abused girls, and youth bereaved by the September 11, 2001 terrorist attacks.[47–49] Attempts have been made to clarify these inconsistencies. In a sample of youth exposed to interpersonal violence, a higher level of salivary cortisol was positively associated with PTSD among individuals with recent traumas (previous year), but in individuals with distal traumas (more than a year prior to assessment) the association was the opposite; the more PTSD symptoms the lower the levels of cortisol.[50] These findings highlight the importance of "time since trauma" when evaluating cortisol levels in PTSD. In addition, Pervandiou and colleagues found that, after a motor vehicle accident, children with PTSD initially had elevated evening salivary cortisol, but that levels normalized in the 6 months after the trauma.[51] Thus, the amount of time that has elapsed since the trauma may be a significant factor in the relationship between cortisol and PTSD.

It has also been suggested that significant variations exist in patterns of cortisol regulation among traumatized youth. For example, a study examining different trauma types found that high morning and afternoon cortisol levels were typical of youth with both physical and sexual abuse.[52] However, those with only physical abuse had lower levels of cortisol in the morning, with a smaller decrease in levels from morning to afternoon. In another study of youth exposed to interpersonal trauma, individuals with posttraumatic symptoms had sharper morning declines and higher evening cortisol levels than nontraumatized youth.[53]

It therefore appears that traumatized young people may display greater fluctuations in cortisol levels throughout the day. In conclusion, it appears that what were thought inconsistencies in the neuroendocrine literature might not be so, as the latest evidence suggests that cortisol levels in traumatized youth may be dependent upon trauma type and duration.

The Role of Neuroimaging

Neuroimaging (structural magnetic resonance imaging [MRI], functional MRI [fMRI], and magnetic resonance spectroscopy [MRS]) studies indicate that abnormalities in brain structure and function are also linked to the pathophysiology of PTSD. Three

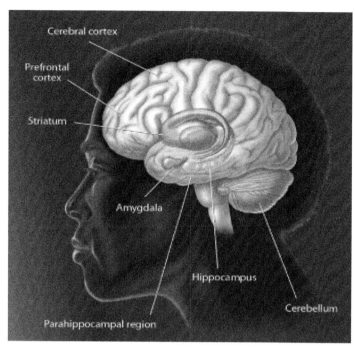

Fig. 1. The amygdala, PFC, and hippocampus. (*Retrieved from* www.sfn.org. Reprinted with permission from the Society for Neuroscience.)

brain regions that are particularly vulnerable to the effects of childhood trauma are the amygdala, prefrontal cortex, and hippocampus (**Fig. 1**).

The amygdala

The amygdala, which is part of the limbic system, is responsible for the processing of emotions and facilitates consolidation of emotional memories.[54] It plays an important role in assessing threatening stimuli.[55] Potentially dangerous stimuli are first processed in the thalamus and either directly or indirectly reach the amygdala where an emotional response will be developed with or without cognitive input. Pediatric neuroimaging studies suggest that there are no amygdala volume differences between traumatized youth with PTSD and healthy controls.[56–58] Although one study found a 5.1% reduction in amygdala volume of maltreated youth compared to healthy controls, when the results were corrected for total brain gray matter, no significant differences remained.[59] Numerous functional imaging studies, utilizing threatening words or faces, have identified hyper-responsiveness of the amygdala in traumatized adults.[60] A similar result was found in one study of trauma0tized youth. In youth exposed to interpersonal trauma, individuals with posttraumatic stress symptoms had increased amygdala activation in response to threatening facial expressions when compared with healthy controls.[61] In this study, 23 medication-naive youth with PTSD symptoms and 23 age- and gender-matched healthy controls underwent fMRI while viewing fearful, angry, sad, happy, and neutral expressions. The PTSD group had greater activation in the early part of the epoch, including greater early phase amygdala activation to angry faces compared to the controls.

The prefrontal cortex

The prefrontal cortex (PFC) is the anterior part of the frontal lobes involved in executive function. Executive function involves operations related to attention regulation, memory processing, and response inhibition.[62]

The majority of the pediatric PTSD structural neuroimaging studies indicate abnormalities of the PFC. Maltreated youth failed to show the typical frontal lobe asymmetry (right > left) seen in controls, mainly due to larger left frontal lobe volume.[59] A follow-up study on a similar sample found reduced white matter volume in the PFC although this was no longer significant after adjustment for intracranial volume.[58] In a study examining the relationship between cortisol and the PFC in children exposed to interpersonal trauma compared to healthy controls, youth with PTSD symptoms had decreased left ventral and left inferior prefrontal gray volumes.[63] In addition, elevated pre-bedtime cortisol levels were associated with reduced left ventral PFC gray volume. The results suggest a potential link between cortisol dysregulation and PFC volume. One study found no PFC differences between traumatized youth and healthy controls.[56]

Within the PFC lies the medial prefrontal cortex (mPFC) which, through its connection with the amygdala, is involved in emotional regulation and the processing of fear.[54] Impairments in this region have also been implicated in pediatric PTSD. De Bellis and colleagues used single-voxel proton MRS (proton MRS) to measure the relative concentration of N-acetylaspartate and creatine, markers of neural integrity, in the anterior cingulate, a specific area within the mPFC.[64] The lower concentration of N-acetylaspartate compared to creatine suggests abnormal neuronal metabolism. In an fMRI task assessing sustained attention and response inhibition, maltreated adolescents with PTSD showed relatively decreased activation of the middle frontal cortex, but increased activation in the mPFC when compared to healthy controls.[65] These findings suggest that traumatized youth with PTSD are not engaging core areas of the PFC to the same extent as healthy individuals.

The hippocampus

The hippocampus is a structure in the limbic system responsible for consolidation of memory.[66] Although adult trauma studies have consistently found reduced hippocampal volumes, findings from a meta-analytic study indicate that hippocampal volumes fail to differ in maltreated children relative to controls based on both cross-sectional child studies and one longitudinal study.[67] More recent longitudinal studies, however, have found differences in the hippocampus of traumatized youths. Carrion and colleagues found that severity of PTSD and cortisol levels, independently, predicted reductions in hippocampal volume over a 12- to 18-month interval.[66] During a memory retrieval task, youth with PTSD showed reduced activation of the right hippocampus compared to nontraumatized controls.[68] Severity of avoidance and emotional numbing symptoms correlated with reduced left hippocampal activation during retrieval in the PTSD group. The inconsistencies found in hippocampal volume between traumatized adults and traumatized youth may be due to developmental processes. A study of rats exposed to early stress and sacrificed at different ages showed that differences in the hippocampus emerged only after young adulthood.[69] Thus, trauma-induced glucocorticoid exposure may damage the hippocampus, but it is possible that decreased hippocampal volume occurs only in later development after chronic trauma exposure.

Neurobiological Studies Supplement Behavioral Studies

Although the behavioral descriptions of the DSM criteria are useful in providing a common language for PTSD, the aforementioned neurobiological studies may be used to supplement these descriptions to further enhance our understanding of the clinical profile of

PTSD. By facilitating the identification of biological risk factors and markers associated with childhood PTSD symptoms, these studies may aid in early detection of individuals susceptible to the disorder. In addition, such studies may help to clarify individual symptom presentations and identify markers associated with resiliency. The core areas targeted in current interventions match the impairments found in these studies. Thus, outcomes from these studies may inform treatment development and implementation. Furthermore, biological markers may assist in tailoring individualized treatments.

BRAIN PLASTICITY

Throughout childhood, brain development occurs during specific stages, termed critical periods, in which a specific brain structure is receptive to input from environmental stimuli and forms rapidly.[70] Experience shapes the extensive formation and organization of neural connections. Failure to form connections results in selective elimination or "pruning" of unused neurons.[71] As discussed, childhood trauma has been linked with alterations in the neurobiological systems involved in brain development and function.[72] Impairments in these systems have been associated with PTSD; however, the brain has the ability to generate new neurons and repair connections in response to novel experiences, thus reversing the negative effects of trauma.[73] The brain is at its most malleable during childhood, so early intervention can be critical. It has been suggested that the use of evidence-based psychotherapy to treat trauma symptoms may improve brain function by promoting cortical neurogenesis.[74]

Adult studies have proven the utility of psychotherapy in improving brain function for a variety of disorders. For example, in a sample of adults with PTSD secondary to a motor vehicle accident, cognitive behavioral therapy (CBT) compared to a waitlist control group was effective in reducing right hemisphere activation, which is associated with avoidance symptoms.[75] Another study found that before treatment, depressed individuals had reduced activation of the dorsolateral PFC, parietal cortex, and striatum but that group CBT helped restore activation of these regions to the same level as healthy controls.[76] Similar studies devoted to youth are now emerging that examine this same interface.[77] For example, a family-based intervention consisting of 22 weekly group sessions and 10 biweekly home visits was successful in altering cortisol levels in preschoolers at risk for conduct problems, compared to healthy controls.[78]

PSYCHOTHERAPEUTIC INTERVENTIONS
Single-Event Trauma

The most widely used treatment for single-event trauma has been CBT.[79] Many variations of trauma-specific CBT interventions exist. However, all share components summarized by the acronym PRACTICE[80]:

Psychoeducation
Relaxation and coping skills
Affective expression and modulation
Cognitive processing
Trauma narrative
In vivo exposure to trauma reminders
Conjoint child–parent sessions
Enhancing safety and future development

The majority of these treatments have been implemented as school-based group interventions.[79]

Table 3	
Single-trauma versus multiple-trauma interventions	
Single Trauma	**Multiple Trauma**
Trauma-focused cognitive behavioral therapy (TF-CBT) Website: TF-CBT.musc.edu	TF-CBT Website: TF-CBT.musc.edu
Multi-Modal Trauma Treatment Protocol (MMTT) Website: www.ccfh.nc.org	Trauma systems therapy (TST) Website: www.aboutourkids.org
Cognitive Behavioral Intervention for Trauma in Schools (CBITS) Website: www.cbitsprogram.org	CBITS Website: www.cbitsprogram.org
Trauma/grief focused therapy Website: www.nctsnet.org	Child–parent psychotherapy (CPP) Website: www.childtrauma.ucsf.edu
Eye movement desensitization and reprocessing (EMDR)	Parent–child interaction therapy (PCIT) Website: www.pcit.org
Play therapy	Intergenerational Trauma Treatment Model (ITTM) Website: theittm.com
Mind–body skills	Cue-centered treatment (CCT) Website: www.elsrp.stanford.edu

- **The Multi-Modal Trauma Treatment Protocol (MMTT)**, an intervention utilizing developmentally sensitive methods, has been successfully implemented in both school and community mental health settings.[81,82]
- **The Cognitive Behavioral Intervention for Trauma in Schools (CBITS)** is a 10-session treatment that has been shown to improve psychosocial functions in youth exposed to violence.[83]
- Several studies of earthquake survivors, victims of the Bosnian war, and victims of community violence, respectively, have found that **trauma/grief focused therapy** resulted in significant reduction of PTSD symptoms.[84–86]
- **Eye movement desensitization and reprocessing (EMDR)** has also been used for the treatment of single-trauma treatment. EMDR is believed to work by helping to reprocess traumatic memories through forming associations with positive information stored in other memory networks.[87] A randomized, controlled trial of EMDR in youth exposed to a natural disaster resulted in a decrease in trauma related memories and their associated symptoms.[87] Other modalities that have been employed in single-trauma intervention include play therapy and mind–body skills.[88,89]

Multiple-Event Trauma

Just as with single-trauma treatment, CBT-based approaches are the most common for multiple-trauma treatment (**Table 3**).

- **Trauma-focused cognitive behavioral therapy (TF-CBT)** combines both individual and parent-child sessions, and consists of the PRACTICE components described previously.[80] TF-CBT has proven efficacious in numerous randomized controlled trials for reduction of PTSD, depression, and other emotional and behavioral difficulties for both single-event and multiple-event traumas.[90–92] Trauma-focused CBT has also been proven to be superior to child-centered therapy in reducing PTSD symptoms, especially hyperarousal and avoidance in youth exposed to intimate partner violence.[93]

- **Trauma systems therapy (TST)** is an individual treatment addressing trauma-related symptoms and the environmental factors perpetuating them.[94] TST has demonstrated improvements in PTSD symptoms, environmental stability, and functioning.[94]

Other treatments for multiple-trauma include parent–child therapies based on psychodynamic theory:

- **Child–parent psychotherapy (CPP)** is a dyadic treatment in which play and other expressive methods are used to repair attachment and regulate traumatic stress.[95]
- **Parent–child interaction therapy (PCIT)** has also been found to improve social, emotional, and behavioral functioning through play therapy and live coaching aimed at improving attachment.[96]
- **The Intergenerational Trauma Treatment Model (ITTM)**, an intervention aimed at monitoring dysfunctional family patterns and altering them, has resulted in improvements in social functioning in traumatized children.[97]

A manual-based hybrid treatment protocol, **The Stanford Cue-Centered Therapy (CCT)**, combines elements of CBT, psychodynamic, expressive, and family therapies and augments these with education in classical conditioning and trauma-related reminders (cues), focusing on how these are linked to current behaviors, emotions, thoughts, and physiological reactions.[98] CCT emphasizes the importance of collaboration between the therapist, child, and caregiver to increase a sense of efficacy and empowerment through knowledge. CCT is divided into four parts:

1. Psychoeducation and coping strategies
2. Incorporating traumas into life narratives involving expression of emotions, filling of memory gaps, identification of cues, correction of cognitive distortions, and integration of the traumas into the greater context of the child's life
3. Gradual exposure to cues while replacing maladaptive behaviors with adaptive ones
4. Consolidation of learned skills.

The AACAP 2010 practice parameters consider trauma-focused therapies to be the first line of treatment for youth with PTSD.[99] The parameters state that these therapies ought to directly address the traumatic experience, include caregivers in the therapy process as agents of change, and focus not only on symptom improvement but also on enhancing functioning, resiliency, and developmental trajectories. The parameters state that, while studies on the efficacy of PTSD interventions are limited, CBT treatments and especially TF-CBT are the most widely researched and accepted. In addition, psychodynamic and family therapies are also suitable.[100] Psychotherapy is considered the first choice of treatment for childhood PTSD, however psychotropic medications such as selective serotonin reuptake inhibitors (SSRIs) may be warranted in situations of severe symptoms, comorbidity, or when psychotherapy is not effective. A review of all psychotropic medication that may be effective in treating childhood PTSD is beyond the scope of this article; however, Wilkinson and Carrion provide such a review.[100]

IMPLICATIONS FOR RESEARCH AND CLINICAL PRACTICE

There is a growing consensus that the current diagnostic model for PTSD is neither sensitive enough nor sufficient for traumatized youth. Research from multiple disciplines suggests a distinction between the manifestations of PTSD in children compared to adults. This research also hints at the crucial role for the accumulation of stressors throughout life in shaping PTSD. The duration of this process of stress accumulation, referred to as "allostatic load," may be more critical than chronological age of the individual for physiologic effects and symptom development. For example, an adult with no previous trauma history may present with a characteristically "young" response (ie, dissociation, high levels of diurnal cortisol, and no markers of stress on brain structures) whereas a child with chronic trauma may demonstrate more typical DSM symptoms, low levels of diurnal cortisol, and insidious effects of cortisol in key brain regions. The posttraumatic period is a dynamic process, exacerbated by the presence of traumamimetic cues and worsening when inadequate or no intervention is available. Vietnam combat veterans who developed PTSD have significantly more history of child maltreatment compared to veterans with no PTSD.[101] While PTSD was not manifested after child maltreatment, this previous history may have started a process that facilitated the development of the disorder after subsequent trauma.

Advancements in the field of neurobiology have aided assessment and treatment by identifying neurobiological risk factors and biomarkers for PTSD. Cortisol abnormalities have been associated with PTSD and appear to be affected by the type and duration of trauma. Impairments in certain brain regions, especially the amygdala, PFC, and hippocampus are also prominent in traumatized youth. Psychotherapeutic interventions have the potential to modulate these negative effects by providing new experiences that repair brain function and promote the growth of neural connections. Current evidence-based treatments employ such methods as emotional and behavioral regulation, cognitive processing, coping strategies, and exposure to traumatic reminders to target the areas identified from neurobiological studies. Future treatment outcome studies should integrate neuroscience with psychotherapy. Such studies will help identify which components of treatment are the most crucial for specific populations. These studies will also inform treatment outcome.

REFERENCES

1. Copleland-Linder N. Posttraumatic stress disorder. Pediatr Rev 2008;29:103–4.
2. Yule W. Post-traumatic stress disorder in children and adolescents. Int Rev Psychiatry 2001;13:194–200.
3. Gillespie CF, Phifer J, Bradley B, et al. Risk and resilience: genetic and environmental influences on development of the stress response. Depress Anxiety 2009;26:984–92.
4. Pynoos RS, Steinberg AM, Piacentini JC. Developmental psychopathology of childhood traumatic stress and intersection with anxiety disorders. Biol Psychiatry 1999; 46:1542–54.
5. American Psychiatric Association. Diagnostic and statistical manual of mental disorders. 3rd edition, text revision (3rd revised edition). Washington, DC: American Psychiatric Press; 1987.
6. American Psychiatric Association. Diagnostic and statistical manual of mental disorders. 4th Edition, text revision (4th revised edition). Washington, DC: American Psychiatric Press; 2000. p. 467.
7. American Psychiatric Association. Trauma and stressor related disorders. Available at: http://www.DSM5.org. Accessed October 14, 2011.

8. Dyregov A, Yule W. A review of PTSD in children. Child Adolescent Ment Health 2006;11:176–84.
9. Perrin S, Smith P, Yule W. Practitioner review: the assessment and treatment of post-traumatic stress disorder in children and adolescents. J Child Psychol Psychiatry 2000;41:277–89.
10. Kletter H, Weems CF, Carrion VG. Guilt and posttraumatic stress symptoms in child victims of interpersonal violence. Clin Child Psychol Psychiatry 2009;14:71–83.
11. Rust JO, Troupe PA. Relationships of treatment of child sexual abuse with school achievement and self-concept. J Early Adolesc 1991;11:420–9.
12. Terr LC. Childhood traumas: an outline and overview. Am J Psychiatry 1991;148: 10–20.
13. Herman JL. Complex PTSD: a syndrome in survivors of prolonged and repeated trauma. J Trauma Stress 1992;5:377–91.
14. McDermott BM. Child and youth emotional trauma: an explanatory model of adverse outcomes. Psychiatry Psychol Law 2004;11:269–79.
15. van der Kolk BA. Developmental trauma disorder: toward a rational diagnosis for children with complex trauma histories. Psychiatr Ann 2005;35:401–8.
16. van der Kolk BA, Roth S, Pelcovitz D, et al. Disorders of extreme stress: the empirical foundation of a complex adaptation to trauma. J Trauma Stress 2005;18:389–99.
17. Tremblay C, Hebert M, Piche C. Type I and type II posttraumatic stress disorder in sexually abused children. J Child Sex Abuse 2000;9:65–90.
18. Suliman S, Mkabile SG, Fincham DS, et al. Cumulative effect of multiple trauma on symptoms of posttraumatic stress disorder, anxiety, and depression in adolescents. Compr Psychiatry 2009;50:121–7.
19. Hagenaars MA, Fisch I, van Minnen A. The effect of trauma onset and frequency on PTSD-associated symptoms. J Affect Disord 2011;132:192–9.
20. Scheeringa MS, Zeanah CH, Myers L, et al. New findings on alternative criteria for PTSD in preschool children. J Am Acad Child Adolesc Psychiatry 2003;42:561–70.
21. American Academy of Child and Adolescent Psychiatry. Practice parameters for the assessment and treatment of children and adolescents with posttraumatic stress disorder. J Am Acad Child Adolesc Psychiatry 1998;37:4s–26s.
22. Broman-Fulks JJ, Ruggerio KJ, Green BA, et al. The latent structure of PTSD among adolescents. J Trauma Stress 2009;22:146–52.
23. Pynoos RS, Steinberg AM, Layne CM, et al. DSM-V PTSD diagnostic criteria for children and adolescents: a developmental perspective and recommendations. J Trauma Stress 2009;22:391–8.
24. Salmon K, Bryant RA. Posttraumatic stress disorder in children: the influence of developmental factors. Clin Psychol Rev 2002;22:163–88.
25. Scheeringa MS, Zeanah CH, Myers L, et al. Predictive validity in a prospective follow-up of PTSD in preschool children. J Am Acad Child Adolesc Psychiatry 2005;44:899–906.
26. Langeland W, Olff M. Psychobiology of posttraumatic stress disorder in pediatric injury patients: a review of the literature. Neurosci Behav Rev 2008;32:161–74.
27. Corapcioglu A, Tural U, Yargic I, et al. Subthreshold post traumatic stress disorder in the survivors of Marmara earthquake. Primary Care Psychiatry 2004;9:137–43.
28. Zhang W, Ross J, Davidson JRT. Posttraumatic stress disorder in callers to the Anxiety Disorders Association of America. Depress Anxiety 2004;19:96–104.
29. Carrion VG, Weems CF, Ray R, et al. Toward an empirical definition of pediatric PTSD: the phenomenology of PTSD symptoms in youth. J Am Acad Child Adolesc Psychiatry 2002;41:166–73.

30. Cortes AM, Saltzman KM, Weems CF, et al. Development of anxiety disorders in a traumatized pediatric population: a preliminary longitudinal evaluation. Child Abuse Negl 2005;29:905–14.
31. Pfefferbaum B. Posttraumatic stress disorder in children: a review of the past 10 years. J Am Acad Child Adolesc Psychiatry 1997;36:1503–11.
32. Nader K, Kriegler JA, Blake DD, et al. Clinician administered PTSD scale, child and adolescent version. White River Junction (VT): National Center for PTSD; 1996.
33. Pynoos R, Rodriguez N, Steinberg A, et al. UCLA PTSD Index for DSM-IV. Los Angeles (CA): UCLA Trauma Psychiatry Service; 1998.
34. Fletcher K. Psychometric review of the Childhood PTSD Interview. In: Stamm BH, editor. Measurement of stress, trauma, and adaptation. Lutherville (MD): Sidran Press; 1996. p. 87–9.
35. Saigh P, Yaski AE, Oberfield RA, et al. The Children's PTSD Inventory: development and reliability. J Trauma Stress 2000;30:369–80.
36. Foa EB, Johnson KM, Feeny NC, et al. The Child PTSD Symptom Scale: a preliminary examination of its psychometric properties. J Clin Child Psychol 2001;30: 376–84.
37. Briere J. Trauma Symptom Checklist for Children (TSCC), professional manual. Odessa (FL): Psychological Assessment Resources; 1996.
38. Bernstein DP, Fink L, Handelsman L, et al. Initial reliability and validity of a new retrospective measure of child abuse and neglect. Am J Psychiatr 1994;151: 1132–6.
39. Pervanidou P. Biology of post-traumatic stress disorder in childhood and adolescence. J Neuroendocrinol 2008;20:632–8.
40. De Bellis MD, Baum AS, Birmaher B, et al. Developmental traumatology: I. biological stress systems. Biol Psychiatry 1999;45:1259–70.
41. Carrion VG, Weems CF, Ray RD, et al. Diurnal salivary cortisol in pediatric posttraumatic stress disorder. Biol Psychiatry 2002;51:575–82.
42. Gunnar MR, Morrison SJ, Chisholm K, et al. Salivary cortisol levels in children adopted from Romanian orphanages. Dev Psychopathol 2001;13:611–28.
43. Bevans K, Cerbone AB, Overstreet S. The interactive effects of elevated mid-afternoon cortisol and trauma history on PTSD symptoms in children: a preliminary study. Psychoneuroendocrinology 2009;34:1582–5.
44. Hart J, Gunnar M, Cicchetti D. Altered neuroendocrine activity in maltreated children related to symptoms of depression. Dev Psychopathol 1996;8:201–14.
45. Kolaitis G, Giannakopoulos G, Liakopoulou M, et al. Predicting pediatric posttraumatic stress disorder after road traffic accidents: the role of parental psychopathology. J Trauma Stress 2011;24:414–21.
46. Suglia SF, Staudenmayer J, Cohen S, et al. Posttraumatic stress symptoms related to community violence and children's diurnal cortisol response in an urban community-dwelling sample. Int J Behav Med 2010;17:43–50.
47. Goenjian AK, Yehuda R, Pynoos RS, et al. Basal cortisol, dexamethasone suppression of cortisol, and MHPG in adolescents after the 1988 earthquake in Armenia. Am J Psychiatry 1996;153:929–34.
48. King JA, Mandansky D, King S, et al. Early sexual abuse and low cortisol. Psychiatry Clin Neurosci 2001;55:71–4.
49. Pfeffer CR, Alternus M, Heo M, et al. Salivary cortisol and psychopathology in children bereaved by the September 11, 2001 terror attacks. Biol Psychiatry 2007; 61:957–65.
50. Weems CF, Carrion VG. The association between PTSD symptoms and salivary cortisol in youth: the role of time since the trauma. J Trauma Stress 2007;20:903–7.

51. Pervanidou P, Kolaitis G, Charitaki S, et al. The natural history of neuroendocrine changes in pediatric posttraumatic stress disorder (PTSD) after motor vehicle accidents: progressive divergence of noradrenaline and cortisol concentrations over time. Biol Psychiatry 2007;62:1095–102.

52. Ciccheti D, Rogosch FA. Diverse patterns of neuroendocrine activity in maltreated children. Dev Psychopathol 2001;13:677–93.

53. Weems CF, Carrión VG. Brief report: diurnal salivary cortisol in youth—clarifying the nature of posttraumatic stress dysregulation. J Pediatr Psychol 2009;34:389–95.

54. Pare D, Collins DR, Pelletier JG. Amygdala oscillations and the consolidation of emotional memories. Trends Cogn Sci 2002;6:306–14.

55. Shin LM, Wright CI, Cannistraro PA, et al. A functional magnetic resonance imaging study of amygdala and medial prefrontal cortex responses to overtly presented fearful faces in posttraumatic stress disorder. Arch Gen Psychiatry 2005;62:273–81.

56. De Bellis MD, Keshavan MS, Clark DB, et al. Developmental traumatology: II. Brain development. Biol Psychiatry 1999;45:1271–84.

57. De Bellis MD, Hall J, Boring AM, et al. A pilot longitudinal study of hippocampal volumes in pediatric maltreatment-related posttraumatic stress disorder. Biol Psychiatry 2001;50:305–9.

58. De Bellis MD, Keshavan MS, Shifflet H, et al. Brain structures in pediatric maltreatment-related posttraumatic stress disorder: a sociodemographically matched study. Biol Psychiatry 2002;52:1066–78.

59. Carrion VG, Weems CF, Eliez S, et al. Attenuation of frontal asymmetry in pediatric posttraumatic stress disorder. Biol Psychiatry 2001;50:943–51.

60. Shin LM, Liberzon I. The neurocircuitry of fear, stress, and anxiety disorders. Neuropsychopharmacology 2010;35:169–91.

61. Garrett A, Carrion VG, Kletter H, et al. Brain activation to facial expressions in youth with PTSD symptoms. Depress Anxiety 2012;29:449–59.

62. Kesler SR, Kent JS, O'Hara R. Prefrontal cortex and executive function impairments in primary breast cancer. Arch Neurol 2011;68:1447–53.

63. Carrion VG, Weems CF, Richert K, et al. Decreased prefrontal cortical volume associated with increased bedtime cortisol in traumatized youth. Biol Psychiatry 2010;68:491–3.

64. De Bellis MD, Keshavan MS, Spencer S, et al. N-Acetylaspartate concentration in the anterior cingulate of maltreated children and adolescents with PTSD. Am J Psychiatry 2000;157:1175–7.

65. Carrion VG, Garrett A, Menon V, et al. Posttraumatic stress symptoms and brain function during a response-inhibition task: an fMRI study in youth. Depress Anxiety 2008;25:514–26.

66. Carrion VG, Weems CF, Reiss AL. Stress predicts brain changes in children: a pilot longitudinal study on youth stress, posttraumatic stress disorder, and the hippocampus. Pediatrics 2007;119:509–16.

67. Woon FL, Hedges DW. Hippocampal and amygdala volumes in children and adults with childhood maltreatment-related posttraumatic stress disorder: a meta-analysis. Hippocampus 2008;18:729–36.

68. Carrion VG, Haas BW, Garrett A, et al. Reduced hippocampal activity in youth with posttraumatic stress symptoms: an fMRI study. J Pediatr Psychol 2010;35:559–69.

69. Andersen SL, Teicher MH. Delayed effects of early stress on hippocampal development. Neuropsychopharmacology 2004;29:1988–93.

70. Pennington BF. How neuropsychology informs our understanding of developmental disorders. J Child Psychol Psychiatry 2009;50:72–8.

71. Sowell ER, Trauner DA, Gamst AJ, et al. Development of cortical and subcortical brain structures in childhood and adolescence: a structural MRI study. Dev Med Child Neurol 2002;44:4–16.
72. De Bellis MD. The psychobiology of neglect. Child Maltreat 2005;10:150–72.
73. Cicchetti D, Cannon TD. Neurodevelopmental processes in the ontogenesis and epigenesis of psychopathology. Dev Psychopathol 1999;11:375–93.
74. De Bellis MD, Thomas LA. Biologic findings of post-traumatic stress disorder and child maltreatment. Curr Psychiatry Rep 2003;5:108–17.
75. Rabe S, Zoellner T, Beauducel A, et al. Changes in brain electrical activity after cognitive behavioral therapy for posttraumatic stress disorder in patients injured in motor vehicle accidents. Psychosom Med 2008;70:13–9.
76. Okamoto Y, Kinoshita A, Onoda K, et al. Functional brain basis of cognition in major depression. Jpn J Psychonomic Sci 2006;25:237–43.
77. Kay J. Toward a neurobiology of child psychotherapy. J Loss Trauma 2009;14:287–303.
78. Brotman LM, Gouley KK, Huang KY, et al. Effects of a psychosocial family-based preventive intervention on cortisol response to a social challenge in preschoolers at high risk for antisocial behavior. Arch Gen Psychiatry 2007;64:172–9.
79. Adler-Nevo G, Manassis K. Psychosocial treatment of pediatric posttraumatic stress disorder: the neglected field of single-incident trauma. Depress Anxiety 2005;22:177–89.
80. Cohen JA, Mannarino AP. Trauma-focused cognitive behavioural therapy for children and parents. Child Adolesc Ment Health 2008;13:158–62.
81. Amaya-Jackson L, Reynolds V, Murray MC, et al. Cognitive-behavioral treatment for pediatric posttraumatic stress disorder: protocol and application in school and community settings. Cogn Behav Pract 2003;10:204–13.
82. March J, Amaya-Jackson L, Murray M, et al. Cognitive behavioral psychotherapy for children and adolescents with post-traumatic stress disorder following a single incident stressor. J Am Acad Child Adolesc Psychiatry 1998;37:585–93.
83. Stein BD, Jaycox LH, Kataoka SH, et al. A mental health intervention for schoolchildren exposed to violence: a randomized controlled trial. JAMA 2003;290:603–11.
84. Goenjian AK, Karayan I, Pynoos RS, et al. Outcome of psychotherapy among early adolescents after trauma. Am J Psychiatry 1997;154:536–42.
85. Layne CM, Pynoos RS, Saltzman WR, et al. Trauma/grief focused group psychotherapy: school-based postwar intervention with traumatized Bosnian adolescents. Group Dyn Theor Res Pract 2001;5:277–90.
86. Saltzman RW, Layne CM, Pynoos RS, et al. Trauma- and grief-focused intervention for adolescents exposed to community violence: results of a school-based screening and group treatment protocol. Group Dyn Theor Res Pract 2001;5:291–303.
87. Chemtob CM, Nakashima J, Carlson JG. Brief treatment for elementary school children with disaster-related posttraumatic stress disorder: a field study. J Clin Psychol 2002;58:99–112.
88. Chemtob C, Nakashima JP, Hamada RS. Psychosocial intervention for postdisaster trauma symptoms in elementary school children: a controlled community field study. Arch Pediatr Adolesc Med 2002;156:211–6.
89. Staples JK, Abdel A, Jamil A, et al. Mind-body skills groups for posttraumatic stress disorder and depression symptoms in Palestinian children and adolescents in Gaza. Int J Stress Manag 2011;18:246–62.
90. Cohen JA, Deblinger E, Mannarino AP, et al. A multisite, randomized controlled trial for children with sexual abuse-related PTSD symptoms. J Am Acad Child Adolesc Psychiatry 2004;43:393–402.

91. Cohen JA, Mannarino AP, Knudsen K. Treating sexually abused children: 1 year follow-up of a randomized controlled trial. Child Abuse Negl 2005;29:135–45.
92. Scheeringa MS, Weems CF, Cohen JA, et al. Trauma-focused cognitive-behavioral therapy for posttraumatic stress disorder in three to six year-old children; a randomized clinical trial. J Child Psychol Psychiatry 2011;52:853–60.
93. Cohen JA, Mannarino AP, Iyengar S. Community treatment of posttraumatic stress disorder for children exposed to intimate partner violence. Arch Pediatr Adolesc Med 2011;165:16–21.
94. Saxe GN, Ellis H, Fogler J, et al. Comprehensive care for traumatized children: an open trial examines treatment using trauma systems therapy. Psychiatr Ann 2005; 53:443–8.
95. Lieberman AF, Van Horn PJ, Ghosh Ippen C. Toward evidence-based treatment: child–parent psychotherapy with preschoolers exposed to marital violence. J Am Acad Child Adolesc Psychiatry 2011;44:1241–8.
96. Thomas R, Zimmer-Gembeck MJ. Accumulating evidence for parent-child interaction therapy in the prevention of child maltreatment. Child Dev 2011;82:177–92.
97. Copping VE, Warling DL, Benner DG, et al. A child trauma treatment pilot study. J Child Fam Stud 2001;10:467–75.
98. Carrion VG, Hull K. Treatment manual for trauma-exposed youth: case studies. Clin Child Psychol Psychiatry 2010;15:27–38.
99. American Academy of Child and Adolescent Psychiatry (AACAP). Practice parameter for the assessment and treatment of children and adolescents with posttraumatic stress disorder. J Am Acad Child Adolesc Psychiatry 2010;49:414–30.
100. Wilkinson J, Carrion VG. When and how to use psychopharmacology for pediatric PTSD. Curr Psychopharmacol, in press.
101. Bremner JD, Southwick SM, Johnson DR, et al. Childhood physical abuse and combat-related posttraumatic stress disorder in Vietnam veterans. Am J Psychiatr 1993;150:235–9.

Panic Disorder and School Refusal

Bryce Hella, PhD[a], Gail A. Bernstein, MD[b],*

KEYWORDS

- Panic disorder • School refusal • Cognitive behavior therapy
- Selective serotonin reuptake inhibitors • Agoraphobia

KEY POINTS

- Adolescents receiving panic control treatment for adolescents reported that psychoeducation and cognitive restructuring were the most helpful components of treatment.
- School refusal is a symptom associated with several psychiatric disorders, separation anxiety disorder among the most common *Diagnostic and Statistical Manual of Mental Disorders, Fifth Edition* diagnosis; however, between 20% to 30% of school-refusing children do not meet criteria for any psychiatric diagnosis.
- Important questions for further work in school refusal include whether avoidance behavior remits after formal education or whether school-refusing children miss a significant amount of work in adulthood.
- Children and adolescents will benefit from the clinician, parents, and school professionals joining together as a multidisciplinary team to successfully implement interventions for school refusal.

INTRODUCTION

The treatment of panic disorder, agoraphobia, and school refusal in children and adolescents has been increasingly studied in recent years. Whereas our knowledge about the presentation, causes, and treatment of panic disorder and agoraphobia in adults has grown, the depth of our knowledge about similar topics in children and adolescents continues to be relatively limited. Although a considerable amount of

Disclosures for Dr Bernstein for the past 3 years: National Institute on Alcohol Abuse and Alcoholism (salary), National Institute of Mental Health (salary), University of Minnesota Academic Health Center (research funding), Minnesota Medical Foundation (research funding), Office of the Dean of the Graduate School at the University of Minnesota (research funding), Springer Publishing (book royalties), and Madison Institute of Medicine (honorarium for presentation).
[a] Susan Myket, PhD, and Associates, 1415 Bond Street, Suite 127, Naperville, IL 60563, USA;
[b] Program in Child and Adolescent Anxiety and Mood Disorders, Division of Child and Adolescent Psychiatry, University of Minnesota Medical School, F256/2B West, 2450 Riverside Avenue Minneapolis, MN 55454, USA
* Corresponding author.
E-mail address: berns001@umn.edu

Child Adolesc Psychiatric Clin N Am 21 (2012) 593–606
http://dx.doi.org/10.1016/j.chc.2012.05.012
1056-4993/12/$ – see front matter © 2012 Elsevier Inc. All rights reserved.

childpsych.theclinics.com

Table 1
DSM-IV-TR criteria for panic disorder (with and without agoraphobia) compared with proposed changes for DSM-V

DSM-IV-TR Criteria:	Proposed DSM-V Changes[a]:

A. Both (1) and (2):
    (1) Recurrent unexpected panic attacks
    (2) At least one of the attacks has been followed by 1 month (or more) of one (or more) of the following:
        a. Persistent concern about having additional attacks.
        b. Worry about the implications of the attack or its consequences (eg, losing control, having a heart attack, "going crazy").
        c. A significant change in behavior related to the attacks.
	A. Recurrent unexpected panic attacks
	    Note: accompanying text will state that cued as well as uncued panic attacks may occur.
	
	B. At least one of the attacks has been followed by 1 month (or more) of the following:
	    1. Persistent concern about having more attacks or their implications (eg, losing control, having a heart attack, "going crazy").
	    2. Significant, maladaptive behavioral changes related to the attacks (eg, agoraphobic avoidance).

B. Presence of agoraphobia (for panic disorder with agoraphobia) or absence of agoraphobia (for panic disorder without agoraphobia).	
C. The panic attacks are not due to the direct physiologic effects of a substance (eg, a drug of abuse, a medication) or a general medical condition (eg, hyperthyroidism).	C. Add cardiopulmonary disorders as another example of an exclusionary medical condition.
D. The panic attacks are not better accounted for by another mental disorder, such as social phobia, specific phobia, obsessive-compulsive disorder, posttraumatic stress disorder, or separation anxiety disorder.	D. Change wording from "not better accounted for" to "not restricted to."

[a] Proposed in Craske and colleagues.[2]
Source: DSM-IV-TR criteria reprinted from American Psychiatric Association. Diagnostic and statistical manual of mental disorders. 4th edition, text revision. Washington (DC): American Psychiatric Association; 2000. p. 211–2. Used with permission. © 2000 American Psychiatric Association.

research exists on school refusal, the findings suggest that current interventions fail to significantly improve school attendance in a substantial number of youths. This article discusses what has been found in the research on child and adolescent panic disorder, agoraphobia, and school refusal. Limitations and future directions are discussed as well as proposed changes to the *Diagnostic and Statistical Manual of Mental Disorders, Fifth Edition* (DSM-V).

PANIC DISORDER AND AGORAPHOBIA

In the *Diagnostic and Statistical Manual of Mental Disorders, Fourth Edition, Text Revision* (DSM-IV-TR) nosology, panic attacks are not considered a diagnostic category.[1] Rather, panic attacks are defined as occurring within the context of panic disorder with or without agoraphobia (**Table 1**). A panic attack is an episode of intense anxiety or panic that peaks within 10 minutes. Four or more distinct physiologic or psychological symptoms are required in order to be considered a panic attack.[1]

Physiologic Symptoms of Panic Attack		Psychological Symptoms of Panic Attack
Heart racing	Chest pain	Fear of dying
Sweating	Nausea	Fear of losing control
Trembling	Dizziness	Derealization/depersonalization
Shortness of breath	Numbness/tingling	
Feeling of choking	Chills/hot flushes	

Data from American Psychiatric Association. Diagnostic Criteria from DSM-IV-TR. Arlington (VA): American Psychiatric Association; 2000.

Agoraphobia is defined as anxiety about being in places where a person may not be able to leave or help may not be available if a panic attack or "paniclike" symptoms occur.[1] These symptoms lead to avoidance of situations (eg, riding on a bus, crossing a bridge), restriction of travel, or insistence on traveling with a companion.

Panic disorder and agoraphobia are relatively rare in children and adolescents. Less than 1% of children and 2% to 4% of adolescents meet criteria for panic disorder.[3] Twelve-month prevalence estimates for panic disorder have been reported to be below 1% in 8- to 15-year-olds.[4] Even when examining clinic-referred youth with other psychiatric disorders (n = 1576; ages 5 to 18), only 2% met criteria for panic disorder.[5] Panic symptoms, however, are reported to be more common than panic disorder. In a community sample of youths and young adults (ages 14 to 24), 13% of the sample reported having a "spell" that resembled a panic attack.[6] Moreover, 4% had experienced a DSM-IV panic attack without the development of panic disorder. Hayward and colleagues[7] studied 754 sixth- and seventh-grade girls and found an association between panic attacks and pubertal stage, independent of age. Overall, 5% of the sample reported at least one four-symptom panic attack. None of the subjects at Tanner stage 1 or 2 reported a history of panic attacks. However, rates of panic attacks were greater with increase in sexual maturity to a rate of 8% for girls at Tanner stage 5. This result suggests that biological factors play a role in the onset of panic attacks. Taken together, results suggest that panic attacks increase over the course of puberty. The most common panic symptoms reported in a sample of adolescents with panic disorder were heart palpitations, chest pains, feeling faint, and trembling.[5] These predominant symptoms are similar to those reported in studies of adults with panic disorder.[2]

Three DSM-IV-TR diagnoses include the term *agoraphobia*. A person can meet criteria for panic disorder with agoraphobia, panic disorder without agoraphobia, and agoraphobia without history of panic disorder. Compared with prevalence rates for panic disorder without agoraphobia, far fewer adolescents meet criteria for panic disorder with agoraphobia (ie, > 1%).[6] On the other hand, agoraphobia without history of panic disorder may occur in as many as 8% of 14- to 24-year-olds without comorbid panic disorder or a history of panic attacks.[8] It has been suggested that the incidence of agoraphobia without panic attacks has been underreported because people with agoraphobia without history of panic disorder are less likely to present for treatment.[9]

The age of onset for panic disorder has been reported to be after puberty,[6] which is later than the usual age of onset of other anxiety disorders in youths.[10] Females are more likely than males to be diagnosed with panic disorder without agoraphobia as well as panic disorder with agoraphobia.[6] Several early risk factors have been found to be associated with panic attacks in adolescents. A parental history of panic disorder and negative affect in childhood are predictors of panic attacks in adolescents.[11] Separation anxiety disorder in childhood has also been associated with later panic disorder.[2,11,12] Another risk factor is history of chronic illness in a parent.[11] It is hypothesized that adolescents who develop panic attacks may develop a learned hypersensitivity to physiologic symptoms because they have witnessed a parent struggle with chronic illness.[11]

In spite of the relatively low prevalence rates of panic disorder (with and without agoraphobia) in children and adolescents, youths with panic disorder are likely to have or to develop comorbid psychiatric disorders. In fact, 48% of 14- to 24-year-olds (n = 42) who reported having a panic attack met criteria for a non–panic-related disorder.[5] In a study of adolescents with panic disorder who were referred to a mood disorders clinic, mood disorders and other anxiety disorders were most commonly comorbid with panic disorder.[5] Results were confounded, however, by the fact that the adolescents in the study were referred to a mood disorder clinic, potentially inflating the likelihood of having a comorbid mood disorder. Adolescents and young adults with panic disorder are at increased risk of suicidal behavior and attempts, even after controlling for comorbid psychiatric disorders and life stressors.[13,14] Effective treatments for panic disorder are important, given the risks associated with having panic disorder.

Biological Factors in Panic Disorder

Individuals with anxiety disorders, particularly panic disorder, exhibit interoceptive sensitivity, which is increased sensitivity to somatic sensations.[15] This is commonly related to awareness of stimuli from the cardiac system.[15] It is believed that the increased sensitivity to internal bodily cues is a precursor to dysfunctional cognitive appraisal of the bodily sensations and a bias toward danger-related and catastrophic thinking associated with panic (eg, "I'm having a heart attack"). Conditioned anxiety responses to interoceptive stimuli are thought to play a key role in the maintenance of panic symptoms.[16]

Several brain structures have been implicated in panic attacks and panic disorder. Perhaps most notably is the amygdala, which has been found to be a major structure implicated in classically conditioned fear.[17] The hippocampus, hypothalamus, thalamus, and medial prefrontal cortex have also been hypothesized as important structures in panic attacks. Gorman and colleagues[17] suggest that people with panic disorder have conditioned sensitivity to somatic discomfort, and the addition of these somatic sensations causes activation of the panic pathways in the brain. During functional magnetic resonance imaging, adults with panic disorder (n = 6) compared with healthy controls (n = 8) exhibited significantly greater activation in the posterior cingulate cortex and the dorsolateral prefrontal cortex when shown threat-related words.[18]

DSM-V Changes to Panic Attacks, Panic Disorder, and Agoraphobia

Changes to the conceptualization of psychiatric disorders have been suggested with the upcoming release of the DSM-V in 2013. Perhaps the most significant proposed change is to examine symptoms using a dimensional rather than a categorical assessment system.[9] The goal of the dimensional system would be to provide a more complete description of a person's symptoms, regardless of whether the symptoms are associated with his or her primary disorder. Moreover, DSM-V revisions will increase clinicians' ability to track treatment progress by implementing severity ratings for each of the patient's symptoms. There is some indication that panic attacks will be a diagnostic specifier or dimensional rating that can be associated with other anxiety, mood, eating, psychotic, and substance use disorders in DSM-V.[2] For example, an individual could receive a diagnosis of major depressive disorder with panic attacks. It is important to note that such changes will not be solidified until the release of the new diagnostic manual and currently represent proposed changes.

In addition to the dimensional changes that have been proposed, changes to the descriptions of panic attacks, panic disorder, and agoraphobia have been suggested. The primary criteria are not likely to change substantially. All panic attack symptoms will likely be retained, as will the number of symptoms required to meet criteria for a panic attack. The idea that panic attacks are "uncued" (ie, happen without known triggers or activating events) will likely remain a defining criterion of panic disorder. However, it is likely that the accompanying text in DSM-V will clarify that persons with panic disorder sometimes experience cued panic attacks, as well as uncued panic attacks.[2] Other proposed changes include combining "persistent concern about having additional attacks" and "worry about the implications of the attack" into one symptom, because they are commonly endorsed together and may not represent separate diagnostic constructs.[2] In addition, it has been suggested that the specifiers "presence of agoraphobia" or "absence of agoraphobia" be removed in favor of a statement that maladaptive behavioral changes such as agoraphobia may be associated with panic attacks.[2] Finally, minor changes to criteria C and D are suggested. Proposed changes for DSM-V are outlined in **Table 1**.[2]

Overall, changes in the DSM-V will attempt to be more developmentally sensitive when symptoms of disorders present differently across the life span. There are some data to indicate that younger adolescents (ages 14–17) may have fewer concerns about "implications" of having future panic attacks than older adolescents and young adults (ages 18–24).[2] However, robust developmental differences have not been established to date; therefore, differences in criteria based on age or developmental stage are not likely to be included for panic disorder.[2]

The definition of agoraphobia has changed throughout different versions of the DSM. Initially, agoraphobia was thought to be akin to a specific phobia of public places until the release of the *Diagnostic and Statistical Manual of Mental Disorders, Third Edition* (DSM-III). At that time, agoraphobia began to be viewed as a "classically conditioned response to situations in which a panic attack has occurred."[8] It has been assumed that the relationship between panic attacks and agoraphobia is that a person first experiences panic or panic attacks, which then progress to agoraphobia. In the revisions made between DSM-III and DSM-IV-TR, agoraphobia continued to be diagnosed only as it relates to panic disorder or panic attacks, and the idea that the two are strongly related was further solidified.[1] Agoraphobia without history of panic disorder is currently diagnosed when the fear of certain situations or places is primarily related to fear of having panic attacks. In other words, a person cannot meet criteria for agoraphobia unless he/she has a primary concern about panic attacks. This diagnosis differs from the *International Statistical Classification of Diseases and Related Health Problems, 10th Revision* diagnosis of agoraphobia, which does not require that agoraphobia occur within the context of panic disorder or paniclike symptoms.[19]

In fact, data suggest that agoraphobia might occur outside of panic disorder.[20] In adults, epidemiologic data suggest that 25% to 85% of people who report agoraphobia do not have co-occurring panic attacks, providing support for this idea.[20] The wide range of prevalence rates reportedly is due to different criteria used in research studies. What is more, a proportion of patients have reported that agoraphobic avoidance preceded panic symptoms, calling into question the temporal association between panic and agoraphobia. Wittchen and colleagues[20] suggest that current criteria limit clinical utility of the diagnoses by unnecessarily restricting agoraphobia to only occurring in the context of panic. They propose that agoraphobia be considered a completely separate entity from panic disorder in DSM-V, and they believe this distinction will help ascertain the true incidence of agoraphobia outside the context of panic attack or paniclike symptoms.

Treatment for Panic Disorder

Psychosocial treatment

Practice parameters for treatment of anxiety disorders in children and adolescents have been outlined elsewhere.[21] Cognitive behavior therapy (CBT) is the primary psychosocial treatment approach for anxiety disorders in adolescents. Specific components of CBT for panic disorder have included educating parents, teaching coping strategies, training in physiologic symptom reduction, challenging negative cognitions, interoceptive exposure, and preventing relapse.

Pincus and colleagues[22] conducted a randomized controlled treatment study of adolescents with panic disorder. The researchers compared 13 adolescents ages 14 to 17 who received panic control treatment for adolescents (PCT-A)[23] with 13 adolescents who engaged in self-monitoring and 20- to 30-minute check-ins with a therapist. Both interventions lasted 11 to 12 weeks. The PCT-A condition consisted of three core components of adult panic control treatment:

1. Restructuring cognitions regarding misinterpretations of physiologic symptoms
2. Breathing retraining
3. Extinguishing the conditioned fear response to physiologic symptoms (eg, increased heart rate, dizziness) by interoceptive exposure.

This treatment consisted of therapist-guided exposure to bodily sensations that often lead to panic (eg, having participants hyperventilate or run up a set of stairs). The investigators revised the adult treatment by changing the language to be more understandable to adolescents and by providing age-appropriate examples. Adolescents receiving the PCT-A showed significantly greater reductions in panic, anxiety, and depressive symptom severity after treatment than participants in the self-monitoring group. Treatment gains for the PCT-A group were maintained at 3- and 6-month follow-up. Small sample size limited the generalizability of the findings. Nevertheless, these results suggest that an 11-session panic disorder treatment might be helpful for adolescents with panic disorder.[22]

Researchers examined whether they could identify key treatment components of PCT-A.[24] Twenty-one adolescents completed PCT-A. Dramatic treatment gains were reported (eg, large reduction in panic attack frequency or significant reduction in anxiety). Participants' average number of panic attacks was greatly reduced following the first session in which psychoeducation was provided. A significant reduction in anxiety was reported after the first cognitive restructuring session, during which participants were taught to thoroughly examine available evidence against their faulty beliefs about panic. What is more, adolescents reported that psychoeducation and cognitive restructuring were the most helpful components of treatment. Taken together, these results provide preliminary evidence suggesting that psychoeducation and cognitive restructuring are the key treatment components for panic disorder in adolescents. Future research should examine these treatment components with a larger sample of adolescents and should include a control group for comparison.

A brief, more intensive treatment approach was devised at Boston University.[25] Given the relative efficacy of several short-term, intensive treatments for other anxiety disorders (eg, obsessive-compulsive disorder, specific phobia), Angelosante and colleagues[25] established a short-term intervention for panic disorder and are in the process of examining treatment outcomes in that modality. The researchers are comparing adolescents with panic disorder who were randomly assigned to one of two treatment groups: 8-day panic treatment with or without a parent training component. Treatment consisted of 6 sessions that occurred over 8 days. Four of the sessions (ie, sessions 1 through 3 and 6) were 2 hours long, whereas two sessions (ie, sessions 4 and 5) were 6 to 8 hours. The longer sessions included extensive interoceptive and in vivo exposures that were therapist-guided and often occurred outside of the therapist's office. Sessions 5 and 6 occurred on a Friday and a Monday so participants could complete exposures on their own over the weekend. The treatment approach, called adolescent panic control treatment with in vivo exposure, is designed to be used in intensive outpatient or inpatient settings, and the goal is to provide a short-term intervention that can be accessed by families that may need to travel in order to receive treatment. A booster session was also included in the treatment protocol and was intended for implementation 1 month after the intensive phase of treatment. Data on the efficacy of the treatment have not been published yet, but this intervention may be a promising treatment approach that could meet the needs for patients requiring a more intensive, quick treatment.

Pharmacotherapy
Selective serotonin reuptake inhibitors (SSRIs) have been shown to reduce panic disorder symptoms in adult patients and have also been examined for use with panic disorder in two small, uncontrolled studies of panic disorder in children and adolescents.[26,27] Renaud and colleagues[26] evaluated 1 child and 11 adolescents with panic disorder (ages 8 to 18 years) in an open label study of SSRIs, some in conjunction with a benzodiazepine, for 6 to 8 weeks with a follow-up period of approximately 6 months. Participants were initially offered fluoxetine. However, if a previous trial of fluoxetine had failed or if they refused this medication, paroxetine or sertraline was prescribed. At the end of the acute treatment phase, the 9 participants who received fluoxetine were at a mean dose of 34.4 mg/d (range of 20 to 60 mg/d), the two on paroxetine were at a dose of 20 mg/d, and one who received sertraline was at 125 mg/d. On the Clinical Global Impression Scale, 75% of participants were rated as "much" to "very much" improved on the SSRIs at posttreatment. In addition, 67% no longer met criteria for panic disorder.

Masi and colleagues[27] conducted a chart review of 18 children and adolescents (ages 7 to 16) who received paroxetine, an SSRI, for panic disorder, during a 2-year period. Medications were individually titrated to between 10 and 40 mg/d. Youths were treated between 2 and 24 months. Eighty-three percent of the participants were classified as treatment responders, meaning that they showed a positive response to treatment (ie, clinician ratings of "markedly improved") based on retrospective ratings made at the time of the chart reviews. One-half the participants in the study were reported to be panic-free after 10 weeks of treatment. The mean length of treatment was 12 months, and 55% of the participants continued with paroxetine for longer than 12 months. The mean medication dosage was 24 mg. Although results from these two studies suggest that SSRIs may be efficacious, the results are tempered by the lack of control groups and lack of blind ratings of symptom improvement.

Data in adults suggest that treatment gains may not be maintained when pharmacologic interventions are discontinued.[28] In a study conducted by Barlow and colleagues,[29] 312 adults (mean age = 37 years) participated in a double-blind study comparing placebo, imipramine (ie, a tricyclic antidepressant), CBT alone, CBT plus placebo, and CBT plus imipramine for treatment of panic disorder. All active interventions were superior to placebo after 3 months of acute intervention (ie, weekly treatment) and 6 months of maintenance (ie, monthly treatment). Six months after treatment was discontinued, the relapse rate of the participants who received imipramine was 25% compared with 4% of participants who received CBT.[29] It was suggested that discontinuing medication for panic disorder is associated with an increase in uncomfortable bodily cues, because participants who were "prescribed" and subsequently discontinued a placebo did not seem to have the same symptom rebound as participants who discontinued active medication.

Implications for Research and Clinical Practice

Overall, data on treatment for panic disorder in adolescents are scarce. There is some evidence to suggest that adolescents benefit from CBT that is implemented much the same way as panic disorder treatment for adults. Pharmacologic interventions may also show promise; however, to the authors' knowledge there have been no randomized, controlled studies comparing medication with placebo in youth with panic disorder. Research on pharmacologic interventions incorporating randomized controlled designs is needed to establish the efficacy of this approach for children and adolescents with panic disorder. There are data to suggest that adults who respond well to pharmacologic interventions in the short term may not maintain treatment gains if medication is discontinued.[28,29] Such a finding has yet to be established in youth but should be the focus of future studies. Future research on treatment of panic disorder in children and adolescents should examine interventions with larger sample sizes, include long-term follow-up data, and examine medication in comparison with psychosocial interventions. Researchers should also examine the presentation of panic attacks and panic disorder in youth compared with adults and potentially update the diagnostic criteria to take into account developmental differences in the presentation across the life span.

SCHOOL REFUSAL

School refusal is not a diagnosable DSM-IV-TR disorder. Instead, it is a term used to describe when children and adolescents refuse to attend entire school days; leave during the school day; protest, plead or tantrum before school; or report somatic symptoms associated with anticipation of school or attendance at school.[30,31] Researchers differentiate between children who fail to attend school because of emotional symptoms (eg, anxiety or depression) and those who do not attend because of disinterest, defiance, or conduct disorder.[30,32] The former group, referred to as "school refusers" and the focus of this section, is thought to have different causative pathways leading to missing school than the latter, referred to as "truants." Data from the Great Smoky Mountain Study, a longitudinal, community-based study of 4500 children, suggested that the overall prevalence rate of anxious school refusers was 1.6% of the study population.[32] This result was compared with 5.8% of the sample being truant school refusers and .5% being mixed (ie, anxious and truant). Age of onset for anxious school refusers (mean age = 12.3 years) was younger than age of onset for truant school refusers (mean age = 14.7 years). Girls and boys were equally likely to be classified as anxious school refusers, whereas boys were twice as likely to be classified as truant school refusers.[32]

School refusal is a symptom associated with several psychiatric disorders. Separation anxiety disorder has been found to be the most common DSM-IV diagnosis associated with school refusal.[33] In a sample of children referred to an outpatient clinic because of school refusal:

- 22% of children had a primary diagnosis of separation anxiety disorder.
- 11% had generalized anxiety disorder.
- 8% were diagnosed with oppositional defiant disorder.
- 5% had major depressive disorder.

On the other hand, not all children with school refusal behavior have comorbid psychiatric disorders. Specifically, between 20% to 30% of school-refusing children do not meet criteria for any psychiatric diagnosis.[32,33]

Moreover, it has been suggested that the function of school refusal behavior has more predictive validity than the associated psychiatric disorder. Kearney and Albano[33] described four primary functions of school refusal. One group of children is reported to avoid "negative affectivity" (eg, depressive or anxious symptoms) triggered by school-related stimuli. A second group of children intends to "escape. . . school-related aversive social and/or evaluative situations".[33(p151)] School-refusing children may also fail to attend school because of positive reinforcement; some children receive attention from family members or other significant people in their lives when staying home from school. For example, children who are at home with a parent may be reinforced by spending time running errands with that person during the school day. The fourth group of children was reported to avoid school because of positive reinforcers outside of the school setting such as unsupervised access to video games. In a study on 222 children referred to an outpatient clinic for school-refusing behavior (ages 5–17), functional behaviors related to school refusal were better predictors of absenteeism than psychiatric symptoms associated with school refusal.[34]

Treatment

Psychosocial treatment

CBT is a well-established treatment option for school refusal.[35] CBT treatment modalities that have been examined for school refusal include child sessions, parent training, and school consultation. Individual child sessions may include teaching strategies to manage stress, examining cognitions about school, building an anxiety or avoidance hierarchy, and setting specific treatment goals to increase exposure to school.[36] Parent sessions have included psychoeducation about school refusal, decreasing factors that maintain school refusal behavior, implementing rewards contingent upon increasing school attendance, and helping to improve the child's confidence. School interventions have included teaching school personnel about psychological issues and introducing school officials to intervention strategies.[36] School-refusing children who engage in CBT show improvement in school attendance and a decrease in psychiatric symptoms and are rated by clinicians as more functional.[35] Interested readers are encouraged to refer to an excellent CBT-based treatment manual for school refusal.[37]

Heyne and colleagues[38] compared treatment outcomes of individual therapy with the child,, adult (ie, parent and teacher) training, and child therapy plus adult training in 61 school-refusing children (age range = 7–14 years). Children receiving individual therapy alone fared less well than children in the parent/teacher training group and the combined treatment group with respect to school attendance, self-reported anxiety symptoms, and parent-reported symptoms.[38] According to study results, there was no additive benefit of including child therapy in the school refusal intervention. In other words, the primary components that seemed to be beneficial were parent and teacher involvement in the intervention. This result suggests that adult intervention (eg, reward/contingency plans, and psychoeducation) may be more beneficial in increasing school attendance and improving psychological functioning than child-focused interventions. These results are surprising, given that roughly 94% of the children in the study had primary anxiety or depression diagnoses (eg, generalized anxiety disorder, specific phobia, major depressive disorder), suggesting that adult reinforcement and encouragement are important regardless of the cause of school refusal.

In a randomized controlled trial, Last and colleagues[39] compared 12 weeks of CBT with educational support in 56 school-refusing children with one or more anxiety disorders. In the educational support condition, psychoeducation and supportive therapy were provided without a specific plan for returning to school. Children in both groups showed improvement in school attendance and a decrease in symptoms of anxiety and depression and were less likely to meet criteria for an anxiety disorder after treatment. The investigators suggest that supportive therapy may offer similar treatment gains for school-refusing children as CBT. To date, these findings have not been replicated, however, and warrant further investigation.

Psychosocial treatment with pharmacotherapy

CBT in combination with medication has been found to be useful in treating school refusal. Bernstein and colleagues[40] conducted a double-blind study comparing imipramine plus CBT with placebo plus CBT in a sample of school-refusing adolescents with comorbid anxiety and major depressive disorders (n = 63, ages 12 to 18). At the end of the 8-week study, teenagers in the imipramine plus CBT group displayed significant improvement in attendance relative to those in the placebo plus CBT group. Fifty-four percent of the imipramine plus CBT group were attending school at least 75% of the time compared with only 17% of the placebo plus CBT group. The low attendance rate posttreatment in the placebo plus CBT group reflects the severe symptoms in this sample of anxious-depressed school refusers and the need for multimodal interventions in treating teenagers with severe school refusal. Both groups displayed a decrease in anxiety and depression, with greater changes occurring for the participants in the imipramine plus CBT versus the placebo plus CBT group.

Pharmacotherapy

Studies on the use of SSRIs to treat anxiety and depression indicate that they are effective treatments for children and adolescents.[21,41-46] However, no studies to date have examined the utility of SSRIs specifically for youth with school refusal. Future research is warranted to examine whether SSRIs, alone or in combination with psychosocial interventions, are efficacious for treatment of school refusal.

Inpatient treatment

Inpatient hospitalization for school refusal was examined by Walter and colleagues[47] in school-refusing adolescents ranging in age from 12 to 18 (n = 147). The adolescents in the study had an average hospital stay of approximately 8 weeks (range 3 to 18 weeks). Participants engaged in inpatient interventions (eg, token economy, individual and family therapy) and specific school refusal interventions (eg, gradual exposure to school, social skills training, parent skills training). Outcome was based on posttreatment school attendance. Specifically, participants were identified as either attending school regularly, attending a "special" school (ie, a school affiliated with the outpatient clinic), or dropping out of school. Two months after the adolescents were discharged, 63% were attending regular school, 31% were attending a special school, and 6% had dropped out of school. These results indicate that the majority of adolescents who engaged in the inpatient treatment program had returned to some form of school; however, school attendance rates (ie, number of days the child attended school) were not reported. Results are tempered by the fact that there was no control group in the study, which is particularly important given the intensity and cost of inpatient hospitalization. Future studies should also include longer follow-up periods after treatment, because it remains to be seen whether treatment gains are maintained.

Summary of the Treatment Literature

Studies reviewed in this article suggest that children and adolescents with school refusal show improvement in attendance and a decrease in anxiety and depressive symptoms with a variety of treatment options.[38–40,47] To further clarify treatment outcomes, Layne and colleagues[48] examined predictors of treatment response in the Bernstein and colleagues[40] sample of anxious-depressed adolescents with school refusal. Outcomes were better if the adolescents' baseline school attendance was higher and the treatment approach combined medication and CBT.[48] In addition, it was found that separation anxiety disorder and avoidant disorder (*Diagnostic and Statistical Manual of Mental Disorders, Third Edition, Revised* diagnosis, which is now replaced by social phobia),[49] predicted less favorable treatment outcomes.[48] Males had higher attendance rates after treatment than females.[48]

Several treatment modalities have been found to improve school attendance and decrease psychological symptoms in school-refusing children. CBT, supportive therapy, medication, and in some cases inpatient hospitalization are related to favorable outcomes for children. Generally speaking, the involvement of parents and school officials is a key component to treatment success. Methodologic weaknesses in some of the school refusal studies include lack of control groups.

Results from treatment studies of school refusal are promising; however, school-refusing children pose a challenge to clinicians. Specifically, many children who undergo treatment for school refusal continue to miss a substantial amount of school. For example, Heyne and colleagues[36] reported that 45% of adolescents who completed outpatient treatment for school refusal were not attending school at all at 2-month follow-up. Last and colleagues[39] reported that 44% of participants were not attending school 95% or more of the time at posttreatment. At 1-year follow-up, Bernstein and colleagues[50] found that anxious-depressed adolescents who had received imipramine or placebo plus CBT for school refusal received a high level of services posttreatment. Specifically, 78% of the adolescents received outpatient therapy, 68% received at least one psychotropic medication trial, 20% had in-home therapy, 20% were hospitalized, and 15% were placed out of their home. In addition, many of the adolescents continued to meet criteria for an anxiety or mood disorder. Specifically, 64% met criteria for an anxiety disorder and 33% met criteria for a depressive disorder at follow-up.

Implications for Research and Clinical Practice

The current treatment approaches for school refusal are efficacious for some but continue to "miss the mark" for a substantial proportion of children. Although there are some data to suggest premorbid functioning and type of disorder may predict treatment outcome,[48] there are still questions about reasons for the lack of treatment response in some youth and substantial rate of relapse in others. In the authors' clinical experience, it has been observed that a proportion of parents may struggle to set limits with their school-refusing child in spite of interventions aimed to address this issue. Future research should examine parent factors that may interfere with treatment progress and serve to maintain school refusal behavior. In addition, prospective studies should be conducted in which school-refusing youth are followed into adulthood to examine long-term outcomes for these children and adolescents. Important questions include whether avoidance behavior remits after formal education or whether school-refusing children miss a significant amount of work in adulthood. It is also possible that some of the underlying reasons for school refusal (eg, being the target of bullying) might not be addressed with the current interventions.

Kearney and Bensaheb[51] have provided guidelines for school professionals, based on CBT intervention strategies. For example, school personnel are advised to facilitate gradual exposure to the school environment, even if it means that the child is not in his or her classroom for the entire day (eg, the child spends part of the day in the school office or arrives for school at lunchtime). Moreover, if a child seeks frequent reassurance, the teacher should attempt to reduce and limit the amount of times per day it is provided (eg, teacher can tell the child once per hour that his or her parents will return at the end of the day and ignore further questions on the topic). If a child requests to leave class to go to the nurse's office, the school staff can help the child identify possible triggers and attempt to get him or her to back to class quickly. The nurse should send the child home only if there is objective evidence of medical illness (eg, elevated temperature). Future research is needed to examine the benefits of school-based interventions. Overall, children and adolescents will benefit from the clinician, parents, and school professionals (eg, teachers, school counselors, and principal) joining together as a multidisciplinary team to successfully implement interventions for school refusal.

REFERENCES

1. American Psychiatric Association. Diagnostic Criteria from DSM-IV-TR. Arlington (VA): American Psychiatric Association; 2000.
2. Craske MG, Kircanski K, Epstein A, et al. Panic disorder: a review of DSM-IV panic disorder and proposals for DSM-V. Depress Anxiety 2010;27(2):93–112.
3. Beesdo K, Knappe S, Pine DS. Anxiety and anxiety disorders in children and adolescents: developmental issues and implications for DSM-V. Psychiatr Clin North Am 2009;32(3):483–524.
4. Merikangas KR, He JP, Brody D, et al. Prevalence and treatment of mental disorders among US children in the 2001-2004 NHANES. Pediatrics 2010;125(1):75–81.
5. Diler RS, Birmaher B, Brent DA, et al. Phenomenology of panic disorder in youth. Depress Anxiety 2004;20(1):39–43.
6. Reed V, Wittchen HU. DSM-IV panic attacks and panic disorder in a community sample of adolescents and young adults: how specific are panic attacks? J Psychiatr Res 1998;32(6):335–45.
7. Hayward C, Killen JD, Hammer LD, et al. Pubertal stage and panic attack history in sixth- and seventh-grade girls. Am J Psychiatry 1992;149(9):1239–43.
8. Wittchen HU, Reed V, Kessler RC. The relationship of agoraphobia and panic in a community sample of adolescents and young adults. Arch Gen Psychiatry 1998; 55(11):1017–24.
9. American Psychiatric Association. DSM-5 development. Arlington (VA): American Psychiatric Association. Available at: http://www.dsm5.org/Pages/Default.aspx; 2010. Accessed December 2, 2011.
10. Carballo JJ, Baca-Garcia E, Blanco C, et al. Stability of childhood anxiety disorder diagnoses: a follow-up naturalistic study in psychiatric care. Eur Child Adolesc Psychiatry 2010;19(4):395–403.
11. Hayward C, Wilson KA, Lagle K, et al. Parent-reported predictors of adolescent panic attacks. J Am Acad Child Adolesc Psychiatry 2004;43(5):613–20.
12. Lewinsohn PM, Holm-Denoma JM, Small JW, et al. Separation anxiety disorder in childhood as a risk factor for future mental illness. J Am Acad Child Adolesc Psychiatry 2008;47(5):548–55.
13. Boden JM, Fergusson DM, Horwood LJ. Anxiety disorders and suicidal behaviours in adolescence and young adulthood: findings from a longitudinal study. Psychol Med 2007;37(3):431–40.
14. Pilowsky DJ, Wu LT, Anthony JC. Panic attacks and suicide attempts in mid-adolescence. Am J Psychiatry 1999;156(10):1545–9.

15. Domschke K, Stevens S, Pfleiderer B, et al. Interoceptive sensitivity in anxiety and anxiety disorders: an overview and integration of neurobiological findings. Clin Psychol Rev 2010;30(1):1–11.
16. Bouton ME, Mineka S, Barlow DH. A modern learning theory perspective on the etiology of panic disorder. Psychol Rev 2001;108(1):4–32.
17. Gorman JM, Kent JM, Sullivan GM, et al. Neuroanatomical hypothesis of panic disorder, revised. Journal of Lifelong Learning in Psychiatry 2004;2(3).
18. Maddock RJ, Buonocore MH, Kile SJ, et al. Brain regions showing increased activation by threat-related words in panic disorder. Neuroreport 2003;14(3):325–8.
19. World Health Organization. The ICD-10 Classification of mental and behavioural disorders: diagnostic criteria for research. Geneva (Switzerland): World Health Organization; 1993.
20. Wittchen HU, Gloster AT, Beesdo-Baum K, et al. Agoraphobia: a review of the diagnostic classificatory position and criteria. Depress Anxiety 2010;27(2):113–33.
21. Connolly SD, Bernstein GA. Practice parameter for the assessment and treatment of children and adolescents with anxiety disorders. J Am Acad Child Adolesc Psychiatry 2007;46(2):267–83.
22. Pincus DB, May JE, Whitton SW, et al. Cognitive-behavioral treatment of panic disorder in adolescence. J Clin Child Adolesc Psychol 2010;39(5):638–49.
23. Hoffman EC, Mattis SG. A developmental adaptation of panic control treatment for panic disorder in adolescence. Cogn Behav Pract 2000;7:253–61.
24. Micco JA, Choate-Summers ML, Ehrenreich JT, et al. Identifying efficacious treatment components of panic control treatment for adolescents: a preliminary examination. Child Fam Behav Ther 2007;29(4):1–23.
25. Angelosante AG, Pincus DB, Whitton SW, et al. Implementation of an intensive treatment protocol for adolescents with panic disorder and agoraphobia. Cogn Behav Pract 2009;16:345–57.
26. Renaud J, Birmaher B, Wassick SC, et al. Use of selective serotonin reuptake inhibitors for the treatment of childhood panic disorder: a pilot study. J Child Adolesc Psychopharmacol 1999;9(2):73–83.
27. Masi G, Toni C, Mucci M, et al. Paroxetine in child and adolescent outpatients with panic disorder. J Child Adolesc Psychopharmacol 2001;11(2):151–7.
28. Otto MW, Deveney C. Cognitive-behavioral therapy and the treatment of panic disorder: efficacy and strategies. J Clin Psychiatry 2005;66(Suppl 4):28–32.
29. Barlow DH, Gorman JM, Shear MK, et al. Cognitive-behavioral therapy, imipramine, or their combination for panic disorder: A randomized controlled trial. JAMA 2000; 283(19):2529–36.
30. King NJ, Bernstein GA. School refusal in children and adolescents: a review of the past 10 years. J Am Acad Child Adolesc Psychiatry 2001;40(2):197–205.
31. Bernstein GA, Victor AM. Separation anxiety disorder and school refusal. In: Dulcan MK, editor. Dulcan's textbook of child and adolescent psychiatry. Washington (DC): American Psychiatric Publishing, Inc; 2010. p. 325–38.
32. Egger HL, Costello EJ, Angold A. School refusal and psychiatric disorders: a community study. J Am Acad Child Adolesc Psychiatry 2003;42(7):797–807.
33. Kearney CA, Albano AM. The functional profiles of school refusal behavior: diagnostic aspects. Behav Modif 2004;28(1):147–61.
34. Kearney CA. Forms and functions of school refusal behavior in youth: an empirical analysis of absenteeism severity. J Child Psychol Psychiatry 2007;48(1):53–61.
35. Suveg C, Aschenbrand SG, Kendall PC. Separation anxiety disorder, panic disorder, and school refusal. Child Adolesc Psychiatr Clin N Am 2005;14(4):773–95, ix.

36. Heyne D, Sauter FM, Van Widenfelt BM, et al. School refusal and anxiety in adolescence: non-randomized trial of a developmentally sensitive cognitive behavioral therapy. J Anxiety Disord 2011;25(7):870–8.
37. Kearney CA, Albano AM. When children refuse school: a cognitive-behavioral approach. 2nd edition. Oxford (UK): Oxford University Press; 2007.
38. Heyne D, King NJ, Tonge BJ, et al. Evaluation of child therapy and caregiver training in the treatment of school refusal. J Am Acad Child Adolesc Psychiatry 2002;41(6): 687–95.
39. Last CG, Hansen C, Franco N. Cognitive-behavioral treatment of school phobia. J Am Acad Child Adolesc Psychiatry 1998;37(4):404–11.
40. Bernstein GA, Borchardt CM, Perwien AR, et al. Imipramine plus cognitive-behavioral therapy in the treatment of school refusal. J Am Acad Child Adolesc Psychiatry 2000;39(3):276–83.
41. Birmaher B, Axelson DA, Monk K, et al. Fluoxetine for the treatment of childhood anxiety disorders. J Am Acad Child Adolesc Psychiatry 2003;42(4):415–23.
42. Emslie GJ, Rush AJ, Weinberg WA, et al. A double-blind, randomized, placebo-controlled trial of fluoxetine in children and adolescents with depression. Arch Gen Psychiatry 1997;54(11):1031–7.
43. Research Unit on Pediatric Psychopharmacology Anxiety Study Group. Fluvoxamine for the treatment of anxiety disorders in children and adolescents. N Engl J Med 2001;344:1279–85.
44. Rynn MA, Siqueland L, Rickels K. Placebo-controlled trial of sertraline in the treatment of children with generalized anxiety disorder. Am J Psychiatry 2001; 158(12):2008–14.
45. Wagner KD, Berard R, Stein MB, et al. A multicenter, randomized, double-blind, placebo-controlled trial of paroxetine in children and adolescents with social anxiety disorder. Arch Gen Psychiatry 2004;61(11):1153–62.
46. Walkup JT, Albano AM, Piacentini J, et al. Cognitive behavioral therapy, sertraline, or a combination in childhood anxiety. N Engl J Med 2008;359:2753–66.
47. Walter D, Hautmann C, Rizk S, et al. Short term effects of inpatient cognitive behavioral treatment of adolescents with anxious-depressed school absenteeism: an observational study. Eur Child Adolesc Psychiatry 2010;19(11):835–44.
48. Layne AE, Bernstein GA, Egan EA, et al. Predictors of treatment response in anxious-depressed adolescents with school refusal. J Am Acad Child Adolesc Psychiatry 2003;42(3):319–26.
49. American Psychiatric Association. Diagnostic Criteria from DSM-III-R. Washington (DC): American Psychiatric Association; 1987.
50. Bernstein GA, Hektner JM, Borchardt CM, et al. Treatment of school refusal: one-year follow-up. J Am Acad Child Adolesc Psychiatry 2001;40(2):206–13.
51. Kearney CA, Bensaheb A. School absenteeism and school refusal behavior: a review and suggestions for school-based health professionals. J Sch Health 2006;76(1):3–7.

Adapting Parent-Child Interaction Therapy to Treat Anxiety Disorders in Young Children

Anthony C. Puliafico, PhD[a],*, Jonathan S. Comer, PhD[b],
Donna B. Pincus, PhD[b]

KEYWORDS

- Anxiety • Parent-child interaction therapy • Parent training • Preschool

KEY POINTS

- As many as 9% of preschoolers suffer from an anxiety disorder, with symptom presentations roughly consistent with anxiety presentations found in older children.
- Early intervention for preschoolers diagnosed with anxiety disorder is critical, given the considerable academic, social, family, and functional impairments associated with these disorders in childhood.
- Accumulating evidence preliminarily supports the clinical utility of treatment adaptation approaches–the developmentally lateral extension of methods for other disorders, as well as the downward extension of methods for the same disorders in older children–to the treatment of early child anxiety.
- Initial research supports the adaptation of Parent-Child Interaction Therapy, a treatment designed to target oppositional and non-compliant behavior in young children, to treat anxiety in young children.

INTRODUCTION

As many as 9% of preschoolers suffer from an anxiety disorder,[1–2] with research showing that preschool anxiety symptom presentations are roughly consistent with

Funding Sources: Dr. Comer: Foundation grant from the Mental Health Initiative (MINT); T-32 Award from the National Institutes of Health (T32 MH016434); K23 award from the National Institutes of Health (K23 MH090247). Dr. Pincus: K-23 award from the National Institute of Mental Health (NIMH: K-23- MH64717).
[a] Department of Psychiatry, Columbia University/New York State Psychiatric Institute, 1051 Riverside Drive Unit 74, New York, NY 10032, USA; [b] Department of Psychology, Boston University, Center for Anxiety and Related Disorders, 648 Beacon Street, 6th Floor, Boston, MA 02115, USA
* Corresponding author.
E-mail address: PuliafiA@nyspi.columbia.edu

anxiety presentations found in older children.[3-4] Early intervention is critical, given the considerable academic, social, family, and functional impairments associated with child anxiety disorders.[5-8] Whereas methods for effectively treating anxiety disorders in children over the age of 7 are well-established,[9-11] our understanding of efficacious treatment options for very young children with anxiety disorders is limited. Supported treatments for children over the age of 7 are cognitive-behavioral in nature and help children to recognize bodily anxiety symptoms, identify and adjust maladaptive cognitions in anxiety-provoking situations, and develop a repertoire of coping strategies. After learning this new set of skills, treatment shifts to an exposure-based format, providing children with systematic opportunities to practice newly acquired skills in increasingly anxiety-provoking situations. Roughly 60% of children over the age of 7 treated with cognitive behavior therapy (CBT) no longer meet diagnostic criteria for an anxiety disorder at posttreatment.[12-15] Treatment gains are typically sustained into adolescence and young adulthood.[16]

A small handful of research groups have recently begun to show support for the use of developmentally sensitive downward extensions of treatments found to work with older youth in controlled trials with preschoolers diagnosed with anxiety disorders.[17-21] These treatments share a focus on parental involvement in treatment, directly targeting parenting practices believed to maintain child anxiety, parental anxiety management, and a high emphasis on the role of parental modeling.

The historically limited focus on treating anxiety disorders in very young children is likely due in part to the fact that supported anxiety treatments for older children rely heavily on strategies and tasks that are beyond the developmental capacities of younger children. Clinical tasks focusing on recognizing bodily anxiety symptoms and identifying and adjusting maladaptive thoughts require sophisticated metacognitive and receptive and expressive language abilities that are not present at earlier developmental stages.[22] Treatment activities in which children reflect on how others might construe feared situations differently require perspective-taking abilities that do not fully emerge until later childhood.[22-23] In addition, the limited organizational skills and restricted attention characteristic of early childhood constrain the ability to assign young children homework tasks,[24] which is a key component of CBT for older children.

The authors outline the treatment programs they have developed that modify parent-child interaction therapy, or PCIT[25-26]—a well-established treatment for early disruptive behavior disorders for the treatment of anxiety disorders presenting in children below age 8, including

- Oppositional defiant disorder
- Conduct disorder
- Attention-deficit/hyperactivity disorder.

Modifying PCIT for the treatment of early child anxiety disorders largely constitutes a developmentally lateral extension of methods and a format found to work with other diagnostic conditions in the same patient age group, rather than a downward extension of methods and formats found to work with older patients affected by the same diagnostic conditions. Accumulating evidence preliminarily supports the clinical utility of both treatment adaptation approaches—in other words, the developmentally lateral extension of methods for other disorders, as well as the downward extension of methods for the same disorders in older children—to the treatment of early child anxiety.[17-21,27-30]

The authors begin with a brief overview of traditional PCIT, followed by an outline of the first modification of PCIT for an anxiety disorder (ie, PCIT for separation anxiety disorder[30]), and then provide an overview of the CALM Program[27] (Coaching Approach behavior and Leading by Modeling) that builds on the initial PCIT modifications for separation anxiety disorder for application to the range of anxiety disorders presenting in early childhood. The authors conclude with a consideration of future directions for the use of modified PCIT methods to treat anxiety disorders in young children.

TRADITIONAL PARENT-CHILD INTERACTION THERAPY FOR DISRUPTIVE BEHAVIOR PROBLEMS

Traditional PCIT[25–26] is a short-term, empirically supported intervention developed for the treatment of disruptive behavior problems in children between the ages of 2 and 8. Drawing on both attachment theory and social learning theory, PCIT incorporates components of play therapy into behavioral parent training, targeting children's maladaptive behavior by modifying parents' behavior. Rather than directly engaging young children who have yet to develop various cognitive developmental abilities, PCIT focuses on reshaping the primary context in which young children's development unfolds—specifically interactions between parent and child.

Parent training emphasizes positive attention, effective communication, problem-solving, and consistency in parent-child interactions. What distinguishes PCIT from neighboring protocols for early disruptive behavior problems is the systematic use of real-time in-session parent coaching from a therapist who monitors naturalistic parent-child interactions from an observation room and provides individualized coaching via a bug-in-the-ear receiver worn by the parent.

Early sessions focus on strengthening a positive and mutually rewarding parent-child relationship (child-directed interaction, or CDI). Parents learn to use selective attention (eg, ignoring undesired behavior, praising desired behavior) as well as incidental teaching (ie, reinforcing the child's spontaneous positive behavior to increase its frequency) to shape the child's behavior. These skills are summarized in the PRIDE skills acronym:

> **Praise:** Frequently praise desired behavior, and specifically state the behavior that is being praised.
> **Reflect:** Repeat statements made by the child.
> **Imitate:** Follow the child's lead during play tasks.
> **Describe:** Narrate aloud the child's behaviors.
> **Enthusiasm:** Express interest in the child's behavior both verbally and nonverbally.

Parents are also discouraged from asking questions, giving commands, and making critical comments while using these positive attending skills, and are encouraged to ignore all unwanted attention-seeking behavior (eg, whining, arguing, yelling). On learning the PRIDE skills, parents practice them during in-session interactions with their child. During these sessions, the therapist coaches parents and tracks their competence in using positive attending skills from session to session.

After parents demonstrate sufficient competence using positive attending and active ignoring skills based on specified mastery criteria,[31] treatment subsequently shifts to focus on effective parent direction and child compliance (parent-directed interaction, or PDI). Parents learn to give commands more effectively, and are taught a specific time-out procedure to use when a child does not comply with instruction. On learning these skills, parents again practice using them during in-session interactions with their child, while being coached by the therapist. The therapist tracks each parent's competency in the use of direct commands and time-out procedures.

When parents demonstrate mastery in these skills, and a child is demonstrating sufficiently improved behavior, termination planning begins.

THE CASE FOR MODIFYING PCIT FOR THE TREATMENT OF EARLY CHILD ANXIETY

PCIT offers a treatment format that targets children's functioning by reshaping parent behavior rather than directly engaging young children with anxiety, most of whom have yet to develop key cognitive developmental capacities. Importantly, research documents the considerable influence parenting has on the development and maintenance of child anxiety.

- Intrusive, overprotective, controlling, and overinvolved parenting is associated with anxiety disorders in youth.[32–37]
- Parents of anxious children grant less autonomy and take over tasks that children can normatively perform independently.
- Anxious children's parents, relative to the parents of their nonanxious peers, are more likely to offer approval of children's avoidance strategies during problem-solving activities.[38]

These parenting behaviors function to limit children's exposure to anxiety-provoking situations and their resolution and deny children mastery opportunities (ie, opportunities to demonstrate for themselves that they can effectively navigate age-appropriate situations).[39]

Because child anxiety is so highly associated with specific *parent* behaviors, an intervention such as PCIT that modifies parent behavior offers promise in treating anxiety in young children. Unlike other parent training interventions, the in-session coaching that occurs in PCIT provides a powerful transfer of skill to parents that can be particularly useful in managing avoidant anxiety-driven behaviors. In recent years, two related treatment programs have adapted PCIT to treat anxiety disorders in children ages 3 to 8. These treatments are described later; please see **Table 1** for a comparison of these treatments with traditional PCIT.

MODIFYING PCIT FOR EARLY SEPARATION ANXIETY DISORDER
Traditional PCIT in the Treatment of Separation Anxiety Disorder

Through a series of studies, Pincus and colleagues[29] investigated the utility, implementation, and efficacy of using traditional PCIT for the treatment of separation anxiety disorder (SAD) in young children, aged 4 through 8. Given that the major aims of PCIT are to target maladaptive parenting styles, increase positive parent-child interaction, promote secure attachment, and improve family functioning, it was initially hypothesized that traditional, unmodified PCIT could effectively ameliorate the problematic parent-child interactions that typically ensue in families with a young child with SAD.[29]

In an initial pilot study using a multiple baseline experimental design,[40] the unmodified PCIT protocol was used to treat three families who each had a young child with a principal diagnosis of SAD. The length of the baseline separation anxiety monitoring phase was staggered, with the first family beginning treatment after a 1-week monitoring phase, the second family after a 2-week monitoring phase, and the third family after a 4-week monitoring phase.

- After PCIT treatment, clinically significant change in separation anxiety was observed on all measures, and disruptive behaviors also decreased.
- Additionally, parents evidenced significant increases in their use of praise and decreases in their questions and criticisms.

Table 1

Comparison of traditional PCIT with PCIT adaptations to treat anxiety

Treatments	Treatment Components (In Order)					
Traditional PCIT	CDI Teach Session (one session, 60 min)	CDI Coach Sessions (until mastery criteria are met)	PDI Teach Session (one session, 60 min)	PDI Coach Sessions (until mastery criteria are met and symptoms are sufficiently improved)		
PCIT Adaptation for Separation Anxiety Disorder	CDI Teach Session (one session, 60 min)	CDI Coach Sessions (until mastery criteria are met) (two or more sessions, until mastery criteria met; 60 min each)	BDI Teach Session (one session, 60 min)	BDI Coach Sessions (two sessions, 60 min each)	PDI Teach Session (one session)	PDI Coach Sessions (until mastery criteria are met and symptoms are sufficiently improved)
CALM Program	CDI Teach Session/Anxiety Psychoeducation Session (one session, 90 min)	CDI Coach Sessions (two sessions)	Exposure Sessions (until CDI mastery criteria are met)	DADS Teach Session (one session, 60 min)	DADS Coach/Exposure Sessions (until mastery criteria are met and symptoms are sufficiently improved)	

- Patients' gains were maintained at 3-month follow up, suggesting that traditional PCIT might be a useful and promising intervention for treatment of young children with SAD and their families.

To continue to assess the feasibility and potential efficacy of standard PCIT for children with SAD, an open pilot trial of standard PCIT was implemented with 10 children (4 girls and 6 boys), aged 4 through 8.[30] The clinical severity of children's SAD was assessed by an independent evaluator at pre- and posttreatment using the Anxiety Disorders Interview Schedule, child and parent versions (ADIS-C/P),[41] and parents also completed self-report measures of their child's anxiety, fear, and avoidance, and monitored their child's separation anxiety symptoms daily. After standard PCIT treatment:

- Parents increased their use of appropriate parenting skills taught during CDI.
- The frequency and severity of children's separation anxiety incidents had decreased.

However, parents reported that their children were still having difficulty entering previously avoided situations and developmentally appropriate activities (eg, birthday parties, play dates) without distress. Although children showed some improvement in the clinical severity of SAD, SAD did not improve to nonclinical levels (below 4 on the 0–8 clinical severity scale of the ADIS-C/P) at posttreatment.

PCIT Adaptations for Separation Anxiety Disorder

To improve on the treatment gains associated with traditional PCIT for SAD, a new component, bravery-directed interaction (BDI), consisting of anxiety education and exposure instruction for parents, was added to standard PCIT and administered between CDI and PDI.[29] (See Pincus and colleagues[30] for a complete description of the process of adapting standard PCIT for preschoolers with SAD.) A recently completed randomized clinical trial tested the efficacy of this modified version of PCIT to treat children aged 4 through 8 with SAD.[28] (Pincus DB, Chase RM, Hardway C, et al: Treatment of childhood separation anxiety using modified parent child interaction therapy: results of a randomized controlled trial. Manuscript in preparation; 2011.) The primary goals of the trial were to evaluate the efficacy of modified PCIT for reducing the frequency and intensity of separation anxious behaviors in young children, and to determine the long-term maintenance of children's improvements at 3, 6, and 12 months following treatment.

In the treatment adapted by Pincus and colleagues,[28] CDI and PDI were implemented according to the standard PCIT manual. The BDI component, developed and added specifically to treat separation anxiety, taught parents

- The cycle of anxiety and factors maintaining anxiety in children
- Ways to apply CDI skills in separation situations
- Appropriate ways to conduct separation exposure practices with their children.

The BDI component occurred after CDI and before PDI. Consistent with CDI and PDI, the BDI phase began with a teaching session in which the therapist taught the parent(s) specific skills, and was followed by sessions in which parents were advised about how to help their child conduct separation anxiety exposure practices.

Thirty-eight young children with a primary diagnosis of SAD (23 girls and 15 boys) and at least one of their parents or caregivers were randomly assigned to one of two study conditions:

1. A treatment condition in which children immediately received modified PCIT
2. An attention-control waitlist (WL) condition in which children waited 9 weeks prior to receiving a full course of the modified PCIT treatment.

To attempt to equate attention between groups, the WL condition attended 30-minute sessions every other week to turn in monitoring and assessment forms and give the therapist updates about the week. A multimodal assessment battery was used to assess child separation anxiety at pretreatment, posttreatment, postwaitlist, and 3, 6 and 12 months follow-up. Results showed that

Children receiving modified PCIT displayed greater improvement than those in the WL group from pre- to posttreatment/postwaitlist on measures of:

- Separation anxiety
- General psychopathology
- Parent-child interaction
- Parenting stress.

These gains were maintained at 3-, 6-, and 12-month follow-up.

Participants in the modified PCIT condition also showed significantly greater reductions in SAD severity compared with those in the WL group. At posttreatment/post waitlist assessment

- 73% of those in the modified PCIT condition no longer met diagnostic criteria for SAD.
- No participants in the WL group were diagnosis-free by postwaitlist.

These findings support the efficacy of a PCIT-adapted treatment for young children with SAD. Current efforts are evaluating the implementation of PCIT modified to treat separation anxiety in community settings.

THE CALM PROGRAM: A PCIT MODIFICATION FOR TREATING THE RANGE OF EARLY ANXIETY DISORDERS
Description of Treatment

The CALM Program[27,42] extended the work of Pincus and colleagues[28–30] to treat young children (ages 3 through 8) with a range of anxiety disorders, including social phobia, generalized anxiety disorder, separation anxiety disorder, and specific phobia.

Similar to Pincus and colleagues' treatment program, the CALM Program. Utilizes the structure and format of PCIT to address symptoms of anxiety through parent behavioral training. Emphasizes in vivo exposure in session. Unlike the Pincus and colleagues model. The majority of treatment sessions involve the in-the-moment coaching of parents in leading their children in exposure situations.

Thus, the CALM Program represents a melding of PCIT with an exposure-based treatment model traditionally used to treat anxiety.

As in PCIT, the CALM Program uses a model in which parents learn behavioral skills and then practice them in session, while receiving live coaching from their therapist.

In the initial treatment session:

- The therapist provides psychoeducation about anxiety and discusses how certain parental behaviors may inadvertently reinforce a child's avoidance of feared situations.
- The therapist teaches parents positive attending skills (ie, PRIDE skills) that will be used to reinforce "brave" behavior.

- Parents are encouraged to actively ignore undesired behavior when interacting with their children, and to avoid questions, commands, and criticisms.
- The therapist gathers information about the child's anxious symptomatology and aids the child's parents in developing an exposure hierarchy. The exposure hierarchy lists situations that the child fears, from least anxiety-provoking to most, and guides the sequences of exposures in subsequent sessions.

Because this initial session covers a substantial amount of material, it is recommended that a double session is scheduled or the content is reviewed over two sessions.

In subsequent treatment sessions:

- The therapist coaches parents in the use of positive attending and active ignoring skills during parent-child interactions.
- During the first two coaching sessions, parents practice using these skills in play-based situations.
- In the third coaching session, in vivo exposures begin in a graded fashion, starting with situations that provoke mild anxiety. Examples of possible exposures include the child interacting with an unfamiliar person, entering a dark room, or coming into close contact with a feared animal. During these sessions, parents are coached to positively attend to their child when s/he approaches the feared object/situation, and to actively ignore any anxiety-driven behaviors such as hiding, whining, or crying. Thus, the parent creates a contingency in which a child facing a feared situation is reinforced with parental positive attention.
- Treatment sessions focus on the coaching of positive attending and active ignoring skills until parents demonstrate mastery of the traditional PCIT PRIDE skills according to therapist coding. (See Eyberg and colleagues[43] for mastery criteria.)

DADS steps:

Once parents achieve mastery in using positive attending and active ignoring skills, they learn a new set of skills known as the DADS steps. DADS stands for

D escribe the feared situation (make at least three descriptive statements).

A pproach the feared situation.

D irect command for child to approach feared situation.

S electively attend to child's approach behavior.

The DADS steps represent a sequence of behaviors for parents to follow when guiding their child through an anxiety-provoking situation. Parents follow this step-by-step sequence until the child begins to approach the feared situation, at which point parents immediately praise the approach behavior. Specifics of the DADS steps can be found elsewhere.[42]

For the remainder of treatment, parents practice the DADS steps, as well as positive attending and active ignoring skills, during increasingly anxiety-provoking exposures. The therapist continues to coach parents during in-session coaching sessions via a discreet bug-in-the ear worn by the parent. Parents are also instructed to practice using the DADS steps as they guide their children through feared situations at home in between sessions. At the end of each treatment session, the therapist and parents identify exposure situations to attempt between sessions. Parents are asked to track their use of the DADS steps during these exposures, whether the child successfully approached the feared situations, and if so, at which step of the DADS sequence the child did so. During sessions, parents' use of the DADS steps is observed and coded to track their competence in using these skills.

Mastery of these skills, along with child's progress in facing feared situations, are used as benchmarks for treatment progress and to determine when treatment should end.

Empirical Support

To date, one formal open trial[27] has been conducted in which seven children ages 3 through 8, along with their parents, completed the CALM Program (two additional families began treatment but withdrew before completing). All participating children met *Diagnostic and Statistical Manual of Mental Disorders* (Fourth Edition)[44] criteria for an anxiety disorder according to the ADIS-C/P at pretreatment assessment.

- The majority of participants met criteria for more than one anxiety disorder.
- 88% of participants met criteria for separation anxiety disorder.
- 33% met criteria for social phobia.
- 22% met criteria for generalized anxiety disorder.
- 11% met criteria for specific phobia.
- 2 participants met criteria for selective mutism.
- 1 participant met for obsessive-compulsive disorder.
- 2 met for oppositional defiant disorder.
- 2 exhibited school refusal behavior.

For research purposes, treatment followed a 12-session format for all participants.

- Session 1 and Session 6 were parent-only sessions dedicated to teaching CDI and DADS skills, respectively. All other sessions involved parent and child.
- Sessions 2 and 3 were dedicated to coaching CDI skills.
- Sessions 4 and 5 involved coaching CDI skills during low-level exposure tasks.
- Sessions 7 through 12 involved live coaching parents in the use of the DADS steps during child exposures to feared situations.

In posttreatment analyses of completing participants, all but one child (85.7%) no longer met criteria for any anxiety disorders. Furthermore, participants exhibited improvement in overall functioning following treatment, with an average increase of 21 points on the Children's Global Assessment Scale from pre- to posttreatment and an average decrease of 2.6 points on the Clinical Global Inventory–Severity. According to intent-to-treat analyses, gains were also considerable, albeit more modest, with 66.7% of participants demonstrating remittance of anxiety disorders. Follow-up data were not collected in the CALM pilot trial.

SUMMARY

Given the substantial individual and societal costs associated with anxiety disorders, treating anxiety at a young age constitutes a matter of great public health importance. Interventions targeting anxiety symptoms in children below age 7 require developmental sensitivity, because young children generally do not possess the cognitive skills needed for traditional cognitive behavior treatment showing support with older youth. With its focus on providing parents with skills to shape their children's behavior, modified parent-child interaction therapy, or PCIT, represents a promising and increasingly supported format with which to target anxiety symptoms in young children.

Recent adaptations of PCIT for anxiety have applied the parent-training format of PCIT to teach parents behavioral methods to reinforce a child approaching feared situations and extinguish avoidance behavior patterns. Like other treatments developed for young children with anxiety disorders,[17-18, 21] PCIT-adapted anxiety treatments emphasize graded exposure to feared situations. Uniquely, these treatments also focus on unobtrusively coaching parents *in session* in the skills they can use in exposure-based situations to reinforce a child's brave behavior. The treatment developed by Pincus and colleagues[30] includes the bravery-directed interaction skills developed specifically to provide parents with skills to apply in exposure-based situations. Building on this work, the CALM Program teaches parents the DADS steps and coaches parents live in using these skills during in-session in vivo exposures.

Implications for Research

Preliminary evidence suggests that these PCIT modifications are associated with a decrease in anxiety symptoms,[27-28] although additional studies are certainly needed to test the efficacies of these interventions against credible comparison treatments, incorporating long-term follow-up evaluations. Future research should also focus on clarifying the relative efficacies of the various components of PCIT-modified treatments. The treatments described previously, along with traditional PCIT, each consist of several treatment components (eg, CDI, PDI, BDI, DADS). It is unclear whether each of these components contributes meaningfully to each treatment's overall efficacy, or whether specific components are primarily responsible for treatment gains. Assessing the efficacies of the various components of these treatments will aid in refining treatments to be more efficient.

There is also a need for future work to examine the transportability of PCIT-adapted treatments to the wide array of settings in which children and families seek treatment. Whereas a setting with a one-way mirror and one-way radio devices is ideal, it is not often feasible for clinicians in the community to have access to these resources. Research suggests that PCIT conducted with the therapist coaching parents from within the treatment room has shown initial support.[45] It will be important to assess the feasibility and efficacy of in-room coaching for the anxiety treatments described previously, and to consider modifications that may enhance in-room coaching.

Implications for Clinical Practice

A broader problem involves access to care. Many families in need of anxiety treatment for young children do not have access to mental health providers with proper behavioral training. Comer and colleagues[46] have begun to assess the clinical utility of Internet-based delivery of PCIT, specifically via webcam-based technology and videoconferencing software. The delivery of PCIT via Internet-based technology directly to families in their homes may represent a promising option for expanding access to care. Because the therapist primarily coaches outside of the therapy room in standard PCIT, the process of live coaching may not vary much. In addition, with Internet-based delivery, the therapist will have the opportunity to observe the family interact and provide coaching in their home environment, which could potentially lead to greater generalization of treatment gains.

To conclude, the modification of PCIT to treat anxiety in young children is a relatively new and promising clinical development. The treatments described in this article represent initial attempts to combine the structure and format of PCIT with an exposure-based treatment model. Of course, further empirical evaluations of these treatments are warranted before conclusions on treatment efficacy and effectiveness can be made. Nevertheless, they represent a potentially valuable, developmentally compatible treatment option for a population—young children with anxiety disorders—for whom treatment options have historically been limited.

REFERENCES

1. Egger HL, Angold A. Common emotional and behavioral disorders in preschool children: presentation, nosology, and epidemiology. J Child Psychol Psychiatry 2006; 47:313–37.
2. Lavigne JV, Gibbons RD, Christoffel KK, et al. Prevalence rates and correlates of psychiatric disorders among preschool children. J Am Acad Child Adolesc Psychiatry 1996;35:204–14.
3. Eley TC, Bolton D, O'Connor TG, et al. A twin study of anxiety-related behaviours in pre-school children. J Child Psychol Psychiatry 2003;44:945–60.
4. Spence SH, Rapee RM, McDonald C, et al. The structure of anxiety symptoms among preschoolers. Behav Res Ther 2001;39:1293–316.
5. Alfano CA, Ginsburg GS, Kingery JN. Sleep-related problems among children and adolescents with anxiety disorders. J Am Acad Child Adolesc Psychiatry 2007;46: 224–32.
6. Grills AE, Ollendick TH. Peer victimization, global self-worth, and anxiety in middle school children. J Clin Child Adolesc Psychol 2002;31:59–68.
7. Kaplow JB, Curran PJ, Angold A, et al. The prospective relation between dimensions of anxiety and the initiation of adolescent alcohol use. J Clin Child Psychol 2001;30: 316–26.
8. Storch EA, Ledley DR, Lewin AB, et al. Peer victimization in children with obsessive-compulsive disorder: relations with symptoms of psychopathology. J Clin Child Adolesc Psychol 2006;35:446–55.
9. Kendall PC, Furr JM, Podell JL. Child-focused treatment of anxiety. In: Weisz JR, Kazdin AE, editors. Evidence-based psychotherapies for children and adolescents. 2nd edition. New York: Guilford Press; 2009. p. 45–60.
10. Ollendick TH, King NJ. Empirically supported treatments for children with phobic and anxiety disorders: current status. J Clin Child Psychol 1998;27:156–67.
11. Silverman WK, Pina AA, Viswesvaran C. Evidence-based psychosocial treatments for phobic and anxiety disorders in children and adolescents. J Clin Child Adolesc Psychol 2008;37:105–30.
12. Kendall PC, Flannery-Schroeder E, Panichelli-Mindel SM, et al. Therapy for youth with anxiety disorders: a second randomized clinical trial. J Consult Clin Psychol 1997;65: 366–80.
13. Kendall PC, Hudson JL, Gosch E, et al. Cognitive-behavioral therapy for anxiety disordered youth: a randomized clinical trial evaluating child and family modalities. J Consult Clin Psychol 2008;76:282–97.
14. Silverman WK, Ollendick TH. Evidence-based assessment of anxiety and its disorders in children and adolescents. J Clin Child Adolesc Psychol 2005;34:380–411.
15. Walkup JT, Albano AM, Piacentini J, et al. Cognitive behavioral therapy, sertraline, or a combination in childhood anxiety. N Engl J Med 2008;359:2753–66.
16. Kendall PC, Safford S, Flannery-Schroeder E, et al. Child anxiety treatment: outcomes in adolescence and impact on substance use and depression at 7.4-year-follow-up. J Consult Clin Psychol 2004;72:276–87.
17. Freeman JB, Choate-Summers ML, Moore PS, et al. Cognitive behavioral treatment for young children with obsessive-compulsive disorder. Biol Psychiatry 2007;61:337–43.
18. Hirshfeld-Becker DR, Masek B, Henin A, et al. Cognitive behavioral therapy for 4- to 7-year-old children with anxiety disorders: a randomized clinical trial. J Consult Clin Psychol 2010;78:498–510.

19. Kennedy SJ, Rapee RM, Edwards SL. A selective intervention program for inhibited preschool-aged children of parents with an anxiety disorder: effects on current anxiety disorders and temperament. J Am Acad Child Adolesc Psychiatry 2009;48:602–9.
20. Cartwright-Hatton S, McNally D, Field AP, et al. A new parenting-based group intervention for young anxious children: results of a randomized controlled trial. J Am Acad Child Adolesc Psychiatry 2011;50:242–51.
21. Waters AM, Ford LA, Wharton TA, et al. Cognitive-behavioral therapy for young children with anxiety disorders: comparison of a child + parent condition to a parent only condition. Behav Res Ther 2009;47:654–62.
22. Flavell JH, Miller PH, Miller SA. Cognitive development. 4th edition. New York: Prentice Hall; 2001.
23. Zhang WW, Zheng J. The development of children's social perspective taking and the differences between perspective taking subtypes. Psychol Sci 1999;22:116–9.
24. Shaw P, Eckstrand K, Sharp W, et al. Attention-deficit hyperactivity disorder is characterized by a delay in cortical maturation. Proc Natl Acad Sci U S A 2007;104:19649–54.
25. Eyberg SM. Parent-child interaction therapy: integrity checklists and session materials [version 2.10]. Gainesville (FL): PCIT International; 2010.
26. McNeil CB, Hembree-Kigin TL. Parent-child interaction therapy. New York: Springer; 2010.
27. Comer JS, Puliafico AC, Aschenbrand SG, et al. A pilot feasibility evaluation of the CALM Program for anxiety disorders in early childhood. J Anxiety Disord 2012;26:40–9.
28. Pincus DB, Chase R, Chow CW, et al. Efficacy of modified parent-child interaction therapy for young children with separation anxiety disorder. Presented at the 44th annual meeting of the Association of Behavioral and Cognitive Therapies. San Francisco, November 2010.
29. Pincus D, Eyberg SM, Choate ML. Adapting parent-child interaction therapy for young children with separation anxiety disorder. Educ Treat Children 2005;28:163–81.
30. Pincus D, Santucci LC, Ehrenreich JT, et al. The implementation of modified parent-child interaction therapy for youth with separation anxiety disorder. Cogn Behav Pract 2008;15:118–25.
31. Eyberg SM, Nelson MM, Duke M, et al. Manual for the dyadic parent-child interaction coding system. 3rd edition. Published 2005. Available at: www.pcit.org. Accessed November 23, 2011.
32. Hudson JL, Comer JS, Kendall PC. Parental responses to positive and negative emotions in anxious and nonanxious children. J Clin Child Adolesc Psychol 2008;37:303–13.
33. McLeod BD, Wood JJ, Weisz JR. Examining the association between parenting and childhood anxiety: a meta-analysis. Clin Psychol Rev 2007;27:155–72.
34. Moore PS, Whaley SE, Sigman M. Interactions between mothers and children: impacts of maternal and child anxiety. J Abnorm Psychol 2004;113:471–6.
35. Rapee RM. Potential role of childrearing practices in the development of anxiety and depression. Clin Psychol Rev 1997;17:47–67.
36. Siqueland L, Kendall PC, Steinberg L. Anxiety in children: perceived family environments and observed family interaction. J Clin Child Psychol 1996;25:225–37.
37. Wood JJ, McLeod BD, Sigman M, et al. Parenting and childhood anxiety: theory, empirical findings, and future directions. J Child Psychol Psychiatry 2003;44:134–51.
38. Dadds MR, Barrett PM, Rapee RM. Family process and child anxiety and aggression: an observational analysis. J Abnorm Child Psychol 1996;24:715–34.

39. Chorpita BF, Barlow DH. The development of anxiety: the role of control in the early environment. Psychol Bull 1998;124:3–21.
40. Choate ML, Pincus DB, Eyberg SM, et al. Parent-child interaction therapy for treatment of separation anxiety disorder in young children: a pilot study. Cogn Behav Pract 2005;12:126–35.
41. Silverman WK, Albano AM. Anxiety disorders interview schedule for DSM-IV, child and parent versions. San Antonio (TX): Psychological Corporation; 1997.
42. Puliafico AC, Comer JS, Albano AM. Coaching approach behavior and leading by modeling: rationale, principals, and a session-by-session description of the CALM Program for early child anxiety. Cogn Behav Pract 2011, in press.
43. Eyberg and colleagues, 2005.
44. American Psychiatric Association. Diagnostic and Statistical Manual of Mental Disorders. 4th edition. Washington, DC: American Psychiatric Association; 1994.
45. Eyberg SM. Tailoring and adapting parent-child interaction therapy to new populations. Educ Treat Children 2005;28(2):197–201.
46. Comer JS, McNeil CB, Eyberg SM. Development of an Internet-delivered protocol for in-home parent-child interaction therapy. Presented at the 45th annual meeting of the Association for Behavioral and Cognitive Therapies. Toronto (ON, Canada), November 2011.

Social Phobia and Selective Mutism

Courtney P. Keeton, PhD*, Meghan Crosby Budinger, MS, LCPC

KEYWORDS

- Selective mutism • Speech • Communication • Shyness • Social phobia
- Social anxiety disorder

KEY POINTS

- Social phobia (SOP) typically onsets in adolescence.
- Selective mutism (SM) typically onsets before age 5 years.
- SOP and SM confer risk for other disorders or ongoing social disability, but more favorable outcomes may be associated with young age and low symptom severity.
- Psychosocial treatments that are considered "probably efficacious" for SOP include Individual Cognitive-Behavioral Therapy (ICBT), Social Effectiveness Training for Children (SET-C), and Group Cognitive-Behavioral Therapy (GCBT) with and without parents.
- Evidence-based treatment approaches for SOP and SM involve behavioral, cognitive, and pharmacologic strategies.
- Selective serotonin reuptake inhibitors (SSRIs) are considered first-line medications for youth with moderate or severe anxiety symptoms.

INTRODUCTION

Social phobia (SOP), which typically onsets in midadolescence, is characterized by persistent fear of scrutiny and avoidance or high distress in social situations. Selective mutism (SM) tends to appear in the preschool years and occurs when children who are capable of speech withhold it in some social situations in which speech is expected, such as at (pre)school or around unfamiliar people (see **Table 1** for Diagnostic and Statistical Manual of Mental Disorders [DSM]-IV Text Revision criteria for SOP and SM in children). Since the publication of DSM-III and subsequent editions in which SOP and SM are classified as distinct disorders, evidence has accumulated regarding their overlapping phenomenology. Despite the discrepant ages of onset, children with SM typically also have SOP diagnosed, and those who recover from SM

The authors have nothing to disclose.
Department of Psychiatry, Johns Hopkins University School of Medicine, 550 North Broadway/ Suite 201, Baltimore, MD 21205, USA
* Corresponding author.
E-mail address: ckeeton@jhmi.edu

Child Adolesc Psychiatric Clin N Am 21 (2012) 621–641
http://dx.doi.org/10.1016/j.chc.2012.05.009
1056-4993/12/$ – see front matter © 2012 Elsevier Inc. All rights reserved.

Table 1
DSM-IV-TR diagnostic criteria of SOP and SM in children

	Social Phobia	Selective Mutism
Primary symptoms	Marked and persistent fear of embarrassment or humiliation in 1 or more social or performance situations with peers. There must be evidence of the capacity for age-appropriate social relationships with familiar people Exposure to the feared social situation almost invariably provokes anxiety, may provoke panic attacks, and may be expressed by crying, tantrums, freezing, or shrinking from social situations with unfamiliar people The child may or may not recognize that their fear is excessive The feared social or performance situations are avoided or else are endured with intense anxiety or distress	Consistent failure to speak in specific social situations where speaking is expected (eg, school) despite speaking in other situations (eg, home)
Impairment	The avoidance, anxious anticipation, or distress in the feared social or performance situation(s) interferes significantly with the person's normal routine, occupational (academic) functioning, or social activities or relationships or there is marked distress about having the phobia	The disturbance interferes with educational or occupational achievement or with social communication
Duration	6 months	1 month (not the first month of school)
Not due to/better accounted for by	Physiologic effects of a substance, a general medical condition, and is not better accounted for by another mental disorder	Lack of knowledge of or discomfort with the primary language, communication disorder, pervasive developmental disorder, schizophrenia, or other psychotic disorder.
Specifier(s)	Generalized: If the fears include most social situations	N/A

Adapted from American Psychiatric Association. Diagnostic and statistical manual of mental disorders, Fourth Edition, Text Revision. Washington, DC: American Psychiatric Association; 2000.

continue to suffer from discomfort in social situations. Also, children with either diagnosis endorse comparable levels of anxiety, comorbidities, family histories of anxiety, and behaviorally inhibited temperaments. In light of their shared typology and the proposed reclassification of SM as a specifier of SOP in DSM-V[1,2] this article focuses on the 2 disorders collectively.

EPIDEMIOLOGY

SOP has the second-highest lifetime prevalence of anxiety disorders after specific phobia.[3] Data using American and German adolescent samples estimates the lifetime prevalence of SOP at 8.6% and 7.3%, respectively.[4,5] Prevalence rates of SOP for girls (9.2% to 9.5%) are higher than that for boys (4.9% to 7.9%).[4,5] Also, the generalized subtype of SOP, characterized by social fears across performance and interpersonal situations, earlier onset, and greater severity, is slightly more common than the nongeneralized subtype, particularly in girls.[4]

Prevalence estimates for SM vary depending on setting but are generally lower than those for SOP. In treatment settings, the prevalence of SM is 0.11% to 0.5%.[6-8] Higher rates, between 0.71% to 2.0%, have been found in community studies conducted in the United States, West Jerusalem, Finland, and Sweden, with higher rates among older children.[9-12] Lower relative prevalence rates in treatment settings and in younger children support the notion that a high percentage of children affected by SM are never seen for treatment[13] and that there is a considerable delay between onset and treatment.[14] Most studies report that SM is more common in females[15,16]; however, others have found comparable rates among boys and girls.[10,13,17] SM occurs at higher rates in bilingual or immigrant children.[9,18]

AGE OF ONSET

In general, anxiety disorders tend to occur earlier than other mental disorders.[3] According to epidemiologic data, SOP onsets between 8 and 15 years, and the generalized subtype onsets earlier.[4,5] Retrospective accounts by adults indicate a median age of onset of 13 to 15.1 years.[19,20] Among youth with the generalized subtype, those with a parent affected by SOP tend to have an earlier age of onset (6 years) compared with youth without an affected parent (11 years).[21] In contrast, SM tends to onset earlier, and the mean age of onset is 2.7 to 3.7 years.[13,17] One study on individuals with SM ages 18 and older reported an average age of onset of 9.4 years.[15]

COURSE

Both SOP and SM tend to onset gradually, often present early on as behavioral inhibition (BI) and run a stable course (for a detailed description of BI see article by Blackford & Pine, in this issue).[13,15,22] In 1 epidemiologic study, of the 8.6% 13- to 18-year-olds meeting lifetime diagnostic criteria for SOP, 87% continued to meet current criteria at the time of the interview, even though more than 60% reported receiving treatment for their disorder.[4] Prospective epidemiologic data showed that adolescents with SOP are 3.6 to 4.9 times as likely to have SOP in young adulthood compared with adolescents without SOP.[23] Moreover, SOP in childhood is associated with subsequent depression, suicidality, and substance abuse.[24-26] Ongoing SOP is associated with functional impairment, such as marital instability and lower educational attainment and income levels.[24,27,28]

Cases of SM onsetting abruptly in response to a stressful event[16,29] are relatively uncommon and may be transient.[15] In one survey study of 153 children and adults with current or lifetime SM, 71.3% reported having SM for 3 or more years, and only one individual had SM for less than a year.[15] For individuals who once had SM but no longer did (64% of total sample), the average age of cessation was 7.6 years; however, more than half reported considerable discomfort in social situations currently.[15] One community-based, case-controlled study found that 28% of elementary school children with SM showed some improvement at a 6-month follow up but that the majority remained significantly impaired in their academic and social functioning compared with their nonaffected peers.[10] A follow-up study of 41 young adults who had SM as children found that 32% showed mild or no improvement in mutism symptoms.[30] More than one-third of the sample (39%) was considered in remission; however, other psychosocial problems, such as depressive/dysphoric mood, were present currently in those who were recovered or mildly impaired (23%). Another study of young adults 13 years after clinical referral reported a remission rate of 58% and high rates of phobic (42.4%) and other disorders at follow-up (eg, substance use disorder, 15.2%; depressive disorder, 9.1%), even when SM had remitted.[31] Overall, SOP and SM are stable disorders that carry risks for continued mental health problems and functional disability.

COMORBIDITY

Both SOP and SM are associated with co-occurring anxiety disorders and symptoms in children.
SOP most commonly co-occurs with[4]:

- Agoraphobia, 32.4%
- Generalized anxiety disorder (GAD), 32%
- Separation anxiety disorder (SAD), 27.4%
- Panic disorder, 27.2%
- Posttraumatic stress disorder, 24.4%
- Specific phobia (SP), 21.5%.

As many as 97% to 100% of children with SM also have SOP diagnosed.[13,32]
SM often co-occurs with[17,33]:

- SAD, 31.5%
- SP, 13%
- GAD, 13%
- High rates of shyness and somatic symptoms.

US epidemiologic data showed that 17.4% of socially anxious adolescents met criteria for a substance use disorder,[4] and data using a community sample showed a significant association between SOP and smoking in boys.[34] Girls with SOP may be less likely to use drugs compared with girls with other anxiety or depressive disorders.[34] There are no data on substance use disorder with SM.

Major depressive disorder (MDD) was diagnosed in 18.7% of adolescents with SOP in an epidemiologic sample.[4] In a primary care sample, lifetime and current MDD were present in 28% and 6% of SOP cases, respectively.[35] Results of an Australian population-based sample showed that 42% of males and 59% of females with SOP also had MDD.[36] There are no data on comorbid SM and MDD.

Children with SM have high rates of elimination problems, such as constipation, enuresis, and encopresis.[13,37] For example, the rate of 33% enuresis or encopresis in 1 sample of SM children[16] was comparable to the rate of 31.5% reported in another study, and this rate was significantly higher than the 9.3% in the control group.[17]

Many children with SM show evidence of delayed speech acquisition or poor articulation, and, when compared with children with SOP, they perform worse on nonverbal tests of language.[38] As many as half the children with SM may have a diagnosable language or communication problem.[16,17]

Whereas some data show no differences in parent- or teacher-reported externalizing behaviors, such as attention deficit-hyperactivity disorder (ADHD), oppositional defiant disorder (ODD), and conduct disorder (CD) among children with SM and healthy controls,[10,33] many studies characterize children with SM as oppositional, aggressive, controlling, or stubborn.[15,39] When compared with children with SOP alone, parents of children with SM and SOP reported significantly higher scores on the delinquency and aggression scales.[40] One study found that 29% of children with SM and SOP had comorbid ODD compared with 5% of those with SOP only.[41] Epidemiologic findings showed that, among adolescents with SOP, 17.8% had comorbid ODD and 16.9% had comorbid CD.[4] Finally, a latent profile analysis of 130 children with SM resulted in 3 distinct groups including an exclusively anxious group, an anxious communication-delayed group, and an anxious mildly oppositional group.[39]

ETIOLOGY

Temperament, familial, and environmental factors contribute to the onset and maintenance of SOP and SM.

Behavioral inhibition is a temperament characterized by shyness, apprehension, and withdrawal. A clear relationship between BI and SOP has been established empirically.[42,43] In one study, children classified as BI at age 21 months and 31 months were significantly more likely to have SOP diagnosed at age 13 (61%) compared with those who had not been classified as BI (27%).[22] Another study found that 17% of 2-, 4-, and 6-year-olds classified as BI also met criteria for SOP, whereas there was no relationship between BI and other mood or anxiety disorders.[44] The association between BI and SM is more speculative and is based on shared features such as reluctance to speak, lifetime shyness, slow-to-warm-up personality, and difficulty responding to novel situations and handling transitions.[15,32,45]

Findings from family, twin, and genotyping studies suggest moderate heritability of SOP. Twin studies estimated that 39% to 65% of the variance in shared phenotypes is caused by genetic effects.[36,46,47] Meta-analytic data of family and twin studies suggest that first-degree relatives of probands with simple phobia, social phobia, or agoraphobia have a 4.1 odds ratio of also having a diagnosable phobia.[48] Also, a longitudinal community-based study found that adolescents of parents with SOP had significantly elevated rates of SOP (9.6%) compared with offspring of parents without SOP (2.1%).[21] Genotyping studies have found an association between SOP and the human serotonin transporter–linked polymorphic region (5-HTTLPR) gene.[49,50] The presence of 2 long 5-HTT alleles, as opposed to 1 or 2 short alleles, is associated with increased serotonin reuptake, which plays an important role in affective regulation.[51] Individuals with SOP and the short allele polymorphism of the 5-HHT gene may have greater anxiety severity, as demonstrated in a genotyping study involving a public speaking task.[50]

There are no genetics studies that include both SAD and SM. However, one study examined several single nucleotide polymorphisms (SNP) of the contactin-associated proteinlike 2 (CNTNAP2) gene in children with SM and young adults with social anxiety-related traits.[52] Variations in CNTNAP2 have been implicated in the developmental language-delayed component of autism and were examined in this study because language deficits also characterize children with SM. Results showed that variation in CNTNAP2, specifically the rs2710102 SNP, is associated with risk for SM in a family-based sample and with behavioral inhibition and social anxiety in a sample of young adults. Findings provided preliminary evidence of a potential shared genetic etiology for autism spectrum disorders and SM, but replication and further investigation is necessary.

Familial aggregation of SM and related symptoms suggests that, like SOP, genetic factors play a role in the etiology. In one study, about 70% of first-degree relatives of children with SM had a history of social anxiety and shyness, and 37% of first-degree relatives had a history of SM.[13] Poor language production, extreme shyness, and speech and language disorders occurred in 78% of first-degree relatives in another sample, with concordance rates of SM in first-degree relatives up to 27%.[30] The rates of avoidant personality disorder and lifetime generalized social phobia among parents of children with SM are higher compared with parents of children without any disorder.[37]

Consistent with suggestions from twin and prospective-longitudinal data that nongenetic environmental variables increase susceptibility to SOP,[21,46] several environmental variables have been linked empirically with both SOP and SM. Many studies have found links between child anxiety and specific parenting behaviors, such as overprotection, criticism, anxious modeling, and lack of warmth and granting of autonomy.[53,54] Parental overprotection and rejection have been linked specifically with adolescent SOP, even when controlling for parental psychopathology.[21] Similarly, parents of children with SM have been rated as significantly more controlling based on parent–child interaction tasks and clinician-administered interviews compared with parents of anxious and nondisordered groups.[33,55] Evidence also suggests that families of children with SOP or SM are less socially active, less involved in recreational activities, and provide fewer opportunities for socialization.[56] Finally, negative life events or trauma may increase a child's risk for both SOP and SM development.[57,58]

ASSESSMENT

Useful methods for the initial diagnosis and ongoing monitoring of SOP and SM include standardized diagnostic interviews, paper-and-pencil questionnaires, and physiologic and behavioral measures.

Diagnostic Interviews

Standardized interviews (**Box 1**) are valuable for soliciting reports from a child and caregiver regarding symptoms, severity, and impairment to make DSM diagnoses. The "gold-standard" interview for pediatric anxiety is the Anxiety Disorders Interview Schedule for DSM-IV (ADIS-IV: C/P),[59] which assesses the full range of Axis I disorders. The ADIS IV: C/P has demonstrated reliability and validity for assessing anxiety symptoms in children ages 6 to 17 and has excellent test-retest and inter-rater reliability.[60–62] The Kiddie Schedule for Affective Disorders and Schizophrenia and Diagnostic Interview for Children and Adolescents do not assess SM, but investigators have added questions to do so.[63,6]

Rating Scales

There are many available parent-, self-, and teacher-report rating scales that assess anxiety in general and include a SOP-specific subscale and others that are unique to SOP or SM. Frequently used anxiety questionnaires with good internal consistency, validity, and test-retest reliability include the Screen for Child Anxiety and Related

---

Box 1
Structured and semistructured diagnostic interviews

- Anxiety Disorders Interview Schedule for DSM-IV (ADIS-IV)[59]

- Kiddie Schedule for Affective Disorders and Schizophrenia–Present and Lifetime Version (K-SADS-PL)[65]

- Diagnostic Interview Schedule for Children-Version 4 (DISC-IV)[66]

- Children's Interview for Psychiatric Syndromes (ChIPS)[67]

- Diagnostic Interview for Children and Adolescents (DICA)[68]

- Diagnostic Interview for Children and Adolescents for Parents of Preschool and Young Children (DICA-PPYC)[64]

- Child and Adolescent Psychiatric Assessment (CAPA)[69]

- Preschool-Age Psychiatric Assessment (PAPA)[70]

Disorders,[71,72] the Multidimensional Anxiety Scale for Children,[73,74] the Spence Children's Anxiety Scale,[74] and the Revised Child Anxiety and Depression Scales.[75–77] Details regarding scales specific to SOP and SM are reported in **Table 2**.

Physiologic and Observational Methods

Physiologic and performance-based methods provide opportunities to objectively assess correlates and behavioral markers of anxiety.[78] Physiologic measures assess the electrocortical system (eg, cortisol reactivity), the cardiovascular system (eg, heart rate variability), electrodermal activity (eg, skin conductance level), and muscle contraction activity (eg, auditory startle reflex), and provide links between autonomic nervous system regulatory activities and behavioral responses. Data are emerging that assesses physiologic arousal in children with SM and SOP; preliminary data found higher arousal levels measured by skin conductance among the SOP group compared with the SM and control groups.[79] Studies measuring the stress hormone cortisol as a physiologic marker of SOP have produced mixed results.[80,81] Blushing has stood out as a correlate of social anxiety in contrast to other autonomic variables.[82] This study, like many others,[83] also showed a discrepancy between subjective reports and actual physiologic responses.

Commonly used observational methods of behavioral assessment include social competence tasks and behavioral assessment tasks. Social competence tasks assess social skill behaviors within various interactions between the child and a same-age peer. In studies of youth with SOP and SM, role-plays involving situations such as starting conversations and offering to help have been rated by observers for social effectiveness and used as a measure of treatment outcome.[40,84] Behavioral assessment tasks assess observed anxiety-related behaviors during laboratory or naturalistic settings. For example, as part of a treatment study of anxious youth, pre- and posttreatment behaviors during a videotaped task were coded across 30-second intervals for a 5-minute period.[85] This method has also been used to rate indicators of BI in young children during videotaped interactions with parents and unfamiliar stimuli.[86]

TREATMENT

Evidence-based treatment approaches for SOP and SM involve behavioral, cognitive, and pharmacologic strategies. Most treatment studies operationalize outcome as

Table 2
Disorder-specific rating scales

Measure	Reporter	Age Range	Subscales/Factors	Sample Item	No. of Items	Response Format	Cronbach α	Clinical Cut off
Social Anxiety Disorder								
Social Anxiety Scale for Children – Revised[135]	Child	6–15	Fear of negative evaluation, Social avoidance of distress in new situations	"I worry about what other children say about me."	22	1 (not at all) to 5 (all the time)	.60–.90[136]	50 (boys) 54 (girls)
Social Anxiety Scale for Adolescents[137]		12–18	Social avoidance of distress in general situations	"I get nervous when I talk to peers I don't know very well."			.70–.91[137,138]	50
Social Phobia and Anxiety Scale for Children[139]	Parent Child	8–17	Assertiveness, public performance, Physical/cognitive symptoms, social encounter, avoidance	"I feel scared when I have to speak or read in front of a group of people."	26	0 (never) to 2 (most of the time or always)	.64–.92[140,141]	18
Leibowitz Social Anxiety Scale for Children & Adolescents[142]	Clinician	NS	Social anxiety, social avoidance, performance anxiety, performance avoidance	"Looking at people you don't know very well in the eyes."	24	Fear/Anxiety: 0 (none) to 3 (severe); Avoidance: 0 (never) to 3 (usually)	.83–.97[143]	30
Selective Mutism								
Selective Mutism Questionnaire[144]	Parent	NS	School situations, social situations with family, other social situations	"My child talks when in clubs, teams, or organized activities outside of school."	17	0 (never) to 3 (always)	.84–.97[144]	NS
School Speech Questionnaire[10]	Teacher	NS	Total score	"When called on by his/her teacher, this student answers verbally"	11	0 (never) to 3 (always)	.94[10]	NS

Abbreviation: NS, not specified.

response rates based on diagnostic recovery rates or ratings of ≤2, "much improved" or "very much improved" on a Clinical Global Impressions–Improvement scale. Comparative trial data suggest that combination treatment with cognitive-behavioral therapy (CBT) plus a selective serotonin reuptake inhibitor (SSRI) produce relatively superior outcomes for children with anxiety disorders, including SOP.[87] However, evidence suggests that a primary diagnosis of SOP is associated with less-favorable outcomes, independent of treatment type, when compared with children with a primary diagnosis of GAD or SAD (Compton S, Peris T, Birmaher B, et al. Predictors and moderators of treatment response in childhood anxiety disorders: results from the CAMS Trial. Submitted for publication).[88]

Psychosocial Treatment

Psychosocial treatments that are considered "probably efficacious"[89] for SOP include individual cognitive-behavioral therapy (ICBT), social effectiveness training for children (SET-C), and group cognitive-behavioral therapy (GCBT) with and without parents.[90] Meta-analytic data suggests that CBT for youth with anxiety disorders including SOP has an effect size of $d = 0.94$.[91] In the absence of randomized, controlled trials (RCTs) for the psychosocial treatment of SM, cognitive and behavioral strategies are considered first-line interventions.[14,92] These treatments are described below, in addition to newly emerging, promising interventions involving cognitive and behavioral strategies, namely, computerized interventions, developmentally modified interventions for preschool-aged children, and intensive summer group programming.

Individual cognitive behavioral therapy

The majority of studies examining the efficacy of ICBT for social anxiety enrolled children with any combination of SOP/avoidant disorder, GAD/overanxious disorder, and SAD, and utilized the 16-session "Coping Cat" manual[93] or its Australian adaptation, the "Coping Koala."[94] Typical CBT components that are represented in these manuals include education about the nature of anxiety and the link between anxious feelings, physiologic arousal, negative thoughts, and avoidant behavior; cognitive restructuring to correct negative automatic thoughts and generate positive self-talk; and behavioral strategies such as modeling, role playing, relaxation training, contingent reinforcement, and graduated exposure. The effectiveness of ICBT with pediatric anxiety disorders (GAD, SOP, and SAD) has been demonstrated across several RCTs showing 53% to 69.8% resolution of anxiety diagnoses after treatment, long-term maintenance of gains up to 7.4 years after treatment, and lowered substance use over time with early successful treatment.[95–98] When SOP is examined as a child's most impairing condition, treatment approaches containing medication appear more effective than ICBT (Compton S, Peris T, Birmaher B, et al. Predictors and moderators of treatment response in childhood anxiety disorders: results from the CAMS Trial. Submitted for publication).

Exposure-based strategies stand out in the SM treatment literature,[92,99,100] but there are no controlled trials of CBT for this population. Manualized anxiety treatment can be adapted for use with SM, involving increased parent training, school collaboration, psychoeducation about SM, and simplifying the cognitive restructuring component for the likely younger age of the SM patient.[92,101,102] Adaptation of the Coping Cat manual is described in a case report involving an 8-year-old girl with SM; adapted strategies include developing rapport with the parent-child dyad with reduced emphasis on the child, shaping communication through praise of spontaneous speech efforts, utilizing parent-only sessions to teach behavior modification strategies such as shaping and creating daily structure, collaborating with the parent to teach coping skills, and utilizing video and audio recordings to implement a gradual hierarchy of speech exercises.[101] In another case report, a modularized CBT manual is adapted for use with an 8-year-old boy with SM; specific strategies include developing an initial rapport through shaping, consistently utilizing teacher and parent reports, offering positive coping statements, and creating an exposure hierarchy based on increasingly distressing speech tasks.[103]

Social effectiveness therapy for children

Social Effectiveness Therapy for Children (SET-C) is a behavioral group treatment targeting SOP through 12 sessions involving psychoeducation for child and parent, social skills training (starting and maintaining conversations), peer generalization experiences (eg, pizza party to practice social skills), and in vivo exposure (eg, reading aloud in front of a group).[104] In the initial RCT involving 67 children age 8 to 12, resolution of SOP was achieved in 67% of the SET-C group and 5% of the study skills comparison group, and treatment gains were maintained at 6-month follow-up.[104] Participants in the SET-C group also showed improvements in social skills and social interaction and decreased social fears, anxiety, and associated psychopathology. SET-C also resulted in significantly greater treatment response rates relative to fluoxetine and control groups in a comparative RCT involving youth age 7 to 17.[84] Both SET-C and fluoxetine were more effective than placebo in reducing symptoms and functional impairment; however, only SET-C participants showed improvements in social skills, social competence, and anxiety in specific social interactions. The long-term efficacy of SET-C for SOP has been shown in 3- and 5-year follow-up studies.[105,106] SET-C has been applied to an individual case of a child with SM.[107] For this 10-year-old, SET-C sessions were adapted to begin with shaping exercises involving vocalizations followed by learning and role-playing a new social skill, and several parent training sessions and school-based interventions were added. Although there were a number of challenges associated with the case, it showed that SET-C could be appropriate for school-age or adolescent youth who have SM and obvious social anxiety or social skills deficits.

Group cognitive behavioral therapy

Like SET-C, other group treatments have emphasized the importance of teaching social skills training in the treatment of SOP. In one study involving 50 children age 7 to 14, GCBT plus social skills training with and without parental involvement was compared with a waitlist control.[108] Treatment involved 12 weekly sessions and 2 follow-up sessions. The CBT condition included the traditional components described above (eg, cognitive restructuring, graduated exposure). The social skills training emphasized eye contact, active listening, joining a group, and assertiveness, and the parental component involved observation of the CBT sessions and learning contingency management and modeling. After treatment, rates of resolved SOP diagnosis were statistically higher in the parent involvement group (87.5%) and no-parent group (58%) compared with the control group (7%). There were also significant improvements in both treatment groups, but not the control group, on self-reports of anxiety symptoms and social worries and parent reports of social skills and social competence. Gains were maintained at 12-month follow-up.

A comprehensive review of other studies using GCBT for anxious youth including those with SOP supports the efficacy of both GCBT and GCBT involving parents.[90] While one randomized study comparing individual and group CBT for anxious youth found that children with high levels of social anxiety responded significantly better to individual treatment,[109] meta-analysis suggests that there are no significant differences between individual and group treatments on diagnostic recovery rates.[90] With regard to SM, an 8-week group treatment focused on psychoeducation, relaxation exercises, and gradual exposure, and rewards resulted in significant increases in speech production across settings for the 5 participants (mean age, 6.1 years).[110] Another GCBT trial emphasizing exposure, social skills training, and speech and language techniques has resulted in speech inside and outside of treatment for the majority of children treated.[111]

Emerging treatments

Computerized or internet-based CBT (iCBT) is a recent advance in the treatment of anxiety that typically incorporates the principles of CBT in self-paced lessons with varying remote support from a clinician. In one case of a 7-year-old with SM, iCBT resulted in significant reductions in anxiety and overall SM symptom severity.[112] A number of controlled studies and preliminary reports investigating iCBT for anxiety have produced favorable outcomes.[113] For example, an RCT using computer-assisted CBT for anxious youth age 7 to 13 resulted in resolution of primary diagnosis in 81% of children compared with 19% in the education support condition.[114] Although these studies included youth with a variety of anxiety disorders, several RCTs using iCBT to treat SOP specifically in adults have produced favorable results including superior outcomes relative to waitlist controls and comparable efficacy to face-to-face CBT.[115–117] Computerized forms of CBT hold the potential to offer advantages including increased availability of empirically based treatment, reduced treatment costs, and privacy.[113,118]

Although participants in the majority of psychosocial treatment studies for anxiety have a mean age of at least 7 years, emerging treatments for young children have been prompted by increasing recognition of anxiety and BI in this population and the early age of onset of SM. In one RCT, 64 children age 4 to 7 with non-SM anxiety disorders (67% with SOP) were assigned to a 20-session developmentally modified version of ICBT or waitlist control.[86] Specific developmental modifications included significant parent involvement and the use of games to teach age-appropriate coping skills. Clinical Global Impressions–Improvement response rates were significantly higher in the ICBT condition (69%) compared with waitlist (32%), and treatment gains were maintained after 1 year. Like some SOP medication treatment studies, when symptom severity predicted poorer response to treatment,[119] higher levels of child BI predicted poorer treatment response. In another study involving young children age 5 to 7 with mixed anxiety (including SOP and SM), a 12-session GCBT involving concurrent child and parent sessions was examined in an open trial.[120] The program incorporated stories, crafts, and other activities to teach typical CBT concepts. Resolution of at least 1 anxiety disorder occurred in 71.9% of children.

One recent report focused exclusively on children with SM and described a behavioral treatment for 7 children aged 3 to 5.[121] Treatment started in the home where the child was most comfortable and then moved to the kindergarten where symptoms were most impairing. The clinician, parents, and teacher utilized communication strategies such as sitting beside rather than across from the child, creating joint attention using an activity the child enjoys, and thinking aloud rather than asking the child direct questions. These strategies were paired with psychoeducation, stimulus fading, and rewards for weekly or twice-weekly sessions for a maximum of 6 months. After 6 months, 6 of 7 children spoke fluently in school. At the 1-year follow-up, 5 out 7 children spoke freely in the classroom.

Finally, a novel treatment approach involving an intensive 1-week summer camp is offered in several locations throughout the United States. In this program, children with SM attend a summer program in a simulated classroom where verbalizations are modeled and reinforced in "real-world" situations representative of a typical school day. Pilot data involving 9 children age 4 to 7 years show promising results, such as increases in spontaneous verbalizations, across the 5-day program. Also, mean increases on the Selective Mutism Questionnaire school subscale from 0.49 at baseline to 1.40 after treatment and 1.75 at a 3-month follow-up demonstrated speech improvement comparable with results found in multiweek behavioral treatments.[122]

Pharmacotherapy

Treatment with medication is recommended for youth when anxiety symptoms are moderate or severe or when psychotherapy is inadequate.[123] SSRIs are considered first-line medications, with safety and acute efficacy demonstrated in RCTs involving fluoxetine,[119] fluvoxamine,[124] paroxetine,[125] and sertraline[87] for the treatment of SOP. Data also support the use of venlafaxine, a selective-norepinephrine reuptake inhibitor for SOP.[126] Data from a large RCT involving youth ages 7 to 17 with GAD, SOP, or SAD showed that, although combination treatment (sertraline and CBT) produced superior outcomes overall when compared with monotherapies and placebo,[87] superior outcomes when SOP is the primary diagnosis were achieved with treatment conditions involving medication (combination or sertraline-only) compared with CBT only and placebo (Compton S, Peris T, Birmaher B, et al. Predictors and moderators of treatment response in childhood anxiety disorders: results from the CAMS Trial. Submitted for publication). All of these studies are reviewed in detail in this issue, and this review focuses on the pharmacotherapy of SM. Two controlled trials involving SM have been conducted[127,128]; however, the majority of pharmacologic support with this population comes from case reports.

SSRI treatment

Fluoxetine is the most studied SSRI for the treatment of SM, and was used in a 12-week RCT involving 15 children age 6 to 11.[127] The mean maximum dose of fluoxetine was 21.4 mg/d. Fluoxetine-treated subjects showed significant improvement across ratings of mutism and anxiety; however, they remained highly symptomatic at the end of 12 weeks, and comparisons with the placebo group were not statistically significant except for parent-reported global improvement. Side effects were minimal (drop in systolic blood pressure), and there were no significant differences in side effects for the placebo and active drug groups. The authors concluded that 12 weeks may be too short a period to find significant changes, that early changes may be less evident at school compared with other settings, and that starting treatment during the summer or early in the school year, before patterns of nonspeaking in the school context have become too entrenched, may be most beneficial. Additionally, dosing may have been conservative given the severity of the patient population.

An open trial of fluoxetine with 21 children (age 5 to 14) with SM found that an optimal response at the end of 9 weeks was achieved with 20 mg/d.[129] Significant pre- to posttreatment changes were found across self- and parent-rated social behavior and anxiety symptoms and clinician-rated global assessment of functioning and overall improvement. Younger children showed the greatest improvements. Several case reports focused on fluoxetine described positive outcomes and few side effects in children in SM.[130] Time to response and treatment duration within the case reports are variable, with some children beginning to speak after only 2 weeks of fluoxetine treatment, and others requiring 6 to 12 weeks to achieve some benefit.

Paroxetine 5 mg/d was given in a case report of an 8-year-old girl with SM, SOP, and separation anxiety with no adverse events.[131] An increase in speaking behaviors occurred 3 weeks into treatment according to parent and teacher report, and the other anxiety disorders resolved. The child was treated for 3 years without relapse of symptoms.

Sertraline was studied in a double-blind, placebo-controlled multiple baseline trial with 5 children, aged 5 to 11, with SM.[128] Children were given 50 mg/d for 2 weeks, then 100 mg/d for 8 to 12 weeks. All participants showed rapid improvements in talking behavior in home and community settings, and 2 of 5 demonstrated improved speech at school. The youngest 2 children no longer met diagnostic criteria at the end of the study.

IMPLICATIONS FOR RESEARCH AND CLINICAL PRACTICE

Although the treatment literature for SOP is well established, there remains a dearth of controlled studies identifying the most effective strategies for SM, including treatment options for very young children. In the absence of scientifically rigorous treatment studies for SM, existing studies paired with its relatedness to SOP suggest great promise in particular for the use of behavioral techniques and SSRIs with this population. Increased awareness and dissemination of SM treatments are needed, an effort being modeled for example by Dr Steven Kurtz, whose "Brave Buddies" intensive summer treatment program is being increasingly adapted for use by others (Boston University's "Brave Bunch" program, "Confident Kids" camp in Michigan, among others). Also, the expected development of a clinician's guide and toolkit for the treatment of SM will offer a valuable resource to clinicians (R. Gallagher, written communication, April 2012). Other resources, such as in-depth descriptions of audio or video self-modeling as a behavioral treatment technique for SM,[132–134] are underrecognized. It is possible that the merge of SM with SOP in DSM-V will explicate their similarities and foster competence and motivation for clinicians in accessing treating strategies for SM. In addition to treatment dissemination, research initiatives should not overlook the reality that a sizeable portion of youth treated for SM or SOP does not respond to evidence-based care. Thus, future research should examine innovative refinements to existing interventions to enhance treatment outcomes and sustainability.

REFERENCES

1. Bogels SM, Alden L, Beidel DC, et al. Social anxiety disorder: Questions and answers for the DSM-V. Depress Anxiety 2010;27(2):168–89.
2. American Psychiatric Association. Diagnostic and statistical manual of mental disorders, Fourth Edition, Text Revision Washington, DC: American Psychiatric Association; 2000.
3. Kessler RC, Ruscio AM, Shear K, et al. Epidemiology of anxiety disorders. Behavioral neurobiology of anxiety and its treatment. New York, NY US: Springer Science + Business Media; 2010. p. 21–35.
4. Burstein M, Jian-Ping H, Gabriela K, et al. Social Phobia and subtypes in the national comorbidity survey-adolescent supplement: prevalence, correlates, and comorbidity. J Am Acad Child Adolesc Psychiatry 2011;50(9):870–80.
5. Wittchen HU, Stein MB, Kessler RC. Social fears and social phobia in a community sample of adolescents and young adults: prevalence, risk factors and co-morbidity. Psychol Med 1999;29:309–23.

6. Carlson JS, Kratochwill TR, Johnston H. Prevalence and treatment of selective mutism in clinical practice: a survey of child and adolescent psychiatrists. J Child Adolesc Psychopharmacol 1994;4(4):281–91.

7. Chavira DA, Stein MB, Bailey K, et al. Child Anxiety in primary care: prevalent but untreated. Depress Anxiety 2004;20(4):155–64.

8. Egger HL, Angold A. Common emotional and behavioral disorders in preschool children: presentation, nosology, and epidemiology. J Child Psychol Psychiatry 2006;47(3/4):313–37.

9. Elizur Y, Perednik R. Prevalence and description of selective mutism in immigrant and native families: a controlled study. J Am Acad Child Adolesc Psychiatry 2003; 42(12):1451–9.

10. Bergman RL, Piacentini J, McCracken JT. Prevalence and description of selective mutism in a school-based sample. J Am Acad Child Adolesc Psychiatry 2002;41(8): 938–46.

11. Kumpulainen K, Räsänen E, Raaska H, et al. Selective mutism among second-graders in elementary school. Eur Child Adolesc Psychiatry 1998;7(1):24–9.

12. Kopp S, Gillberg C. Selective mutistn: a population-based study: a research note. J Child Psychol Psychiatry 1997;38(2):257–62.

13. Black B, Uhde TW. Psychiatric characteristics of children with selective mutism: a pilot study. J Am Acad Child Adolesc Psychiatry 1995;34(7):847–56.

14. Viana AG, Beidel DC, Rabian B. Selective mutism: a review and integration of the last 15 years. Clin Psychol Rev 2009;29(1):57–67.

15. Ford MA, Sladeczek IE, Carlson J, et al. Selective mutism: phenomenological characteristics. School Psychology Quarterly 1998;13(3):192–227.

16. Steinhausen H-C, Juzi C. Elective mutism: an analysis of 100 cases. J Am Acad Child Adolesc Psychiatry 1996;35(5):606–14.

17. Kristensen H. Selective mutism and comorbidity with developmental disorder/delay, anxiety disorder, and elimination disorder. J Am Acad Child Adolesc Psychiatry 2000;39(2):249–56.

18. Bradley S, Sloman L. Elective mutism in immigrant families. J Am Acad Child Psychiatry 1975;14:510–4.

19. Kessler RC, Berglund P, Demler O, et al. Lifetime prevalence and age-of-onset distributions of DSM-IV disorders in the national comorbidity survey replication. Arch Gen Psychiatry 2005;62:593–602.

20. Grant BF, Hasin DS, Blanco C, et al. The epidemiology of social anxiety disorder in the United States: results from the National Epidemiologic Survey on Alcohol and Related Conditions. J Clin Psychiatry 2005;66(11):1351–61.

21. Lieb R, Wittchen H-U, Höfler M, et al. Parental psychopathology, parenting styles, and the risk of social phobia in offspring: a prospective-longitudinal community study. Arch Gen Psychiatry 2000;57(9):859–66.

22. Schwartz CE, Snidman N. Adolescent social anxiety as an outcome of inhibited temperament in childhood. J Am Acad Child Adolesc Psychiatry 1999;38(8):1008–15.

23. Pine DS, Cohen P, Gurley D, et al. The risk for early-adulthood anxiety and depressive disorders in adolescents with anxiety and depressive disorders. Arch Gen Psychiatry 1998 1998;55(1):56-64.

24. Stein MB, Kean YM. Disability and quality of life in social phobia: epidemiologic findings. Am J Psychiatry 2000;157(10):1606.

25. Crum RM, Pratt LA. Risk of heavy drinking and alcohol use disorders in social phobia: a prospective analysis. Am J Psychiatry 2001;158(10):1693.

26. Beesdo K, Bittner A, Pine DS, et al. Incidence of social anxiety disorder and the consistent risk for secondary depression in the first three decades of life. Arch Gen Psychiatry 2007;64(8):903–12.
27. Kessler RC, Chiu WT, Demler O, et al. Prevalence, severity, and comorbidity of 12-month DSM-IV disorders in the National Comorbidity Survey Replication. Arch Gen Psychiatry 2005;62(6):617–27.
28. Katzelnick DJ, Greist JH. Social anxiety disorder: an unrecognized problem in primary care. J Clin Psychiatry 2001;62(Suppl 1):11–6.
29. Anyfantakis D, Botzakis E, Mplevrakis E, et al. Selective mutism due to a dog bit trauma in a 4-year-old girl: a case report. J Med Case Reports 2009;3.
30. Remschmidt H, Poller M, Herpertz-Dahlmann B, et al. A follow-up study of 45 patients with elective mutism. Eur Arch Psychiatry Clin Neurosci 2001;251(6): 284–96.
31. Steinhausen H-C, Wachter M, Laimbock K, et al. A long-term outcome study of selective mutism in childhood. J Child Psychol Psychiatry 2006;47(7):751–6.
32. Dummit ES, Klein RG, Tancer NK, et al. Systematic assessment of 50 children with selective mutism. J Am Acad Child Adolesc Psychiatry 1997;36(5):653–60.
33. Buzzella BA, Ehrenreich-May J, Pincus DB. Comorbidity and family factors associated with selective mutism. Child Dev Res 2010;2011:1–9.
34. Wu P, Goodwin RD, Fuller C, et al. The relationship between anxiety disorders and substance use among adolescents in the community: specificity and gender differences. J Youth Adolesc 2010;39(2):177–88.
35. Chavira DA, Stein MB, Bailey K, et al. Comorbidity of generalized social anxiety disorder and depression in a pediatric primary care sample. J Affect Disord 2004; 80(2-3):163–71.
36. Mosing MA, Gordon SD, Medland SE, et al. Genetic and environmental influences on the co-morbidity between depression, panic disorder, agoraphobia, and social phobia: a twin study. Depress Anxiety 2009;26(11):1004–11.
37. Chavira DA, Shipon-Blum E, Hitchcock C, et al. Selective mutism and social anxiety disorder: All in the family? J Am Acad Child Adolesc Psychiatry 2007; 46(11):1464–72.
38. Manassis K, Fung D, Tannock R, et al. Characterizing selective mutism: is it more than social anxiety? Depress Anxiety 2003;18(3):153–61.
39. Cohan SL, Chavira DA, Shipon-Blum E, et al. Refining the classification of children with selective mutism: a latent profile analysis. J Clin Child Adolesc Psychol 2008; 37(4):770–84.
40. Yeganeh R, Beidel DC, Turner SM, et al. Clinical distinctions between selective mutism and social phobia: an investigation of childhood psychopathology. J Am Acad Child Adolesc Psychiatry 2003;42(9):1069–75.
41. Yeganeh R, Beidel DC, Turner SM. Selective mutism: more than social anxiety? Depress Anxiety 2006;23(3):117–23.
42. Hirshfeld-Becker DR, Masek B, Henin A, et al. Cognitive-behavioral intervention with young anxious children. Harv Rev Psychiatry 2008;16(2):113–25.
43. Muris P, van Brakel AML, Arntz A, et al. Behavioral inhibition as a risk factor for the development of childhood anxiety disorders: a longitudinal study. J Child Family Studies 2011;20(2):157–70.
44. Biederman J, Hirshfeld-Becker DR, Rosenbaum JF, et al. Further evidence of association between behavioral inhibition and social anxiety in children. Am J Psychiatry 2001;158(10): 1673–9.
45. Scott S, Beidel DC. Selective mutism: an update and suggestions for future research. Curr Psychiatry Rep 2011;13(4):251–7.

46. Kendler KS, Karkowski LM, Prescott CA. Fears and phobias: reliability and heritability. Psychol Med 1999;29(03):539–53.

47. Beatty MJ, Heisel AD, Hall AE, et al. What can we learn from the study of twins about genetic and environmental influences on interpersonal affiliation, aggressiveness, and social anxiety?: A meta-analytic study. Communication Monographs 2002; 69(1):1.

48. Hettema JM, Annas P, Neale MC, et al. A twin study of the genetics of fear conditioning. Arch Gen Psychiatry 2003;60(7):702–8.

49. Stein MB, Chartier MJ, Kozak MV, et al. Genetic linkage to the serotonin transporter protein and 5HT[sub]2A[/sub] receptor genes excluded in generalized social phobia. Psychiatry Res 1998;81(3):283–91.

50. Furmark T, Tillfors M, Garpenstrand H, et al. Serotonin transporter polymorphism related to amygdala excitability and symptom severity in patients with social phobia. Neurosci Lett 2004;362(3):189–92.

51. Lesch K-P, Bengel D, Heils A, et al. Association of anxiety-related traits with a polymorphism in the serotonin transporter gene regulatory region. Science 1996; 274(5292):1527–31.

52. Stein MB, Yang B-Z, Chavira DA, et al. A common genetic variant in the neurexin superfamily member CNTNAP2 is associated with increased risk for selective mutism and social anxiety-related traits. Biol Psychiatry 2011;69(9):825–31.

53. Ginsburg GS, Schlossberg MC. Family-based treatment of childhood anxiety disorders. Int Rev Psychiatry 2002;14(2):143–54.

54. Ronald MR. Potential role of childrearing practices in the development of anxiety and depression. Clin Psychol Rev 1997;17(1):47–67.

55. Edison SC, Evans MA, McHolm AE, et al. An investigation of control among parents of selectively mute, anxious, and non-anxious children. Child Psychiatry Hum Dev 2011;42(3):270–90.

56. Bruch MA, Heimberg RG. Differences in perceptions of parental and personal characteristics between generalized and nongeneralized social phobics. J Anxiety Disord 1994;8(2):155–68.

57. Hackmann A, Clark DM. Recurrent images and early memories in social phobia. Behav Res Ther 2000;38(6):601.

58. Andersson CB, Thomsen PH. Electively mute children: an analysis of 37 Danish cases. Nord J Psychiatry 1998;52(3):231–8.

59. Silverman WK, Albano AM. The anxiety disorders interview schedule for DSM-IV-child and parent versions. San Antonio, TX: Graywind Publications, A Division of The Psychological Corporation; 1996.

60. Silverman WK, Rabian B. Test-retest reliability of the DSM-IIIâ€;R childhood anxiety disorders symptoms using the Anxiety Disorders Interview Schedule for Children. J Anxiety Disord 1995;9(2):139–50.

61. Silverman WK, Saavedra LM, Pina AA. Test-retest reliability of anxiety symptoms and diagnoses with anxiety disorders interview schedule for DSM-IV: Child and parent versions. J Am Acad Child Adolesc Psychiatry 2001;40(8):937–44.

62. Grills AE, Ollendick TH. Multiple informant agreement and the Anxiety Disorders Interview Schedule for Parents and Children. J Am Acad Child Adolesc Psychiatry 2003;42(1):30–40.

63. Sørensen MJ, Nissen JB, Mors O, et al. Age and gender differences in depressive symptomatology and comorbidity: an incident sample of psychiatrically admitted children. J Affect Disord 2005;84(1):85–91.

64. Ezpeleta L, la Osa Nd, Granero R, et al. The diagnostic interview of children and adolescents for parents of preschool and young children: psychometric properties in the general population. Psychiatry Res 2011;190(1):137–44.
65. Kaufman J, Birmaher B, Brent D, et al. Schedule for affective disorders and schizophrenia for school-age children-present and lifetime version (K-SADS-PL): initial reliability and validity data. J Am Acad Child Adolesc Psychiatry 1997;36(7): 980–8.
66. Shaffer D, Fisher P, Lucas CP, et al. NIMH diagnostic interview schedule for children version IV (NIMH DISC-IV): description, differences from previous versions, and reliability of some common diagnoses. J Am Acad Child Adolesc Psychiatry 2000; 39(1):28–38.
67. Weller EB, Weller RA, Fristad MA, et al. Children's interview for psychiatric syndromes (ChIPS). J Am Acad Child Adolesc Psychiatry 2000;39(1):76–84.
68. Reich W. Diagnostic interview for children and adolescents (DICA). J Am Acad Child Adolesc Psychiatry 2000;39(1):59–66.
69. Angold A, Costello EJ. The Child and Adolescent Psychiatric Assessment (CAPA). J Am Acad Child Adolesct Psychiatry 2000;39(1):39–48.
70. Egger H, Angold A. The Preschool Age Psychiatric Assessment (PAPA): a structured parent interview for diagnosing psychiatric disorders in preschool children. In: DelCarmen-Wiggins R, Carter A, eds. Handbook of infant, toddler, and preschool mental assessment. New York: Oxford University Press; 2004. p. 223–3.
71. Birmaher B, Khetarpal S. The screen for child anxiety related emotional disorders (SCARED): scale construction and. J Am Acad Child Adolesc Psychiatry 1997;36(4): 545.
72. Birmaher B, Brent DA, Chiappetta L, et al. Psychometric properties of the Screen for Child Anxiety Related Emotional Disorders (SCARED): a replication study. J Am Acad Child Adolesc Psychiatry 1999;38(10):1230–6.
73. March JS, Parker JDA. The Multidimensional Anxiety Scale for Children (MASC): Factor structure, reliability and validity. J Am Acad Child Adolesc Psychiatry 1997; 36(4):554.
74. Spence SH. A measure of anxiety symptoms among children. Behav Res Ther 1998;36(5):545–66.
75. Chorpita BF, Yim L, Moffitt C, et al. Assessment of symptoms of DSM-IV anxiety and depression in children: a revised child anxiety and depression scale. Behav Res Ther 2000;38(8):835–55.
76. Chorpita BF, Moffitt CE, Gray J. Psychometric properties of the Revised Child Anxiety and Depression Scale in a clinical sample. Behav Res Ther 2005;43(3): 309–22.
77. Weems CF, Costa NM. Developmental differences in the expression of childhood anxiety symptoms and fears. J Am Acad Child Adolesc Psychiatry 2005;44(7): 656–63.
78. Vasey MW, Lonigan CJ. Considering the Clinical utility of performance-based measures of childhood anxiety. J Clin Child Psychol 2000;29(4):493–508.
79. Beidel DC, Trombly TN, Cassisi J, et al. Psychophysiological assessment of selective mutism. Anxiety Disorders Association of America. Baltimore, MD; 2010.
80. Martel FL, Hayward C, Lyons DM, et al. Salivary cortisol levels in socially phobic adolescent girls. Depression Anxiety (1091-4269) 1999;10(1):25–7.
81. Beaton EA, Schmidt LA, Ashbaugh AR, et al. Low salivary cortisol levels among socially anxious young adults: preliminary evidence from a selected and a non-selected sample. Personality and Individual Differences 2006;41(7):1217–28.

82. Hofmann SG, Moscovitch DA, Kim H-J. Autonomic correlates of social anxiety and embarrassment in shy and non-shy individuals. Int J Psychophysiol 2006; 61(2):134–42.
83. Anderson ER, Hope DA. The relationship among social phobia, objective and perceived physiological reactivity, and anxiety sensitivity in an adolescent population. J Anxiety Disord 2009;23(1):18–26.
84. Beidel DC, Turner SM, Sallee FR, et al. SET-C versus fluoxetine in the treatment of childhood social phobia. J Am Acad Child Adolesc Psychiatry 2007;46(12): 1622–32.
85. Kendall PC, Flannery-Schroeder E, Panichelli-Mindel SM, et al. Therapy for youths with anxiety disorders: a second randomized clinical trial. J Consult Clin Psychol 1997;65(3):366–80.
86. Hirshfeld-Becker DR, Masek B, Henin A, et al. Cognitive Behavioral therapy for 4- to 7-year-old children with anxiety disorders: a randomized clinical trial. J Consult Clin Psychol 2010;78(4):498–510.
87. Walkup JT, Albano AM, Piacentini J, et al. Cognitive behavioral therapy, sertraline, or a combination in childhood anxiety. N Engl J Med 2008;359(26):2753–66.
88. Crawley SA, Beidas RS, Benjamin CL, et al. Treating socially phobic youth with CBT: differential outcomes and treatment considerations. Behav Cogn Psychother 2008; 36(4):379–89.
89. Chambless DL, Hollon SD. Defining empirically supported therapies. J Consult Clin Psychol 1998;66(1):7–18.
90. Silverman WK, Pina AA, Viswesvaran C. Evidence-based psychosocial treatments for phobic and anxiety disorders in children and adolescents. J Clin Child Adolesc Psychol 2008;37(1):105–30.
91. Ishikawa S-i, Okajima I, Matsuoka H, et al. Cognitive behavioural therapy for anxiety disorders in children and adolescents: a meta-analysis. Child and Adolescent Mental Healt. 2007;12(4):164–72.
92. Cohan SL, Chavira DA, Stein MB. Practitioner Review: psychosocial interventions for children with selective mutism: a critical evaluation of the literature from 1990-2005. J Child Psychol Psychiatry 2006;47(11):1085–97.
93. Kendall PC. Coping cat workbook. Ardmore, PA: Workbook Publishing; 1990.
94. Barrett PM, Dadds MR, Rapee RM. Coping Koala Workbook: School of Applied Psychology, Griffith University; 1991.
95. Kendall PC. Treating anxiety disorders in children: results of a randomized clinical trial. J Consult Clin Psychol 1994;62(1):100–10.
96. Kendall PC, Southam-Gerow MA. Long-term follow-up of a cognitive–behavioral therapy for anxiety-disordered youth. J Consult Clin Psychol 1996;64(4):724–30.
97. Kendall PC, Safford S, Flannery-Schroeder E, et al. Child anxiety treatment: outcomes in adolescents and impact on substance use and depression at 7.4-year follow-up. J Consult Clin Psychol 2004;72(2):276–87.
98. Barrett PM, Dadds MR, Rapee RM. Family treatment of childhood anxiety: a controlled trial. J Consult Clin Psychol 1996;64(2):333–42.
99. McHolm AE, Cunningham CE, Vanier MK. Helping your child with selective mutism: Practical steps to overcome a fear of speaking. Oakland (CA): New Harbinger Publications; 2005.
100. Kearney CA. Helping children with selective mutism and their parents: a guide for school-based professionals. New York (NY): Oxford University Press; 2007.
101. Hudson JL, Krain AL, Kendall PC. Expanding horizons: adapting manual-based treatments for anxious children with comorbid diagnoses. Cognitive and Behavioral Practice 2001;8(4):338–45.

102. Grover RL, Hughes AA, Bergman RL, et al. Treatment modifications based on childhood anxiety diagnosis: demonstrating the flexibility in manualized treatment. J Cog Psychother 2006;20(3):275–86.

103. Reuther ET, Davis TE III, Moree BN, et al. Treating selective mutism using modular CBT for child anxiety: a case study. J Clin Child Adolesc Psychol 2011;40(1):156–63.

104. Beidel DC, Turner SM, Morris TL. Behavioral treatment of childhood social phobia. J Consult Clin Psychol 2000;68(6):1072–80.

105. Beidel DC, Turner SM, Young B, et al. Social effectiveness therapy for children: three-year follow-up. J Consult Clin Psychol 2005;73(4):721–5.

106. Beidel DC, Turner SM, Young BJ. Social effectiveness therapy for children: five years later. Behav Ther 2006;37(4):416–25.

107. Fisak BJ Jr, Oliveros A, Ehrenreich JT. Assessment and behavioral treatment of selective mutism. Clinical Case Studies 2006;5(5):382–402.

108. Spence SH, Donovan C. The treatment of childhood social phobia: the effectiveness of a social skills training-based, cognitive-behavioural intervention, with and without parental involvement. J Child Psychol Psychiatry 2000;41(6):713.

109. Manassis K, Mendlowitz SL, Scapillato D, et al. Group and individual cognitive-behavioral therapy for childhood anxiety disorders: a randomized trial. J Am Acad Child Adolesc Psychiatry 2002;41(12):1423–30.

110. Sharkey L, Mc Nicholas F, Barry E, et al. Group therapy for selective mutism—a parents' and children's treatment group. J Behav Ther Exp Psychiatry 2008;39(4):538–45.

111. Mendlowitz S, Monga S. Breaking the silence: utilizing cognitive behavioral therapy (CBT) in selective mutism paper presented at Anxiety Disorders Association of America. Baltimore (MD), 2010.

112. Fung DSS, Manassis K, Kenny A, et al. Web-based CBT for selective mutism. J Am Acad Child Adolesc Psychiatry 2002;41(2):112–3.

113. Kendall PC, Khanna MS, Edson A, et al. Computers and psychosocial treatment for child anxiety: recent advances and ongoing efforts. Depress Anxiety 2011;28(1):58–66.

114. Khanna MS, Kendall PC. Computer-assisted cognitive behavioral therapy for child anxiety: Results of a randomized clinical trial. J Consult Clin Psychol 2010;78(5):737–45.

115. Andrews G, Davies M, Titov N. Effectiveness randomized controlled trial of face to face versus Internet cognitive behaviour therapy for social phobia. Aust N Z J Psychiatry 2010;45(4):337–40.

116. Carlbring P, Gunnarsdottir M, Hedensjo L, et al. Treatment of social phobia: randomised trial of internet-delivered cognitive–behavioural therapy with telephone support. Br J Psychiatry 2007;190:123–8.

117. Hedman E, Andersson G, Ljótsson Bn, et al. Internet-based cognitive behavior therapy vs. cognitive behavioral group therapy for social anxiety disorder: a randomized controlled non-inferiority trial. PLoS Clin Trials 2011;8(3):1–10.

118. Hedman E, Andersson E, Ljótsson Bn, et al. Cost-effectiveness of Internet-based cognitive behavior therapy vs. cognitive behavioral group therapy for social anxiety disorder: Results from a randomized controlled trial. Behav Res Ther 2011;49(11):729–36.

119. Birmaher B, Axelson DA, Monk K, et al. Fluoxetine for the treatment of childhood anxiety disorders. J Am Acad Child Adolesc Psychiatry 2003;42(4):415.

120. Monga S, Young A, Owens M. Evaluating a cognitive behavioral therapy group program for anxious five to seven year old children: a pilot study. Depression Anxiety (1091-4269). 2009;26(3):243–50.

121. Oerbeck B, Johansen J, Lundahl K, et al. Selective mutism: a home-and kindergarten-based intervention for children 3–5 Years: a pilot study. Clin Child Psychol Psychiatry 2011. [Epub ahead of print].

122. Kurtz SMS. Brave Buddies: Intensive real-world group treatment of selective mutism. Paper presented at the annual meeting of the Selective Mutism Group. Chicago (IL), July 2001.

123. Connolly SD, Bernstein GA. Practice parameter for the assessment and treatment of children and adolescents with anxiety disorders. J Am Acad Child Adolesc Psychiatry 2007;46(2):267–83.

124. Fluvoxamine for the treatment of anxiety disorders in children and adolescents. N Engl J Med 2001;344(17):1279–85.

125. Wagner KD, Berard R, Stein MB, et al. A multicenter, randomized, double-blind, placebo-controlled trial of paroxetine in children and adolescents with social anxiety disorder. 2004;61:1153-62.

126. March JS, Entusah AR, Rynn M, et al. A randomized controlled trial of venlafaxine ER versus placebo in pediatric social anxiety disorder. Biol Psychiatry 2007;62(10): 1149–54.

127. Black B, Uhde TW. Treatment of elective mutism with fluoxetine: a double-blind, placebo-controlled study. J Am Acad Child Adolesc Psychiatry 1994;33(7):1000–6.

128. Carlson JS, Kratochwill TR, Johnston HF. Sertraline treatment of 5 children diagnosed with selective mutism: a single-case research trial. J Child Adolesc Psychopharmacol 1999;9(4):293–306.

129. Dummit ES III, Klein RG, Tancer NK, et al. Fluoxetine treatment of children with selective mutism: an open trial. J Am Acad Child Adolesc Psychiatry 1996;35(5): 615–21.

130. Kaakeh YS, Janice L. Treatment of selective mutism: focus on selective serotonin reuptake inhibitors. Pharmacotherapy 2008;28(2):214–24.

131. Lehman RB. Rapid resolution of social anxiety disorder, selective mutism, and separation anxiety with paroxetine in an 8-year-old girl. J Psychiatry Neurosci 2002;27(2):124–5.

132. Blum NJ, Kell RS, Starr HL, et al. Case study: audio feedforward treatment of selective mutism. J Am Acad Child Adolesc Psychiatry 1998;37(1):40–3.

133. Kehle TJ, Madaus MR, Baratta VS, et al. Augmented self-modeling as a treatment for children with selective mutism. J School Psychol 1998;36(3):247–60.

134. Dowrick PW. A review of self modeling and related interventions. Applied and Preventive Psychology 1999;8(1):23–39.

135. La Greca AM, Dandes SK, Wick P, et al. Development of the Social Anxiety Scale for Children: reliability and concurrent validity. J Clin Child Psychol 1988;17(1):84–91.

136. Ginsburg GS, La Greca AM, Silverman WK. Social anxiety in children with anxiety disorders: relation with social and emotional functioning. J Abnormal Child Psychol 1998;26(3):175–85.

137. La Greca AM, Lopez N. Social anxiety among adolescents: linkages with peer relations and friendships. J Abnorm Child Psychol 1998;26(2):83–94.

138. Inderbitzen-Nolan HM, Walters KS. Social anxiety scale for adolescents: normative data and further evidence of construct validity. J Clin Child Psychol 2000; 29(3):360–71.

139. Beidel DC, Turner SM, Morris TL. A new inventory to assess childhood social anxiety and phobia: The Social Phobia and Anxiety Inventory for Children. Psychol Assess 1995;7(1):73–9.
140. Aune T, Stiles TC, Svarva K. Psychometric properties of the social phobia and anxiety inventory for children using a non-American population-based sample. J Anxiety Disord 2008;22(6):1075–86.
141. Storch EA, Masia-Warner C, Dent HC, et al. Psychometric evaluation of the Social Anxiety Scale for Adolescents and the Social Phobia and Anxiety Inventory for Children: construct validity and normative data. J Anxiety Disord 2004;18(5):665–79.
142. Masia CL, Hoffman SG, Klein RG, et al. The Liebowitz Social Anxiety Scale for Children and Adolescents (LSAS-CA); 1999.
143. Masia-Warner C, Storch EA, Pincus DB, et al. The Liebowitz Social Anxiety Scale for Children and Adolescents: an initial psychometric investigation. J Am Acad Child Adolesc Psychiatry 2003;42(9):1076–84.
144. Bergman RL, Keller ML, Piacentini J, et al. The development and psychometric properties of the Selective Mutism Questionnaire. J Clin Child Adolesc Psychol 2008;37(2):456–64.

Anxiety in the Pediatric Medical Setting

Bela Gandhi, MD[a],*, Shannon Cheek, MD[a], John V. Campo, MD[b]

KEYWORDS

- Anxiety • Chronic disease • Differential diagnosis • Gastrointestinal diseases
- Somatoform disorders

KEY POINTS

- Children with chronic physical illness are at increased risk to develop anxiety disorders.
- Anxiety can predispose to physical health problems and negatively impact the course of comorbid physical disease.
- Children with comorbid anxiety and general medical disorders have greater functional impairment than would be expected with either disorder alone.
- The possibility that a child's anxiety symptoms may be directly caused by physical disease should always be considered.
- Risks associated with the use of psychoactive medications in physically ill children are poorly understood because randomized controlled trials have typically excluded youth with chronic physical diseases.
- Given the heightened risk of physically ill youth to experience adverse medication effects and drug-drug interactions, cognitive behavior therapy may be appealing as a first line treatment.

INTRODUCTION

Although it is well-known that children and adolescents with anxiety disorders are at heightened risk to develop other anxiety, mood, and substance abuse disorders across the lifespan,[1–3] the relationship between pediatric anxiety disorders and physical health is less well-understood, but appreciation of the importance of this relationship is growing. Advances in pediatric medicine, improved sanitation, and better social support services have increased the importance of addressing the relationship between anxiety and physical health. This priority is especially true

The authors have nothing to disclose.
[a] Department of Psychiatry, The Ohio State University and Nationwide Children's Hospital, 700 Children's Drive, Columbus, OH 43205, USA; [b] Department of Psychiatry, The Ohio State University and Nationwide Children's Hospital, The Ohio State University Wexner Medical Center, OSU Harding Hospital, 1670 Upham Drive, Columbus, OH 43210, USA
* Corresponding author.
E-mail address: bela.gandhi@nationwidechildrens.org

Child Adolesc Psychiatric Clin N Am 21 (2012) 643–653
http://dx.doi.org/10.1016/j.chc.2012.05.013
1056-4993/12/$ – see front matter Published by Elsevier Inc.

childpsych.theclinics.com

because chronic physical health conditions are increasingly common, with approximately 1% to 3% of children and adolescents in the United States having significant functional impairment due to a chronic physical health condition.[4] Because most of these chronic conditions do not have a specific cure, they require longitudinal management and are characterized by variable courses of symptoms, potential physical and psychosocial limitations, and the need for daily treatment regimens.

Physical conditions such as asthma, diabetes, and epilepsy can be predisposing, precipitating, and/or comorbid with anxiety symptoms and disorders, and comorbid anxiety may complicate the course of a coexisting physical disease (eg, needle phobia in diabetes).[5] In addition, previously undiagnosed physical disease can present with symptoms of anxiety (eg, temporal lobe epilepsy presenting with panic symptoms),[6] and anxiety disorders may present or be associated with medically unexplained physical symptoms such as functional abdominal pain, headache, and fatigue.[7] This article describes anxiety and its association with physical disease, outlines assessment, and presents a treatment overview including psychotherapy and pharmacotherapy.

AGE-APPROPRIATE VERSUS PATHOLOGIC ANXIETY

Challenges exist in distinguishing "normal" from "pathologic" fear and anxiety, and there is some controversy regarding whether anxiety disorders differ from "normal" fears and worries by kind or degree.[3] Modern conceptualizations have emphasized a dimensional view and have focused on perturbations of the neural fear circuit and the importance of the amygdala in detecting and responding to threat.[8] Normal fear can be viewed as an appropriate response to realistic danger, with pathologic fear and anxiety being judged excessive or inappropriate to context. Practically, transient worries and fears are common in children and adolescents, but are considered pathologic only when associated with significant impairment, distress, and persistence. Discerning developmentally appropriate fears and worries from excessive, inappropriate, and impairing anxiety can be especially challenging in pediatric medical settings, where physically ill children and their families are often faced with out of the ordinary and potentially threatening experiences, including painful diagnostic tests and procedures, hospitalization, surgery, and exposure to medications.[9]

ANXIETY AND PHYSICAL DISEASE

With the advent of the biomedical model, physicians began to differentiate illness, the subjective and symptomatic suffering of patients, from disease, which was primarily understood as a biophysical reality documented by the presence of observable tissue damage or changes known as pathologic conditions.[10] A major focus of modern medical assessment thus involves determining if a given illness can be adequately explained by the presence of a known disease. This approach may be valid even when the presenting symptoms are considered representative of a mental disorder. The relationship between anxiety disorders and physical health is complex and bidirectional, yet despite efforts to maintain an integrative view of health as a unitary construct that cannot be parsed into physical and mental health, clinicians typically struggle with a "practical dualism" in the day-to-day care of patients.[11] The term *somatopsychic* has been applied in circumstances where a mental disorder seems to be the consequence of preexisting physical disease. Conversely, when so-called mental symptoms and disorders seem to predispose to, cause, or perpetuate physical disease, the relationship between mental disorders and physical disease has been conceptualized as *psychosomatic*. Although these terms are used throughout this discussion for practical and heuristic purposes, it is important to emphasize that such categorizations are reductionistic and dualistic, and that the relationship between anxiety disorders, physical symptoms, and general medical conditions is a dynamic and iterative one.

Somatopsychic Considerations

The first step in the differential diagnosis of a given symptom or complaint is typically a search for unrecognized physical disease. Although most children and adolescents presenting with cognitive and physical symptoms consistent with an anxiety disorder will not be found to suffer from causal physical disease, clinicians should nevertheless entertain the hypothesis that anxiety might be caused, exacerbated, or perpetuated by an unrecognized general medical condition.[6] This is an important point to emphasize, because behavioral health professionals, although having little difficulty accepting that mental disorders are commonly underdiagnosed and undertreated in general medical settings, are vulnerable to overlooking the often important relationship between anxiety and physical disease in traditional mental health settings.

Dietary factors and medications are perhaps the most common somatic causes of anxiety symptoms.[11] A careful dietary history is particularly useful, because it may reveal excessive ingestion of caffeinated beverages or "energy" drinks and identify a potentially reversible cause of anxiety.[12] Anecdotally, monosodium glutamate has also been suspected of generating anxiety symptoms.[6] Symptoms of anxiety can develop as a direct effect of a medication or substance or as a withdrawal reaction, and have been associated with intoxication with drugs of abuse such as amphetamines, cocaine, marijuana, and hallucinogens (eg, phencyclidine), as well as with withdrawal from alcohol, barbiturates, benzodiazepines, and opiates.[11] Anxiety symptoms such as panic are not uncommon in association with the use of cannabis, particularly with initial use.[13] A variety of medications, including anabolic steroids, corticosteroids, anticholinergics, angiotensin-converting enzyme inhibitors, beta adrenergic agonists and other asthma medications, decongestants such as pseudoephedrine, dopamine receptor agonists, procaine derivatives, thyroid medications, antirejection drugs such as tacrolimus, and selective serotonin reuptake inhibitors (SSRIs) have been associated with the onset of anxiety.[14] Symptoms of anxiety, restlessness, and agitation may also be prominent in the development of serotonin syndrome.[15]

Certain general medical conditions have been directly associated with the development of anxiety.[6] Of the endocrine disorders associated with anxiety, hyperthyroidism is likely the most common, and the associated symptoms may be difficult to differentiate from those of a primary anxiety disorder. Pediatric patients with thyrotoxicosis may present with symptoms of anxious dysphoria, hyperactivity, irritability, and decreased attention, with symptoms predating the diagnosis of thyrotoxicosis by approximately 6 to 12 months.[3] Anxiety symptoms will typically resolve when the underlying thyroid disorder is treated but may also respond to treatment with beta-blockers. In situations of new onset anxiety, anxiety resistant to treatment, or anxiety presenting with prominent physical findings such as tachycardia, fine tremor, diaphoresis, exophthalmos, and hyperreflexia, consideration should be given to hyperthyroidism and thyroid function tests obtained. Other potential physical causes of anxiety include hypoxia and hypoglycemia, although insulin secreting tumors as a cause of the latter are exceptionally rare. Similarly, the catecholamine secreting tumor known as pheochromocytoma, as well as tumors of the parathyroid and adrenal glands, have been associated with physical and cognitive symptoms of anxiety, including episodic panic attacks, but are also quite rare.[2] Anxiety has been associated with the acute porphyrias.[16] Panic attacks have been associated with complex partial seizures, which can present with symptoms of fear, depersonalization, dizziness, and paresthesias.

Psychosomatic Considerations

Conversely, anxiety may predispose to physical symptoms, complaints, and disease across the lifespan, as well as perpetuate and interfere with the course of physical health problems. Symptoms of anxiety and emotional arousal may also be misperceived by patients as being indicative of undiagnosed and potentially life-threatening physical disease. This tendency is particularly common in the case of panic disorder, where panic attacks typically feature the sudden onset of physical symptoms such as palpitations, tachycardia, shortness of breath, sweating, and tremor. Challenging the common notion of the "worried well," a growing body of literature suggests that anxiety disorders are associated with elevated levels of inflammation, a heightened risk for premature aging and early mortality, an elevated risk of developing general medical conditions such as hypertension and cardiovascular disease, and negative effects on the course of comorbid physical disorders such as coronary artery disease.[17–19] Anxiety may thus impact the course of pediatric physical illness by directly altering the pathophysiology of the disease process (eg, associated elevations in cytokines and autonomic activation), by fostering maladaptive health behaviors (eg, inadequate sleep, dietary indiscretion, or substance abuse) and by medical nonadherence.[9]

The presence of a chronic physical illness seems to be a significant risk factor for developing an anxiety disorder, and anxiety symptoms are especially common in children and adolescents with chronic physical illnesses, with as many as 40% reporting anxiety symptoms.[5,9,20] The nature of the relationship between anxiety and general medical conditions often seems to be bidirectional, and children with chronic physical disease and concurrent anxiety disorders have greater functional impairment than would be expected with either an anxiety disorder or a general medical condition alone.[9]

The relationship between asthma and anxiety is illustrative. Asthma and allergic conditions such as atopic dermatitis are particularly common among children with anxiety disorders,[21] and children with asthma tend to report higher levels of anxiety than unaffected peers.[22,23] Adolescents with asthma and comorbid anxiety and depressive disorders experienced higher health service costs and had more ambulatory and emergency department visits than adolescents with asthma who were free of emotional disorders.[24] The physical symptoms of anxiety, particularly panic anxiety, and asthma may overlap. Panic anxiety may be triggered by the stress and sense of threat associated with an asthma attack and/or can develop in response to hypoxia, hyperventilation, and hypercapnia. Episodes of repeated respiratory distress and medications used to treat asthma may also predispose to or precipitate anxiety, and heightened levels of anxiety may in turn lead to an increase in the frequency and severity of asthma attacks.[2] The presence of comorbid anxiety and depression increases the functional burden experienced by youth with asthma,[25] and also increases the likelihood that asthmatic adolescents will smoke cigarettes.[26] Finally, anxiety may also predispose to vocal cord dysfunction, where patients exhibit inspiratory wheezing over the larynx in the absence of concurrent asthma and wheezing over the lungs.[27]

Epilepsy is also commonly associated with anxiety, and children with seizure disorders frequently experience comorbid anxiety disorders.[28] Caplan and colleagues[29] used self-reports and standardized psychiatric interviews to assess 171 children with epilepsy and found that 33% of affected children reported mood and anxiety symptoms compared with 6% of children without epilepsy; of the 33% who reported mood and anxiety symptoms, 63% met the criteria for an anxiety disorder.[29] Jones and colleagues[30] completed a similar study with 53 children ages 8 to 18 with new onset epilepsy (<1 year duration), and found that *Diagnostic and Statistical Manual of Mental Disorders, Fourth Edition* anxiety disorders were reported by 36%

of children with epilepsy compared with 22% of healthy controls. The presence of anxiety has been associated with increased seizure frequency in epileptic children, as well as treating with multiple anticonvulsants.[31]

Acute and chronic physical illnesses and their associated treatments are likely to be experienced as stressors by affected children and their families. This potential stress includes a spectrum of interventions and procedures perceived as threatening, from relatively simple procedures such as blood draws and intravenous line placement to dramatic and potentially lifesaving treatments such as bone marrow and solid organ transplantation.[32,33] Symptoms of posttraumatic stress disorder (PTSD) in medically traumatized children may predict medical nonadherence,[5] and can persist into adulthood in a subset of patients.[34] Children who survive life-threatening illnesses and who are treated in critical care settings seem to be especially vulnerable to develop PTSD, with point prevalences across studies ranging from 10% to 28%.[35]

ANXIETY AND FUNCTIONAL SOMATIC SYMPTOMS

Functional somatic symptoms (FSS) are physical symptoms and complaints that are medically unexplained after routine medical assessment. FSS are commonly associated with the presence of anxiety symptoms and disorders in childhood and adolescence, and the higher the number of FSS, the greater the likelihood of comorbid anxiety symptoms and disorder, suggesting an apparent "dose-response" relationship between FSS and anxiety.[7] Strong, reciprocal associations exist between FSS and anxiety across the lifespan, with early onset anxiety being associated with FSS later in life and vice versa. Functional abdominal pain (FAP) is quite common, impairing, and associated with other FSS and anxiety disorders in affected children.[36,37] One study using standardized psychiatric interviews delivered by an examiner blind to physical health status identified a concurrent anxiety disorder in 79% of children and adolescents with FAP presenting in primary care consisting of the following: separation anxiety disorder (43%), generalized anxiety disorder (31%), and social phobia (21%).[36] Mothers of children with FAP were also significantly more likely to report anxiety and depressive symptoms and disorders, as well as higher levels of FSS, than the mothers of pain-free children.[38]

From the biomedical perspective, anxiety disorders are no less "medically unexplained" than FSS, but current psychiatric nosology includes many FSS in the diagnostic criteria for specific anxiety disorders.[39] Because emotions and feelings are not equivalent and seem to be managed by different brain regions,[8] it may be that cognitive symptoms of anxiety and FSS may be derivative of the same emotional process, regardless of whether cognitive symptoms of anxiety are recognized and acknowledged by the patient.

ASSESSMENT IN THE MEDICAL SETTING

If an anxiety disorder is suspected in the medical setting, further evaluation should be done with the child and the parent.[9] At this time, there is no specific assessment tool available to evaluate anxiety in the pediatric medical setting so assessment should be conducted in keeping with existing practice parameters for the psychiatric assessment of physically ill children.[40] Clinicians should have a high index of suspicion for unrecognized anxiety in patients presenting with FSS in general medical settings, including the emergency department, because somatic symptoms can be a key feature of anxiety disorders and generate concerns regarding unrecognized life-threatening disease. The task of clinicians is twofold. The first task is to distinguish pathologic anxiety from age-appropriate fears and worries. The second task is to determine the relationship between any observed symptoms of anxiety and comorbid physical symptoms and diseases. The onset and duration of specific cognitive and somatic symptoms of anxiety should be examined and an attempt made to identify a temporal relationship between symptoms of anxiety and the course of the comorbid general medical condition. Inquiry should be made regarding recent and past stressors and traumas, including medical traumas as well as academic problems, family issues, maltreatment, and difficulties with peers such as bullying. There is no substitute for a comprehensive psychiatric and medical history, as well as review of the medical record, medication list, laboratory and other diagnostic tests and procedures, and a directed physical examination when appropriate. As noted previously, anxiety may be the direct consequence of a substance, medication, or physical disease, or may predispose a particular patient to physical illness or disease.

TREATMENT OVERVIEW

The psychiatric diagnostic workup should be reviewed in the context of the child's overall health status, with the goal being shared decision-making and meaningful informed consent. According to the American Academy of Child and Adolescent Psychiatry's Practice Parameter for anxiety disorders, treatment should be "multimodal," and begins with psychoeducation about developmentally normal anxiety, anxiety disorders, and treatment options, which include psychotherapy, pharmacotherapy, or a combination of the two.[41] Although there is considerable evidence supporting several treatments for pediatric anxiety disorders, existing randomized controlled trials (RCTs) have excluded most patients with comorbid physical diseases such as diabetes. Despite a lack of large RCTs addressing the treatment of anxiety in physically ill youth, there is no evidence that proven treatments for anxiety are any less likely to work in youth with comorbid physical illness than in their physically healthy counterparts.

Psychoeducation should explore the potential impact of anxiety and its treatment on the comorbid physical disorder, and informed consent should include the potential impact of treatment and known adverse effects on comorbid physical conditions and their management. Development of a multimodal treatment plan should take place within the context of a partnership between the treating professionals, the patient, and the family, and ideally should include the patient's managing primary care physician or specialist, as well as relevant school personnel such as teachers and school nurses.[40]

Psychotherapy

Psychotherapeutic approaches are often the first treatment considered, especially in the context of mild to moderate anxiety.[42] Cognitive behavior therapies (CBTs), including group CBT interventions, have been reasonably well-studied, and existing evidence supports the efficacy of problem-specific cognitive behavior interventions for a variety of childhood and adolescent anxiety disorders.[43] Common components of CBT include psychoeducation about anxiety and its treatment, somatic management skills training, cognitive restructuring, exposure, and relapse prevention planning. The Coping Cat program is perhaps the best studied manual-based CBT protocol for pediatric anxiety and has been shown to be efficacious in a number of trials, including the Child/Adolescent Anxiety Multimodal Study.[44] Modifications of CBT programs have been created to help address anxiety and somatic symptoms, with some studies showing that effective treatment of anxiety leads to decreases in associated somatic symptoms.[45–47] A modified CBT protocol based on the Coping Cat program that was applied to pediatric patients with anxiety and somatic symptoms in the specialty pediatric medical setting was found to be a promising and feasible intervention to reduce anxiety symptoms and associated physical distress.

The Treatment for Anxiety and Physical Symptoms program (TAPS) used the CBT techniques in the Coping Cat program but focused the techniques on somatic symptoms and pain and highlighted the relationship of these symptoms with anxiety. For example cognitive restructuring is focused on cognitions about physical symptoms, exposures and coping skills such as diaphragmatic breathing are used to target these symptoms, and there are three separate parent sessions to provide psychoeducation, parenting skills, and support.[47]

Pharmacotherapy

The risks associated with the use of psychoactive drugs in the physically ill child are poorly understood given that RCTs have typically excluded youth with chronic physical diseases. Clinicians should individualize treatment and carefully consult prescribing information for each agent considered for use, as well search the medical literature with regard to the use in association with a given physical condition. Details related to the use of medications under consideration should be reviewed, including potential adverse effects, drug interactions, dosing, time to effect, need for monitoring, and any apparent uncertainties. Physically ill youth are likely at greater risk for both pharmacodynamic and pharmacokinetic drug-drug interactions, with the most common pharmacokinetic drug-drug interactions relevant to pediatric psychopharmacology being related to the biotransformation of highly lipid soluble drugs by the cytochrome enzyme system. It is especially important that all prescription and nonprescription medications, contraceptives, and herbal remedies are reviewed and consideration given to known drug-drug interactions.

SSRIs have proven efficacy in the treatment of common pediatric anxiety disorders and are considered the first line pharmacotherapy option in pediatric anxiety because of both effectiveness and side effect profile.[44,48,49] Some clinicians prefer to prescribe SSRIs only when anxiety is moderate to severe, in the presence of comorbid depression, when CBT has been ineffective in producing remission, or when impairment from anxiety makes participation in CBT difficult.

SSRI medications have been associated with a number of potential adverse effects, which are most often dose-related and short lived,[49] but some adverse effects of SSRIs may be especially important to consider in physically ill children and adolescents. Alterations in platelet function produced by SSRIs are important to consider in patients bleeding disorders, low platelet counts, or being treated with nonsteroidal antiinflammatory agents.[50] The US Food and Drug Administration recently recommended that the maximum daily dose of citalopram should be reduced from 60 mg to 40 mg because of concerns over dose-dependent prolongation of the QT interval,[51] although there have been some recent reviews questioning the clinical significance of these findings.[52] Prolongation of the QT interval can predispose to arrhythmias including multifocal ventricular tachycardia or torsades de pointes, with the risk potentially being greater in patients with a history of congenital long QT syndrome, congestive heart failure, bradyarrhythmias, hypokalemia, or hypomagnesemia.[51] Other antidepressants such as venlafaxine and duloxetine have been associated with increases in blood pressure, but these effects have not been especially well-studied in youth. SSRIs have also been anecdotally associated with reductions in glucose levels early in the treatment of diabetic patients, suggesting the need to be vigilant for potential hypoglycemia during SSRI initiation.[50] Physically ill patients treated with SSRIs and multiple other medications will also be at heightened risk of serotonin syndrome, because certain medications will increase the risk of serotonin syndrome when administered in combination with SSRIs (eg, dextromethorphan, sumatriptan).[50]

Benzodiazepines are also used to manage anxiety in children and adolescents, most often as short-term adjuncts to the SSRIs.[41] The goal is most often to achieve a rapid reduction in symptoms that may allow initial symptom relief, improved participation in CBT, and/or great ability to tolerate initiation of SSRI treatment. Side effects of benzodiazepines are typically tolerable if the dose is carefully managed, with the most common side effects being drowsiness and sedation. Use of benzodiazepines can sometimes lead to disinhibition, as well as increased aggression, irritability, incoordination, cognitive impairment, and amnesia. Although respiratory depression at typical dosages is typically not of clinical significance in otherwise healthy patients, use in patients with pulmonary disease and respiratory failure requires careful attention and monitoring.[50] Benzodiazepines seem to be most dangerous in such patients when used at higher doses, when administered parenterally, or when given in combination with other drugs that can depress respiratory drive such as opiates. The SSRIs and the anxiolytic nonbenzodiazepine buspirone should be considered prior to benzodiazepines in the chronic management of anxiety in patients with respiratory disorders.

Because of the possible relationship between serotonergic neurotransmission and gut sensation, as well as observed associations between anxiety and functional abdominal pain, the SSRI citalopram was evaluated as a treatment for FAP in an open label study of 25 affected children and adolescents, with 21 (84%) of the treated youth exhibiting a favorable treatment response based on clinician ratings of much or very much improved.[53] Improvements in child and parent ratings of abdominal pain were accompanied by improvements in ratings of anxiety, depression, and other somatic symptoms. Results of a randomized, placebo-controlled trial of citalopram for pediatric FAP are pending. Two published RCTs of the tricyclic antidepressant (TCA) amitriptyline for pediatric FAP produced mixed results, with a recent review concluding that there is no convincing evidence for the efficacy of TCAs in pediatric FAP.[54] No significant differences were found between low-dose amitriptyline (10 to 20 mg/d) and placebo over 4 weeks in a study that randomized 90 children and adolescents with FAP.[55] A smaller study of 33 adolescents with FAP randomized to amitriptyline or placebo over 13 weeks found improvements in quality of life for the amitriptyline group compared with placebo, but was compromised by methodologic weaknesses that included multiple testing and small sample size.[56] Past reports of sudden death in association with the use of TCAs in children, their potential for lethality in overdose, and the absence of proven efficacy in the treatment of both FAP and pediatric depression[57] make it difficult to confidently recommend TCAs for youth with anxiety and FSS. Although there are numerous antidepressant medications worthy of consideration in the management of anxiety in the presence of physical symptoms, including venlafaxine and duloxetine, mirtazapine is a novel antidepressant that may be of special interest, particularly for patients with gastrointestinal complaints, given its ability to block the serotonin 5-HT$_3$ receptor relevant to nausea and gastrointestinal discomfort.[50]

SUMMARY POINTS

- Children with chronic physical illness are at increased risk to develop anxiety disorders.
- Anxiety can predispose to physical health problems and negatively impact the course of comorbid physical disease.
- Children with comorbid anxiety and general medical disorders have greater functional impairment than would be expected with either disorder alone.

- The possibility that a child's anxiety symptoms may be directly caused by physical disease should always be considered.
- Risks associated with the use of psychoactive medications in physically ill children are poorly understood because RCTs have typically excluded youth with chronic physical diseases.
- Given the heightened risk of physically ill youth to experience adverse medication effects and drug-drug interactions, CBT may be appealing as a first line treatment.

REFERENCES

1. Pine DS, Cohen P, Gurley D, et al. The risk for early-adulthood anxiety and depressive disorders in adolescents with anxiety and depressive disorders. Arch Gen Psychiatry 1998;55:56–64.
2. Woodward LJ, Fergusson DM. Life course outcomes of young people with anxiety disorders in adolescence. J Am Acad Child Adolesc Psychiatry 2001;40(9):1086–93.
3. Klein RG. Anxiety disorders. J Child Psychol Psychiatry 2009;50(1–2):153–62.
4. Gortmaker SL, Walker DK, Weitzman M, et al. Chronic conditions, socioeconomic risks, and behavioral problems in children and adolescents. Pediatrics 1990;85: 267–76.
5. Pao M, Bosk A. Anxiety in medically ill children/adolescents. Depress Anxiety 2011; 28:40–9.
6. Campo JV. Medical issues in the care of child and adolescent inpatients. In: Bellack A, Hersen M, editors. Handbook of behavior therapy in the psychiatric setting. New York: Plenum Publishing Corporation; 1993. p. 373–406.
7. Campo JV. Annual research review: functional somatic symptoms and associated anxiety and depression–developmental psychopathology in pediatric practice. J Child Psychol Psychiatry 2012;53(5):575–92.
8. LeDoux JE. The emotional brain. New York: Simon & Schuster; 1996.
9. Ramsawh H, Chavira D, Stein M. The burden of anxiety disorders in pediatric medical settings: prevalence, phenomenology and a research agenda. Arch Pediatr Adolesc Med 2010;164:965–72.
10. Weiner H, Fawzy FI. An integrative model of health, disease, and illness. In: Cheren S, editor. Psychosomatic medicine: theory, physiology, and practice, vol. 1. Madison (CT): International University Press; 1989; p. 9–44.
11. Schiffer RB, Klein RF, Sider RC. The medical evaluation of psychiatric patients. New York: Plenum Medical Book Co.; 1998.
12. Seifert SM, Schaechter JL, Hershorin ER, et al. Health effects of energy drinks on children, adolescents, and young adults. Pediatrics 2011;127(3):511–28.
13. Thomas H. Psychiatric symptoms in cannabis users. Br J Psychiatry 1993;163: 141–9.
14. Drugs that may cause psychiatric symptoms. Med Lett Drugs Ther 2008;1301:100.
15. Birmes P, Coppin D, Schmitt L, et al. Serotonin syndrome: a brief review. CMAJ 2003;168(11):1439–42.
16. Millward LM, Kelly P, King A, et al. Anxiety and depression in the acute porphyrias. J Inherit Metab Dis 2005;28(6):1099–107.
17. O'Donovan A, Tomiyama AJ, Lin J, et al. Stress appraisals and cellular aging: a key role for anticipatory threat in the relationship between psychological stress and telomere length. Brain Behav Immun 2012;26(4):573–9.
18. Player MS, Peterson LE. Anxiety disorders, hypertension, and cardiovascular risk: a review. Int J Psychiatry Med 2011;41(4):365–77.

19. Roy-Byrne PP, Davidson KW, Kessler RC, et al. Anxiety disorders and comorbid medical illness. Gen Hosp Psychiatry 2008;30(3):208–25.
20. Danzer C, Swendsen J, Maurice-Tison S, et al. Anxiety and depression in juvenile diabetes: a critical review. Clin Psychol Rev 2003;23:787–800.
21. Chavira DA, Garland AF, Daley S, et al. The impact of medical comorbidity on mental health and functional health outcomes among children with anxiety disorders. J Dev Behav Pediatr 2008;29(5):394–402.
22. Katon WJ, Richardson L, Lozano P, et al. The relationship of asthma and anxiety disorders. Psychosom Med 2004;66(3):349–55.
23. Katon W, Lozano P, Russo J, et al. The prevalence of DSM-IV anxiety and depressive disorders in youth with asthma compared with controls. J Adolesc Health 2007;41(5): 455–63.
24. Richardson LP, Russo JE, Lozano P, et al. The effect of comorbid anxiety and depressive disorders on health care utilization and costs among adolescents with asthma. Gen Hosp Psychiatry 2008;30(5):398–406.
25. McCauley E, Katon W, Russo J, et al. Impact of anxiety and depression on functional impairment in adolescents with asthma. Gen Hosp Psychiatry 2007;29(3):214–22.
26. Bush T, Richardson L, Katon W, et al. Anxiety and depressive disorders are associated with smoking in adolescents with asthma. J Adolesc Health 2007;40(5):425–32.
27. Gavin, LA, Wamboldt M, Brugman S, et al. Psychological and family characteristics of adolescents with vocal cord dysfunction. J Asthma 1998;35:409–17.
28. Ekinci O, Titus JB, Rodopman AA, et al. Depression and anxiety in children and adolescents with epilepsy: prevalence, risk factors, and treatment. Epilepsy Behav 2009;14(1):8–18.
29. Caplan R, Siddarth P, Gurbani S, et al. Depression and anxiety disorders in pediatric epilepsy. Epilepsia 2005;46:720–30.
30. Jones JE, Watson R, Sheth R, et al. Psychiatric comorbidity in children with new onset epilepsy. Dev Med Child Neurol 2007;49:493–7.
31. Oguz A, Kurul S, Direk E. Relationship of epilepsy-related factors to anxiety and depression scores in epileptic children. J Child Neurol 2002;17(1):37–40.
32. Mintzer LL, Stuber ML, Seacord D, et al. Traumatic stress symptoms in adolescent organ transplant recipients. Pediatrics 2005;115(6):1640–4.
33. Stuber ML, Shemesh E. Post-traumatic stress response to life-threatening illnesses in children and their parents. Child Adolesc Psychiatr Clin N Am 2006;15(3):597–609.
34. Stuber ML, Meeske KA, Krull KR, et al. Prevalence and predictors of posttraumatic stress disorder in adult survivors of childhood cancer. Pediatrics 2010;125(5): e1124–34.
35. Davydow DS, Richardson LP, Zatzick DF, et al. Psychiatric morbidity in pediatric critical illness survivors: a comprehensive review of the literature. Arch Pediatr Adolesc Med 2010;164(4):377–85.
36. Campo JV, Bridge J, Ehmann M, et al. Recurrent abdominal pain, anxiety, and depression in primary care. Pediatrics 2004;113(4):817–24.
37. Egger H, Costello E, Erkanli A, et al. Somatic complaints and psychopathology in children and adolescents: stomachaches, musculoskeletal pains and headaches. J Am Acad Child Adolesc Psychiatry 1999;38:852–60.
38. Campo JV, Bridge J, Lucas A, et al. Physical and emotional health of mothers of youth with functional abdominal pain. Arch Pediatr Adolesc Med 2007;161(2):131–7.
39. American Psychiatric Association. Diagnostic and statistical manual of mental disorders. 4th edition. Washington (DC): American Psychiatric Association; 2000.

40. DeMaso DR, Martini DR, Cahen LA, et al. Practice parameter for the psychiatric assessment and management of physically ill children and adolescents. J. Am. Acad Child Adolesc Psychiatry 2009;48(2):213–33.
41. Connolly SD, Bernstein GA, and the Workgroup on Quality Issues. Practice parameter for the assessment and treatment of children and adolescents with anxiety disorders. J. Am Acad Child Adolesc Psychiatry 2007;46(2):267–83.
42. Compton SN, March JS, Brent D, et al. Cognitive-behavioral psychotherapy for anxiety and depressive disorders in children and adolescents: an evidence-based medicine review. J Am Acad Child Adolesc Psychiatry 2004;43:930–59.
43. James A, Soler A, Weatehrall R. Cognitive behavioural therapy for anxiety disorders in children and adolescents. Cochrane Database Syst Rev 2005;19:CD004690.
44. Walkup JT, Albano AM, Piacentini J, et al. Cognitive behavioral therapy, sertraline, or a combination in childhood anxiety. N Engl J Med 2008;359(26):2753–66.
45. Kendall PC, Pimentel S. On the physiological symptom constellation in youth with generalized anxiety disorders. J Anxiety Disord 2003;17:211–21.
46. Sanders M, Shepard R, Cleghorn G, et al. The treatment of recurrent abdominal pain in children: a controlled comparison of cognitive-behavioral family intervention and standard pediatric care. J Consult Clin Psychol 1994;62:306–14.
47. Warner CM, Reigada LC, Fisher PH, et al. CBT for anxiety and associated somatic complaints in pediatric medical settings: an open pilot study. J Clin Psychol Med Settings 2009;16:169–77.
48. Research Unit on Pediatric Psychopharmacology Anxiety Study Group. Fluvoxamine for the treatment of anxiety disorders in children and adolescents. N Engl J Med 2001;344:1279–85.
49. Rynn M, Regan J. Anxiety disorders. In: Findling R, editor. Clinical manual of child and adolescent psychopharmacology. Washington (DC): American Psychiatric Publishing, Inc; 2008. p. 143–88.
50. Campo JV. Disorders primarily seen in general medical settings. In: Findling R, editor. Clinical manual of child and adolescent psychopharmacology. Washington, DC: American Psychiatric Publishing, Inc; 2008. p. 375–413.
51. US Food and Drug Administration. FDA drug safety communication: abnormal heart rhythms associated with high doses of Celexa (citalopram hydrobromide). Published 2011. Available at: http://www.fda.gov/Drugs/DrugSafety/uscm269086.htm. Accessed February 23, 2012.
52. Howland R. A critical evaluation of the cardiac toxicity of citalopram. J Psychosoc Nurs Ment Health Serv 2011;49:13–6.
53. Campo JV, Perel J, Lucas A, et al. Citalopram treatment of pediatric recurrent abdominal pain and comorbid internalizing disorders: an exploratory study. J Am Acad Child Adolesc Psychiatry 2004;43(10):1234–42.
54. Kaminski A, Kamper A, Thaler K. Antidepressants for the treatment of abdominal pain-related functional gastrointestinal disorders in children and adolescents. Cochrane Database Syst Rev 2011;7:CD008013.
55. Bahar R, Collins B, Steinmetz B, et al. Double-blind placebo controlled trial of amitriptyline for the treatment of irritable bowel syndrome in adolescents. J Pediatrics 2008;152:685–9.
56. Saps M, Youssef N, Miranda A, et al. Multicenter, randomized placebo-controlled trial of amitriptyline in children with functional gastrointestinal disorders. Gastroenterology 2009;137:1261–9.
57. Geller B, Reising D, Leonard HL, et al. Critical review of tricyclic antidepressant use in children and adolescents. J Am Acad Child Adolesc Psychiatry 1999;38:513–6.

School-Based Anxiety Treatments for Children and Adolescents

Kathleen Herzig-Anderson, PhD[a], Daniela Colognori, PsyD[a],
Jeremy K. Fox, PhD[a], Catherine E. Stewart, BA[a],
Carrie Masia Warner, PhD[a,b,*]

KEYWORDS

- Anxiety • School-based treatment • Children • Adolescents • Dissemination

KEY POINTS

- School-based empirically supported treatments for anxiety disorders are a promising avenue for providing necessary intervention to distressed youth who would otherwise never receive treatment.
- Sustaining such programs in school settings should be viewed as a multiple-stage process, from integration of the program into the institution and maintenance of the intervention to responding to institutional change and ownership of the program by the school.
- Given the scarce resources available to schools, additional research on embedding programs into the school culture and maximizing existing resources is essential to enhancing the sustainability of school-based interventions for anxiety disorders and reaching youth in need.

Anxiety disorders are common among children and adolescents; however, anxious youth are rarely identified.[1] Unlike disruptive behavior disorders, anxiety disorders often go unnoticed by teachers and parents because clinically anxious youth are generally compliant, follow rules, and do not draw attention. Therefore, it is not surprising that anxious youth are the least likely among youth with psychiatric disorders to receive treatment.[2] Furthermore, even when youth access services, it is unclear what type of treatment they receive. Although several empirically supported

This work was supported by NIMH Grant No. R01MH081881 awarded to Carrie Masia Warner, PhD.

The authors have nothing to disclose.

[a] Anita Saltz Institute for Anxiety and Mood Disorders, NYU Child Study Center, Department of Child and Adolescent Psychiatry, NYU Langone Medical Center, One Park Avenue, 8th Floor, New York, NY 10016, USA; [b] Nathan S. Kline Institute for Psychiatric Research, 140 Old Orangeburg Road, Orangeburg, NY 10962, USA

* Corresponding author. NYU Child Study Center, Department of Child and Adolescent Psychiatry, One Park Avenue, 8th floor, New York, NY 10016.

E-mail address: carrie.masia@nyumc.org

Child Adolesc Psychiatric Clin N Am 21 (2012) 655–668

http://dx.doi.org/10.1016/j.chc.2012.05.006

treatments for anxious youth exist,[3–5] more than 80% of community-based treatment for anxious youth is not supported by scientific evidence.[6,7] There are also many barriers to treatment in traditional settings (eg, community clinics and independent clinicians), including stigma, long waitlists, and high costs.[8] Taken together, these factors underscore the importance of exploring alternative venues and methods for identifying and treating youth with anxiety disorders.

ADVANTAGES OF SCHOOL-BASED TREATMENT

Schools are viewed as a promising avenue for providing mental health services to children and adolescents. Schools are already the main point-of-entry into the mental health service system for youth,[9–12] with one study showing that more than 70% of mental health treatment for youth is provided by schools.[10] In addition, because schools offer relatively convenient and inexpensive services, barriers to accessing specialty care, such as financial and transportation difficulties, can be eliminated.[13,14] For example, school-based mental health clinics have been found to increase service utilization for both low-income adolescents[15] as well as adolescents enrolled in a health maintenance organization.[16] In light of common stigmas associated with mental health care, school-based treatment may also promote more positive attitudes toward mental health services among youth,[17,18] especially when offered among a variety of other routine educational and counseling services. Access to treatment in schools may normalize mental health care and may therefore increase the likelihood of students in need receiving treatment.

For these reasons, school-based treatments are receiving increasing attention as a venue to address the unmet mental health needs of youth, particularly those with anxiety disorders.[19] School-based treatments are particularly appropriate for anxiety disorders as schools provide unique opportunities for identification of anxious youth, treatment, and generalization of skills. For example, youth may display significant anxiety in academic and social settings at school that is not apparent or easily triggered in a more comfortable home environment with family support.[20] Schools are also optimal for the treatment of anxiety disorders, as there are ample opportunities to help students confront the many anxiety-provoking situations present at school. Specifically, exposure exercises at school could focus on exams and tests for youth with generalized anxiety disorder and achievement-oriented worries. Socially anxious youth may be helped to face negative evaluation fears associated with public speaking, performance in gym and music classes, and approaching unfamiliar peers and authority figures. Additionally, peers and teachers may be enlisted to assist in exposures to feared situations. In sum, these factors indicate that schools are advantageous settings for the treatment of anxiety disorders in children and adolescents.

Although schools are ideal venues for anxiety disorder treatment in youth, only in recent years has the transportability of efficacious cognitive-behavioral treatments for anxiety disorders to schools been evaluated. This article will review four school-based treatments for anxiety disorders that have shown promise in controlled trials (see **Table 1** for an overview and **Table 2** for links to treatment manuals). This will be followed by a discussion of issues and challenges related to delivering anxiety treatments in a school environment and important areas for future research.

COOL KIDS
Treatment Description

The Cool Kids Program: School Version[21] is an eight-session cognitive-behavioral intervention for anxiety symptoms in children, which was adapted for the school

Table 1
School-based treatments for anxiety

Treatment	Number and Length of Sessions	Format	Treatment Components	Parent/Teacher Components	Overview of Effectiveness in Schools	Implementation Strengths and Limitations
Cool Kids[21]	Eight 1-hour sessions	Group	Psychoeducation, cognitive restructuring, graduated exposure, coping with bullying, social skills, assertiveness	Two parent information sessions on parenting strategies and ways for parents to manage their own anxiety	Significantly greater decreases in self- and teacher-reported anxiety when compared to waitlist control	Strengths: • Group format • Includes dealing with bullying, social skills, and assertiveness components. Limitations: • Unknown if superior to attention control or other treatments. • Use of community mental health workers is unsustainable.
Baltimore Child Anxiety Treatment Study in the Schools (BCATSS)[24–26]	Ten 45-minute sessions[24] or twelve 35-minute sessions[25]	Group[24] and individual[25,26]	Psychoeducation, cognitive restructuring, graduated exposure, self-reward, contingency management, relaxation skills, problem solving, relapse prevention	Up to three sessions include parents to provide parenting strategies and psychoeducation.	Significantly greater decreases in self- and clinician-rated anxiety compared to attention-support control in one small study. Another small study found no difference compared to usual care.	Strengths: • Includes self-reward, contingency management, and problem solving. • Shown to be effective with urban African American youth. Limitations: • No teacher components • Individual format[25,26]

(continued on next page)

Table 1
(continued)

Treatment	Number and Length of Sessions	Format	Treatment Components	Parent/Teacher Components	Overview of Effectiveness in Schools	Implementation Strengths and Limitations
Cognitive-Behavioral Intervention for Trauma in Schools (CBITS)[28]	Ten 1-hour sessions	Group	Psychoeducation, cognitive restructuring, graduated exposure, processing of traumatic memories, relaxation skills, social problem-solving skills, adaptive coping skills	Two parent education meetings, one teacher education meeting	Two studies found significantly greater reductions in PTSD symptoms compared to waitlist control. One study found significantly greater reductions in depressive symptoms compared to waitlist control.	Strengths: • Includes social problem-solving skills, processing traumatic memories, and adaptive coping skills. • Shown to be effective with minor adaptations for urban multicultural populations. Limitations: • Unknown whether it is more effective than attention control. • Use of school-based psychiatric social workers is not a model most schools have the resources to replicate.

Support for Students Exposed to Trauma (SSET[33], an adaptation of CBITS)	Ten 45-minute sessions (one class period)	Group	Psychoeducation, cognitive restructuring, graduated exposure, processing traumatic memories, relaxation skills, adaptive coping, problem solving	Parent phone calls. Can be implemented by teachers.	Small improvements found in PTSD and depressive symptoms at 3-month follow-up in one study.	Strengths: • Designed to be implemented by teachers and school counselors. Limitations: • Only one study without enough power to determine if modest results are significant • No significant parent component
Skills for Academic and Social Success (SASS)[35]	Twelve 40-minute sessions	Group	Psychoeducation, cognitive restructuring, graduated exposure, social skills, peer generalization (through social events)	Two parent meetings including psychoeducation and parenting strategies, two teacher meetings	Significantly greater number of students were classified as responders to treatment compared to waitlist and attention control.	Strengths: • Inclusion of social skills and peer generalization social events Limitations: • To date, shown to be effective only when implemented by clinical psychologists, although study examining SASS in school counselors is underway.

Table 2
Webpages for available treatment manuals

Treatment	Availability	Webpage
Cool Kids[21]	For purchase	http://www.centreforemotionalhealth.com.au/pages/resources-products.aspx
Baltimore Child Anxiety Treatment Study in the Schools (BCATSS)[24–26]	Not available	—
Cognitive-Behavioral Intervention for Trauma in Schools (CBITS)[28]	Free	http://cbitsprogram.org/
Support for Students Exposed to Trauma (SSET[33]; an adaptation of CBITS)	Free	http://www.rand.org/pubs/technical_reports/TR675.html
Skills for Academic and Social Success (SASS)[35]	Not available	—

environment from previous group treatments for anxiety disorders.[22] Sessions focus on core cognitive-behavioral treatment (CBT) components, such as psychoeducation, cognitive restructuring, and graduated exposure to anxiety-provoking situations. Additionally, Cool Kids includes sessions on assertiveness, coping with bullying, and social skills. Treatment sessions last about 1 hour each and are conducted during the school day in groups of eight to ten children. Two parent information sessions address parenting strategies as well as concepts taught to the children, which parents are encouraged to use to manage their own anxiety.

Evidence for Cool Kids

Mifsud and Rapee[21] evaluated Cool Kids in a sample of 91 children (ages 9–10) by randomizing nine schools in low-income communities in Australia to either Cool Kids or a waitlist control.[21] Students scoring in the clinical range of the Revised Manifest Anxiety Scale,[23] a self-report measure of anxiety, were selected to participate. Groups were co-led by a school counselor and an experienced community mental health worker. Compared to the control, children in the Cool Kids condition showed significantly greater decreases in self- and teacher-reported anxiety both at post-treatment and 4-month follow-up. This study suggests that Cool Kids is a promising school-based intervention; however, since delivery by experienced community mental health workers is not a sustainable model, further research is needed to evaluate its effectiveness when delivered only by school-based providers.

BALTIMORE CHILD ANXIETY TREATMENT STUDY IN THE SCHOOLS
Treatment Description

Baltimore Child Anxiety Treatment Study in the Schools (BCATSS)[24–26] is designed to provide mental health treatment for inner-city adolescents with anxiety disorders as an integrated part of established school-based mental health clinics. The treatment was adapted from a previously supported group CBT program.[5,27] The BCATSS program was tailored for the school environment and an urban, lower socioeconomic status, predominantly African American population (eg, examples were changed to be culturally relevant). Based on feedback from school mental health professionals, BCATSS was implemented individually during 12 weekly sessions (35 minutes each).[25] This CBT program is comprised of psychoeducation, relaxation skills, problem solving, cognitive restructuring, relapse prevention and graduated in-vivo exposures to feared situations reinforced by self-reward and contingency contracts. The *BCATSS* intervention has a modular approach, allowing the clinician flexibility in choosing which core CBT skills ("modules") to deliver in a particular session based on the needs of the student.[25] Optional parent sessions (one to three) were also added to increase involvement.[26]

Evidence for BCATSS

The BCATSS treatment has been evaluated in two small randomized controlled trials. Preliminary support for Ginsburg and Drake's[24] adaptation of group CBT for a predominantly inner-city African American population was demonstrated in a small randomized controlled study ($N = 12$) comparing BCATSS to an attention-support control in 14- to 17-year-old adolescents diagnosed with generalized anxiety disorder, social phobia, specific phobia, and/or agoraphobia. Two advanced psychology graduate students with training in CBT implemented the program. Results showed that self- and clinician-rated anxiety symptoms were significantly lower after treatment in the CBT group compared to the control group. In addition, 80% of the control group continued to meet criteria for an anxiety disorder after treatment, versus only 25% of the CBT group.

The second randomized controlled trial[25,26] compared the BCATSS CBT program to usual care (UC) in a small study of 7- to 17-year-old ($M = 10.28$) inner-city African American youth with anxiety disorders ($N = 32$). Therapists were school-based master's and doctoral level clinicians, trained primarily in social work, counseling, or psychology. Because there was only one clinician per school, the same clinician implemented both conditions.[25] Clinicians were explicitly instructed to exclude CBT techniques in the usual care condition and instead implement nonspecific strategies, such as art and supportive therapy.[26] Results showed no differences across conditions at post-treatment, with 50% of CBT participants and 46% of UC participants no longer meeting criteria for an anxiety disorder. Similar results were found at 1-month follow-up: 42% of participants in the CBT group and 57% in the UC group no longer met criteria for an anxiety disorder. A central methodologic limitation was that CBT-trained clinicians also delivered usual care, resulting in poor treatment differentiation across conditions. Per review of 25% of UC therapy sessions, 56% contained CBT techniques, despite ongoing coaching to exclude these components. In addition, although the authors rated how much of the module content (eg, psychoeducation, exposure) was delivered (adherence), they did not report how skillfully these specific techniques were conducted (competence). Therefore, it is possible that the implementation quality impacted treatment outcome. Another possibility is that novice therapists may be more effective with structured rather than flexible treatments, as the latter may require more expertise to determine the appropriate module to deliver. Clearly, several questions remain unanswered, and thus additional research examining the value of modular treatments may be necessary.

COGNITIVE-BEHAVIORAL INTERVENTION FOR TRAUMA IN SCHOOLS
Treatment Description

Cognitive-Behavioral Intervention for Trauma in Schools (CBITS)[28] is a school-based group treatment developed for youth ages 10 to 15 with clinically significant symptoms of posttraumatic stress disorder (PTSD) and depression secondary to trauma exposure (excluding sexual abuse). CBITS was designed to be implemented by mental health clinicians in an urban multicultural environment. CBITS is generally comprised of ten one-hour weekly group treatment sessions (five to eight students per group), one to three individual sessions, two optional parent education meetings, and one teacher education meeting.[28,29] The treatment elements of CBITS include psychoeducation, relaxation, adaptive coping skills, cognitive restructuring techniques, graduated imaginal exposure to traumatic memories, processing of traumatic memories, and social problem solving skills. Imaginal exposure through writing and drawing is initially conducted in individual sessions and subsequently in the group. CBITS sessions present skills using a combination of didactic presentation, developmentally appropriate examples, worksheets, and games. The focus of treatment is the generalization of concepts learned in treatment sessions to real-life situations by applying them to a given child's specific difficulties.[28]

Evidence for CBITS

Two randomized controlled trials have shown support for CBITS compared to a waitlist control in youth with clinically significant PTSD symptoms secondary to exposure to community violence.[28,30] In both studies, CBITS was implemented by psychiatric social workers based in the school districts' mental health clinic. The first study ($N = 199$) found that third through eighth graders (mean age = 11.4 years; $SD = 1.7$) with clinically elevated PTSD symptoms participating in CBITS had significantly lower PTSD symptoms post-treatment compared to waitlist control.[30] Small adaptations for this study included reducing group sessions from ten to eight and increasing parent sessions from two to four, which focused on themes of loss and separation common to immigration. Similarly, Stein and colleagues[28] found that sixth graders ($N = 126$) participating in CBITS reported significantly greater reductions in PTSD and depressive symptoms compared to those in the waitlist control group three months and six months post-treatment. These two studies provide evidence for the effectiveness of CBITS for PTSD symptoms when implemented in urban multicultural schools.

The feasibility of school-based group CBITS compared to clinic-based individual Trauma Focused-Cognitive-Behavioral Therapy (TF-CBT) was supported by an investigation of fourth to eighth graders ($N = 118$) with elevated PTSD symptoms 15-months post-Hurricane Katrina in New Orleans.[31] Three components of CBITS were not delivered in this study due to resource and time limitations: the individual session prior to the start of group, teacher informational meetings and in two of the three schools, parent meetings. The CBITS treatment was implemented by school-based mental health professionals, while TF-CBT was conducted by social workers and psychologists employed at a community mental health center.[32] Although youth in both treatment groups showed clinically significant improvements in PTSD symptoms at 10-month follow-up, CBITS was far more accessible to participants as 98% of youth randomized to CBITS were enrolled in treatment compared to only 23% of youth assigned to TF-CBT. This highlights the greater ability of school-based treatments to reach and retain distressed youth compared to treatments delivered in traditional community mental health settings.

Support for Students Exposed to Trauma

Support for Students Exposed to Trauma (SSET),[33] an adaptation of CBITS, was designed to be implemented by school counselors and teachers to increase accessibility. SSET delivers the components of CBITS in 10 weekly group sessions utilizing a lesson plan format and omits the individual and parent meetings included in CBITS. SSET showed superiority to a waitlist control in 76 sixth to eighth graders scoring at least 11 on the Child PTSD Symptom Scale [34] (ie, moderate to high PTSD symptoms) subsequent to exposure to violence within the last year. Students in the SSET group showed small improvements in PTSD and depressive symptoms at 3-month follow-up. While these decreases appeared to be more substantial than those of the waitlist control, the small sample size limited the statistical power to detect effects. Although additional studies are needed, these preliminary findings suggest that SSET is a feasible intervention for PTSD symptoms that can be delivered by school personnel.

SKILLS FOR ACADEMIC AND SOCIAL SUCCESS
Treatment Description

Skills for Academic and Social Success (SASS)[35] is a school-based group CBT program for adolescents with social anxiety disorder adapted from Social Effectiveness Therapy for Children (SET-C), an efficacious group treatment for children with social anxiety disorder.[3,36] Like SET-C, SASS focuses on gradual exposure, social skills, and peer generalization. However, SASS includes adaptations for adolescents (eg, addition of realistic thinking) and the school environment (eg, shorter sessions, involvement of teachers). SASS consists of 12 weekly 40-minute (ie, one class period) group sessions, two individual meetings, two parent meetings, two teacher meetings, four social events with outgoing peers, and two booster sessions. Social skills training includes initiating and maintaining conversations, nonverbal behaviors (eg, maintaining good eye contact), and assertiveness. Graduated in vivo exposures to feared social situations are often integrated into the school environment, for example, volunteering to answer a question in class, talking with a teacher, or giving an oral presentation. Individual meetings focus on setting goals and problem solving any obstacles to treatment. To increase generalization of skills and exposure to real-world settings, the four social events are conducted with group members and outgoing peers together in settings adolescents often spend time in, such as bowling or laser tag. Parent meetings include psychoeducation, parenting strategies including preventing their child's avoidance, and rewarding nonanxious behavior. Teacher meetings focus on the goals of SASS, education regarding social anxiety, and enlisting teachers' help with classroom exposures.

Evidence for SASS

Support for SASS has been provided by two randomized controlled trials. The first investigation compared SASS to a waitlist control in urban parochial high school students with social anxiety disorder ($N = 35$).[37] Groups were co-led by a clinical psychologist and a psychology graduate student. Results found that 94% of SASS participants were classified as responders based on their improved functioning at post-treatment, versus only 12% of the control group. In addition, 67% of SASS participants, compared to only 6% of controls, no longer met criteria for social anxiety disorder post-treatment. Lower clinician-rated diagnostic severity and self-reported social anxiety and social avoidance were found for the SASS group at post-treatment and 9-month follow-up.

The second trial examined the specific efficacy of SASS compared to a credible attention control in adolescents aged 14 to 16 ($N = 36$) with a primary diagnosis of social anxiety disorder.[1] The attention control group, equal in time and adult attention, included relaxation training and four social events without outgoing peers. Results demonstrated superiority of SASS, with more than 82% of SASS participants classified as responders, compared to 7% of those in the attention control. Importantly, only 41% of SASS participants continued to meet criteria for social anxiety disorder post-treatment, while all control participants still qualified for the disorder.

Students receiving SASS also exhibited greater overall improvement and lower clinician-rated social anxiety severity at post-treatment and 6-month follow-up.

Currently, Masia Warner and colleagues are conducting a large, federally funded, randomized controlled trial of SASS implemented by school guidance counselors to investigate its transportability to school settings.[38] This study will examine whether school personnel without specialized training in CBT can effectively deliver a cognitive-behavioral intervention. Positive findings would highlight the potential effectiveness of a more sustainable model of evidence-based care delivered by school personnel to reach underserved youth with social anxiety disorder.

Summary of School-Based Anxiety Treatments

Studies of school-based treatment programs for anxiety disorders in youth suggest promise for effectively delivering these evidence-based programs in schools. However, several gaps in our current knowledge exist. One shortcoming has been the reliance on specialized mental health clinicians to deliver interventions, which is costly and resource intensive. Researchers have called for training school-based personnel (eg, school counselors and teachers) to deliver these evidence-based interventions, but it remains unknown whether they can do so effectively. In addition, surprisingly few investigations of school-based anxiety treatments have investigated the impact of intervention on academic and other school-related variables upon which schools are evaluated (eg, grades, standardized test scores, attendance). Overall, many questions remain regarding methods to facilitate successful implementation and sustainability of school-based mental health programs. The following section focuses on several areas requiring additional exploration, such as the integration of treatments into school culture, improving identification of anxious youth, and the utilization of school-based personnel as treatment providers.

IMPLICATIONS FOR RESEARCH AND PRACTICE
School Culture and Context

Efforts to increase the accessibility of evidence-based treatments to youth with anxiety disorders may be bolstered by a better understanding of factors affecting the ability of schools to adopt and sustain mental health programs. Consideration of school context, such as school climate, resources, and the impact of educational accountability, will likely influence whether schools will accept and prioritize these treatments.[39] Because schools' main focus is education, future studies providing evidence that school-based treatments positively affect academics and other variables aligning with school values are essential to increasing uptake and sustainability of school-based treatments. Further research on methods to better integrate mental health programs into the school culture may also improve the acceptability of programs to important stakeholders, such as school administrators. For example, incorporating treatment components into the general classroom curriculum has been found to increase program sustainability for universal intervention programs.[40] Applying this concept to targeted students with anxiety disorders, such as evaluating integration of school-based programs into existing student services (eg, guidance counseling) or extracurricular activities (eg, club format), may also increase feasibility. Finally, future research should examine optimal methods to maximize schools' existing resources to manage students' mental health needs. For instance, Ringeisen and colleagues[39] suggest replacing the current individualized case management approach to school-based mental health care with a model combining classroom-based intervention and as-needed group treatment or consultation from specialized clinicians. This innovative model, along with other methods to improve integration of mental health services into the existing school culture, is critical to increasing long-term sustainability of school-based mental health programs.

Identification of Clinically Anxious Students

Another essential area for future study will be testing methods for enhancing recognition or detection of youth with anxiety disorders. Research on the ability of school personnel to identify youth with internalizing disorders has focused mostly on teachers rather than more specialized personnel such as counselors, and findings have been inconclusive. Not surprisingly, teachers are generally more likely to recognize externalizing behaviors than internalizing problems such as anxiety and depression.[41,42] There is some evidence to suggest that youth are more likely to access services when school personnel (eg, teachers, school counselors) are made aware of their anxiety rather than parents or other adults.[43] This indicates that research on educating and training school personnel in the identification of anxiety, through observation or school-wide screenings, is critical to increasing early detection and treatment.[44,45] Studies examining the accuracy and sensitivity of self-report measures in predicting anxiety disorders would clarify the effectiveness and efficiency of utilizing these measures in school-wide screenings to identify anxious youth. Of course, a challenge of improving methods for identifying anxious youth is the resulting increase in referrals for mental health care, which schools may not be equipped to handle. This highlights the importance of increasing the availability of mental health care providers through school-based treatments.

School-Based Treatment Providers

To date, the majority of investigations of school-based interventions have been implemented by mental health clinicians employed by research teams. Because the costs and feasibility of hiring mental health clinicians are prohibitive for most schools, there is a significant need to establish the effectiveness of school-based interventions for anxiety disorders when delivered by school personnel. With specialized training, supervision, and support, school guidance counselors may be ideal candidates to be trained in the implementation of mental health interventions. School counselors are present in all high schools, typically comprise a large team, and enter their profession to assist and guide youth.[46] Furthermore, a recent national survey revealed that 90% of guidance counselors wanted reductions in administrative tasks and caseloads to increase time for assisting students and receiving training.[47] This indicates that guidance counselors may be open to opportunities to receive training in school-based treatments, especially because guidance counselors are routinely asked to manage their students' emotional needs.

However, the literature has shown that efficacious treatments delivered in research settings often show reduced effectiveness in clinical settings.[48] It has been theorized that treatment fidelity, defined as adequate adherence to a treatment manual and competence in delivery,[49] is related to treatment outcome.[50] Further research is needed to document this relationship and to identify what levels of fidelity are sufficient for treatment response, which has the potential to inform training approaches and supervision. The ongoing study by Masia Warner and colleagues examining whether school counselors can effectively implement a group CBT program for adolescents with social anxiety disorder will contribute to this gap in the literature.

SUMMARY

School-based empirically supported treatments for anxiety disorders are a promising avenue for providing necessary intervention to distressed youth who would otherwise never receive treatment. Sustaining such programs in school settings should be viewed as a multiple-stage process, from integration of the program into the institution and maintenance of the intervention to responding to institutional change and ownership of the program by the school.[51] Given the scarce resources available to schools, additional research on embedding programs into the school culture and maximizing existing resources is essential to enhancing the sustainability of school-based interventions for anxiety disorders and reaching youth in need.

REFERENCES

1. Masia Warner C, Fisher PH, Shrout PE, et al. Treating adolescents with social anxiety disorder in school: an attention control trial. J Child Psychol Psychiatry 2007;48: 676–86.
2. Merikangas KR, He J, Burnstein M, et al. Service utilization for lifetime mental disorders in U.S. adolescents: results of the national comorbidity survey-adolescent supplement (NCS-A). J Am Acad Child Psychiatry 2011;50(1):32–44.
3. Beidel DC, Turner SM, Morris TL. Behavioral treatment of childhood social phobia. J Consult Clin Psychol 2000;68:643–50.
4. Kendall PC. Treating anxiety disorders in children: results of a randomized clinical trial. J Consult Clin Psychol 1994;62:100–10.
5. Silverman WK, Kurtines WM, Ginsberg GS, et al. Treating anxiety disorders in children with group cognitive-behavioral therapy: a randomized clinical trial. J Consult Clin Psychol 1999;67(6):995–1003.
6. Labellarte MJ, Ginsburg GS, Walkup JT, et al. The treatment of anxiety disorders in children and adolescents. Biol Psychiatry 1999;46:1567–78.
7. Collins KA, Westra HA, Dozois DJ, et al. Gaps in accessing treatment for anxiety and depression: challenges for the delivery of care. Clin Psychol Rev 2004;24:583–616.
8. Owens PL, Hoagland K, Horwitz SM, et al. Barriers to children's mental health services. J Am Acad Child Adolesc Psychiatry 2002;41:731–8.
9. Costello EJ, Angold A, Burns BJ, et al. The great smoky mountains study of youth: goals, design, methods and the prevalence of DSM-III-R disorders. Arch Gen Psychiatry 1996;53:1129–36.
10. Burns BJ, Costello EJ, Angold A, et al. Children's mental health service use across service sectors. Health Affairs 1995;14(3):147–59.
11. Farmer EM, Burns BJ, Phillips SD, et al. Pathways into and through mental health services for children and adolescents. Psychiatr Serv 2003;54:60–6.
12. Leaf PJ, Alegria M, Cohen P, et al. Mental health service use in the community and schools: results from the four-community MECA study. J Am Acad Child Adolesc Psychiatry 1996;35:889–96.
13. Catron T, Harris, VS, Weiss B. Posttreatment results after 2 years of services in the Vanderbilt school-based counseling project. In: Epstein MH, Kutash K, Duchnowski A, editors. Outcomes for children and youth with emotional and behavioral disorders and their families: programs and evaluation best practices. Austin (TX): PRO-ED; 1998. p. 633–40.
14. Wu P, Hoven CW, Bird HR, et al. Depressive and disruptive disorders and mental health service utilization in children and adolescents. J Am Acad Child Adolesc Psychiatry 1999;38:1081–90.

15. Juszczak L, Melinkovich P, Kaplan D. Use of health and mental health services by adolescents across multiple delivery sites. J Adolesc Health 2003;32(6):108–18.
16. Kaplan D, Calonge B, Guernsey B, et al. Managed care and school-based health centers: use of health services. Arch Pediatr Adolesc Med 1998;152:25–33.
17. Nabors LA, Reynolds MW. Program evaluation activities: outcomes related to treatment for adolescents receiving school-based mental health services. Children's Services: Social Policy, Research, and Practice 2000;3:175–89.
18. Weist MD. Challenges and opportunities in expanded school mental health. Clin Psychol Rev 1999;19:131–5.
19. Masia Warner C, Nangle DW, Hansen DJ. Bringing evidence-based child mental health services to the schools: general issues and specific populations. Educ Treat Child 2006;29:165–72.
20. Kendall PC, Puliafico AC, Barmish AJ, et al. Assessing anxiety with the child behavior checklist and the teacher report form. J Anxiety Disord 2007;21:1004–15.
21. Mifsud C, Rapee RM. Early intervention for childhood anxiety in a school setting: outcomes for an economically disadvantaged population. J Am Acad Child Adolesc Psychiatry 2005;44:996–1004.
22. Rapee RM. Group treatment of children with anxiety disorders: outcome and predictors of treatment response. Aust J Psychol 2000;52:125–9.
23. Reynolds CR, Richmond OB. What I think and feel: a revised measure of children's manifest anxiety. J Abnorm Child Psychol 1978;6:271–80.
24. Ginsburg GS, Drake KL. School-based treatment for anxious African-American adolescents: a controlled pilot study. J Am Acad Child Adolesc Psychiatry 2002;41: 768–75.
25. Ginsburg G, Becker K, Kingery J, et al. Transporting CBT for childhood and anxiety disorders into inner-city school based mental health clinics. Cogn Behav Pract 2008;15:148–58.
26. Ginsburg GS, Becker KD, Drazdowski TK, et al. Treating anxiety disorders in inner city schools: results from a pilot randomized controlled trial comparing CBT and usual care. Child Youth Care Forum 2012;41:1–19.
27. Ginsburg G, Silverman W, Kurtines W. Cognitive-behavioral group therapy. In: Eisen A, Kearney C, Schaefer C, editors. Clinical handbook of anxiety disorders in children and adolescents. Northvale (NJ): Jason Aronson; 1995. p. 521–49.
28. Stein BD, Jaycox LH, Kataoka SH, et al. A mental health intervention for schoolchildren exposed to violence: a randomized controlled trial. JAMA 2003;290:603–11.
29. Jaycox LH, Morse LK, Tanielian T, et al. How schools can help students recover from traumatic experiences: a tool kit for supporting long-term recovery 2006. Available at: http://www.rand.org/pubs/technical_reports/TR413.html. Accessed May 16, 2012.
30. Kataoka S, Stein BD, Jaycox LH, et al. A school-based mental health program for traumatized latino immigrant children. J Am Acad Child Adolesc Psychiatry 2003; 42(3):311–8.
31. Jaycox LH, Cohen JA, Mannarino AP, et al. Children's mental health care following Hurricane Katrina: a field trial of trauma-focused psychotherapies. J Trauma Stress 2010;23:223–31.
32. Cohen JA, Jaycox LH, Walker DW, et al. Treating traumatized children after hurricane Katrina: Project Fleur-de Lis. Clin Child Fam Psychol Rev 2009;21;55–64.
33. Jaycox LH, Langley AK, Stein BD, et al. Support for students exposed to trauma: a pilot study. School Ment Health 2009;1:49–60.
34. Foa EB, Treadwell K, Johnson K, et al. The Child PTSD Symptom Scale: A preliminary examination of its psychometric properties. J Clin Child Psychol 2001;30;376–84.

35. Masia C, Beidel DC, Fisher PH, et al. Skills for academic and social success. New York: New York University School of Medicine; 1999.
36. Beidel DC, Turner SM, Toung, B et al. Social effectiveness therapy for children: three-year follow-up. J Consult Clin Psychol 2005;73:721–5.
37. Masia Warner C, Klein RG, Dent HC, et al. School-based intervention for adolescents with social anxiety disorder: results of a controlled study. J Abnorm Child Psychol 2005;33:707–22.
38. Masia Warner C, Ryan J, Colognori D, et al. Adapting treatment of social anxiety disorder for delivery in schools: training school counselors to deliver a cognitive-behavioral intervention. In: R. Gallagher, Chair. How to keep from getting schooled: dissemination and implementation of empirically-based programs for children and adolescents in educational settings. Symposium presented at the 45th annual meeting of the Association for Behavioral and Cognitive Therapies. Toronto, ON, November 2011.
39. Ringeisen H, Henderson K, Hoagwood K. Context matters: schools and the "Research to Practice Gap" in children's mental health. School Psych Rev 2003; 32(2): 153–68.
40. Rones M, Hoagwood K. School-based mental health services: a research review. Clin Child Fam Psychol Rev 2000;3(4):223–41.
41. Burnett-Zeigler I, Lyons JS. Youth characteristics associated with intensity of service use in a school-based mental health intervention. J Child Fam Stud 2011. DOI: 10.1007/s10826-011-9555-z.
42. Loades ME, Mastroyannopoulou K. Teachers' recognition of children's mental health problems. Child Adolesc Ment Health 2010;15(3):150–6.
43. Colognori D, Ryan JL, Fox JK, et al. Mental health service utilization in a community sample of socially anxious adolescents. In: Masia Warner C, Ryan J, Co-Chairs. Mental health service utilization in youth: deficiencies of availability, awareness, and use of evidence-based treatments. Symposium presented at the 45th annual meeting of the Association for Behavioral and Cognitive Therapies. Toronto, ON, November 2011.
44. Weist MD, Myers CP, Hastings E, et al. Psychosocial functioning of youth receiving mental health services in the schools versus community mental health centers. Commun Ment Health J 1999;35:69–81.
45. Husky MM, Sheridan M, McGuire L, et al. Mental health screening and follow-up care in public high schools. J Am Acad Child Adolesc Psychiatry 2011;50(9):881–91.
46. Evans SW. Mental health services in schools: utilization, effectiveness and consent. Clin Psychol Rev 1999;19:165–78.
47. Bridgeland J, Bruce M. National survey of school counselors: counseling at a crossroads 2011. Available at: http://media.collegeboard.com/digitalServices/pdf/nosca/11b_4230_NarReport_BOOKLET_WEB_111104.pdf. Accessed December 27, 2011.
48. Weisz JR, Donenberg GR, Han SS, et al. Bridging the gap between laboratory and clinic in child and adolescent psychotherapy. J Consult Clin Psychol 1995;63(5):688–701.
49. Perepletchikova F, Hilt LM, Chereji E, et al. Barriers to implementing treatment integrity procedures: surveys of treatment outcome researchers. J Consult Clin Psychol 2009;77:212–8.
50. Hogue A, Henderson CE, Dauber S, et al. Treatment adherences, competence, and outcome in individual and family therapy for adolescent behavior problems. J Consult Clin Psychol 2008;76:544–55.
51. Altman DG. Sustaining interventions in community systems: on the relationship between researchers and communities. Health Psychol 1995;14(6):526–36.

Targeting Parental Psychopathology in Child Anxiety

Hilary B. Vidair, PhD[a,b,*], Cassie N. Fichter, MS[a],
Kristin L. Kunkle, MS[a], Angelo S. Boccia, MA[c]

KEYWORDS

- Child anxiety treatment • Parental psychopathology • Parental anxiety
- Parental depression • Family cognitive-behavioral therapy

KEY POINTS

- Children of parents with psychopathology (ie, anxiety or depression) are at significantly higher risk for developing anxiety disorders than children of parents without psychopathology.
- Existing top-down studies assessing child anxiety and emotional constructs lend some support to the notion that successfully treating parental depression can improve child anxiety, although changes may take up to 1 year.
- Anxious parents whose symptoms were addressed in family-based cognitive-behavioral therapy or adjunct treatment did not improve more than anxious parents whose families received only child treatment. Therefore, the impact of effectively treating parental anxiety in addition to child treatment has not been investigated.
- Given that aspects of parental psychopathology and behavior may impact child anxiety, it is important to develop a family-based treatment paradigm that goes beyond FCBT to attend to parent and child needs equally.

INTRODUCTION

Children of parents with psychopathology (ie, anxiety or depression) are at significantly higher risk for developing anxiety disorders than children of parents without psychopathology.[1–7] These children are also at significantly greater risk for depressive and behavioral disorders, school problems, increased medical utilization,

The authors have nothing to disclose.
[a] Clinical Psychology Doctoral Program, Long Island University, Post Campus, 720 Northern Boulevard, Brookville, NY 11548, USA; [b] Department of Psychiatry, Columbia University College of Physicians and Surgeons, 1051 Riverside Drive, New York, NY 10032, USA; [c] Doctoral Program in Clinical Psychology, Department of Psychology, Temple University, 1701 North 13th Street, Philadelphia, PA 19122, USA
* Corresponding author. Clinical Psychology Doctoral Program, Long Island University, Post Campus, 720 Northern Boulevard, Brookville, NY 11548.
E-mail address: hilary.vidair@liu.edu

outpatient mental health treatment, and more continuous treatment over time.[3,4,6–9] They also commonly exhibit poor family and social functioning.[10]

The increased risk of anxiety in children of parents with psychopathology is a significant public health problem, as early-onset is associated with a variety of difficulties later in life, including adult anxiety and depression, substance dependence, suicide, educational underachievement, and low psychosocial functioning.[11–14] The development of anxiety disorders in children whose parents have their own psychopathology may actually be a precursor for the development of depression during adolescence and young adulthood. In a longitudinal study following children of depressed parents, Weissman and colleagues[6,7] found that the highest risk for the onset of an anxiety disorder was in childhood, while the peak time for the incidence of major depressive disorder was between the ages of 15 and 20. This suggests that children experiencing anxiety disorders are at high risk for developing depression later in life.

Rates of Parental Psychopathology and Child Anxiety in Treatment-Seeking Families

Although many studies have assessed lifetime rates of parental psychopathology in children with anxiety, few have focused solely on times when both parent and child have a current diagnosis and when either is seeking treatment. From a top-down perspective, Beidel and Turner[15] found that children of parents with an anxiety and/or depression diagnosis recruited in an anxiety clinic were more than five times more likely to have an anxiety disorder than children of normal controls. Pilowsky and colleagues[16] found that among mothers entering medication treatment for major depression, 16% of their children met criteria for an anxiety disorder. From a bottom-up perspective, almost 75% of children presenting for anxiety treatment were found to have at least one parent with his or her own current anxiety disorder as compared to 38% of control children.[17] In addition, self-reported parental anxiety and depressive symptoms have been significantly associated with receiving a child anxiety diagnosis during child evaluation.[18]

Child Anxiety Treatment Outcomes When Parents Have Their Own Psychopathology

Several studies have indicated that children of parents with their own current psychopathology have significantly worse treatment outcomes for anxiety disorders than children of parents without psychopathology.[19–24] Southam-Gerow and colleagues[25] found that higher levels of maternal depressive symptoms predicted poorer child response to treatment for an anxiety disorder. Similarly, Rapee[26] found that paternal symptoms of anxiety predicted higher levels of child anxiety at post-treatment and 12-month follow-up.

Some evidence suggests that children's anxiety treatment outcomes may be specific to the type of parental diagnosis. For example, Cooper and colleagues[22] found that children of mothers with social phobia did worse than other children, whereas children of mothers with generalized anxiety disorder (GAD) did as well as their peers.

Differential child treatment outcomes have also been found between maternal and paternal symptoms. Rapee[26] found that higher levels of paternal anxiety, but not maternal anxiety or parental depression, predicted poorer child outcomes. Similarly, Liber and colleagues[27] found that paternal anxiety, depression, rejection, and high maternal warmth (but not maternal anxiety or depression) were significantly predictive of child treatment failure.

Greater family dysfunction, parental frustration, maternal parenting stress, and paternal somatization have also been significantly associated with less favorable child anxiety treatment outcomes.[28]

Some studies, however, do not support findings that parental psychopathology is associated with poorer child response to anxiety treatment. Thienemann and colleagues[29] and Victor and colleagues[30] found no effects of maternal psychopathology on child treatment outcomes. Toren and colleagues[31] found that children of mothers with an anxiety disorder actually improved more than children of mothers without an anxiety disorder. Taken together, these studies suggest that parental psychopathology seems to have a negative effect on child treatment outcomes, though this finding is not always replicated.

Does Treating Parental Psychopathology Improve Child Anxiety?

Based on the high risks related to having a parent with psychopathology, it appears that the next logical step is to determine if treating parents alone or in conjunction with their children has an effect on child anxiety outcome. Gunlicks and Weissman[32] conducted a review of studies that followed children longitudinally when their parents were in treatment for depression. They found initial evidence of a relationship between successful parent treatment and improvements in child outcomes; however, there was no specific focus on changes in child anxiety. Reviews of child anxiety treatment studies with active parent involvement have addressed parental psychopathology, but have been more focused on comparing family-focused treatment to individual treatment.[33–35]

The aim of this article is to review the current evidence base to determine if treating parental psychopathology is associated with improvements in child anxiety. To our knowledge, this is the first article to summarize both top-down and bottom-up studies examining the impact of treating the parent on child anxiety outcomes. A secondary aim of this article is to examine the influence of anxiogenic and depressogenic parental behaviors on child anxiety. Parents with anxiety and depression have been found to be more critical, overcontrolling, avoidant, and less positive and accepting toward their children than parents without psychopathology.[36–38] These anxiogenic and depressogenic parental behaviors have also been associated with higher levels of child anxiety.[39–43] It is important to determine if these behaviors serve as a mechanism of transmission between parent and child outcomes and if they need to be targeted in treatment. We conclude with comments on the state of the current literature and implications for research and clinical practice.

TOP-DOWN STUDIES ASSESSING THE TREATMENT OF PARENTAL PSYCHOPATHOLOGY ON CHILD ANXIETY

A top-down approach implies that parents with psychopathology are identified and treated while their children are followed to determine if parental treatment impacts child outcomes. The following review comprises top-down studies of parents with a current disorder that measured child anxiety diagnoses or anxiety/emotional/internalizing symptoms; studies that solely assessed child depressive diagnoses or symptoms are excluded. Furthermore, this review includes only studies of parents who initiated treatment after baseline data collection and who received a specified treatment for a given period of time. We began with studies in the review by Gunlicks and Weissman,[32] conducted a similar search, and consulted with experts in the area, but found no additional articles that met this inclusion criteria. Few top-down studies have explored how treating parental psychopathology affects child anxiety or related constructs, and those that do focus on parents with mood disorders. **Table 1** provides main findings from the studies reviewed.

Table 1
Top-down studies for treatment of parental depression with assessment of child anxiety

Study, n, Child Age, Parental Disorder	Anxiety-Related Child Domains	Conditions	Parent Outcome	Child Outcome	Follow-Up
Modell et al[44] n = 24; 4–14 y maternal MDD	Anxiety symptoms (PR)	Antidepressant treatment; 1–2 months	33% reduction in depressive symptoms	Symptoms decreased by 20%, correlated with improvement in maternal depression. However, change was accounted for mostly by conduct, learning, and impulsive–hyperactive problems.	N/A
Weissman et al[47] n = 151; 7–17 y maternal MDD	Anxiety disorder (D) Internalizing symptoms (PR)	Medication treatment; 3 months	33% of mothers remitted	Maternal depression remission was associated with reduction in child diagnoses and symptoms, but not specifically anxiety disorders. Children of remitted mothers had larger decreases in internalizing symptoms than those of nonremitted mothers.	1 year: Anxiety disorders in children of early remitting mothers decreased, but not for children of nonremitting mothers, and intermittently for those of late remitting mothers.[52] 1 year after remission: Internalizing symptoms decreased for children of early and late-remitting mothers[53].
Forman et al[46] n = 176; 6 months maternal MDD	Infant emotionality (O) Infant/child emotionality (PR) Internalizing symptoms (PR)	IPT vs WL vs nondepressed; 4 months	IPT > WL for parenting stress	Infant outcomes were not associated with reductions in maternal depression. No significant effects of maternal treatment group on infant emotionality.	18 months: No significant effects of mothers who recovered on child emotionality or internalizing symptoms.
Byrne et al[45] n = 260; 4–16 y parental dysthymia	Emotional symptoms (PR)	Medication vs IPT vs both; 6 months	Greater than 40% reduction in depressive symptoms	N/A	2-years: Children of treatment responders showed more improvement in emotional problems than those of nonresponders.

Abbreviations: D, diagnostic; IPT, interpersonal psychotherapy; MDD, major depressive disorder; N/A, not applicable; O, observation; PR, parent report; WL, waitlist.

Top-Down Treatment Studies for Parental Depression with Assessment of Child Anxiety and Emotional Symptoms

Three studies have assessed the relationship between response to parental treatment for mood disorders and changes in children's anxiety or emotional (ie, internalizing) symptoms.

1. An initial research study found that improvements in maternal depression symptoms after 1 to 2 months of antidepressant treatment were significantly associated with reductions in maternal reports of overall child problems; however, changes in child anxiety and psychosomatic symptoms did not contribute to overall child behavioral change.[44]
2. A second study explored how parental response to 6 months of interpersonal psychotherapy and/or medication for dysthymia could impact children's emotional symptoms.[45] At 2-year follow-up, children of parents responding to treatment showed significant improvement in emotional symptoms as compared to those of nonresponders.
3. In contrast, a third study found that maternal reductions in postpartum depression after 4 months of interpersonal psychotherapy did not impact child emotionality or internalizing symptoms.[46] In addition, reductions in depression were not associated with changes in maternal responsiveness (eg, depressogenic behaviors such as acceptance and sensitivity). The authors suggested, in this study, that the relationship between infant and mother was formed within the context of maternal depression, making it difficult for mothers to create a positive relationship with their infants as they recovered.

Findings related to child anxiety are difficult to discern from these studies, as they did not focus on this construct specifically.

Top-Down Treatment Study for Parental Depression with Assessment of Child Anxiety Disorders

Only one large research study has assessed the impact of effectively treating maternal depression on child anxiety disorders. Weissman and colleagues[47] assessed children of mothers participating in STAR*D (Sequenced Treatment Alternatives to Relieve Depression), a multisite study comparing the effectiveness and acceptability of treatment options for depression.[48–50] Thus, an ancillary study of STAR*D was formed named STAR*D Child.[16] Maternal major depressive disorder was treated with medication and child psychopathology was assessed in relation to mothers' state of remission.[47]

STAR*D Child findings showed that after 3 months:

- Remission of maternal depression was significantly associated with reductions in child diagnoses and symptoms overall.
- Children of remitted mothers who also had an anxiety disorder did not show change in their rates of anxiety disorders (rates of child anxiety disorders remained at 12%).[47]
- Conversely, children of depressed mothers who did not remit demonstrated increases in their rates of anxiety disorders (from 17% to 25%).
- Children's reports of maternal acceptance (ie, warmth, care, attention) partially mediated the relationship between maternal depression remission and improvement in children's internalizing symptoms.[51] It appears that children observed changes in their mothers' depressogenic behavior in a short time; however, children's reports of parental control and family relationship variables were not

associated with improvements in maternal depression. The authors suggested that these variables may need direct intervention or may take longer to change.

Two additional STAR*D Child studies provide follow-up data on these mothers and their children. One year after treatment initiation, Pilowsky and colleagues[52] compared children of early remitters (first 3 months after initiation), later remitters (after 3 months), and nonremitters. Findings showed that overall symptoms significantly decreased in children of early and late remitters but not in children of nonremitters. In addition, anxiety and depressive disorders in children of early remitting mothers decreased significantly over time, while such change was not found among children of nonremitting mothers, and found only intermittently among late remitting mothers. Wickramaratne and colleagues[53] examined changes in child symptoms during the year after mothers' remission of depression or for the following 2 years when mothers remained depressed. Findings showed significant decreases in child internalizing symptoms in mothers who remitted, but not in those whose mothers remained depressed. In both of these follow-up studies, maternal depression remission preceded child improvement, suggesting that improvements in maternal depression led to better child anxiety outcomes. Child treatment also did not appear to bias results, as there were no significant differences in the percentage of children who received their own care by maternal remission status.[52,53]

In summary, among top-down studies:

- Few address the effects of parental treatment on child anxiety.
- None focus on the treatment of parental anxiety disorders.
- Methodologies vary widely, making it difficult to draw definitive conclusions.[32]
- Treating depression in parents of school-age children is associated with improvements in overall child outcomes.
- Improvements in parental depression likely precede improvements in child anxiety, yet may take up to 1 year to become apparent.
- Not treating parents may have detrimental effects on child anxiety.
- Only two studies assessed some type of depressogenic parental behavior. It is not clear if such behaviors mediate the relationship between maternal depression and children's internalizing symptoms.

Although more top-down research is needed, this preliminary evidence suggests that providing parents with treatment for depression likely has utility in helping their children's anxiety. However, the impact of depressogenic parental behavior on child outcome warrants further attention.

STUDIES FOCUSED ON FAMILY COGNITIVE-BEHAVIORAL TREATMENT FOR CHILD ANXIETY

Several studies focused on treating child anxiety have assessed the effects of including parents in family-based cognitive-behavioral therapy (FCBT). FCBT is defined here as an intervention that includes some type of active parental involvement in their child's treatment for anxiety. This involvement has ranged from teaching parents strategies such as removing reinforcement of their child's anxious behavior and reducing family conflict, to providing treatment for parents' own internalizing symptoms.[33] This differs from more passive parental involvement in individual child cognitive-behavioral therapy (ICBT), in which parents' participation is limited to receiving brief updates on child-progress and homework assignments. We review the results of randomized clinical trials (RCTs) that compared FCBT to ICBT for children and adolescents who met diagnostic criteria for separation anxiety disorder (SAD), social phobia (SOP), overanxious disorder/generalized anxiety disorder (OAD/GAD), or simple/specific phobia (SP). We began with relevant studies from Silverman and colleagues'[54] review and conducted an updated search of the journals they reviewed to ensure inclusion of recent FCBT RCTs. One pilot study that treated both parent and child anxiety is also reviewed.[55] We have grouped these studies based on the extent to which parental symptoms were measured and whether management of parental psychopathology was identified as a target variable within the intervention.

FCBT RCTs for Child Anxiety with No Assessment of Parental Psychopathology

A review of FCBT RCTs that include an active parental component but neither assess nor target parental psychopathology reveals mixed findings. One study found that active involvement of parents in their child's anxiety treatment leads to more favorable outcomes than ICBT.[28] Others found nonsignificant differences between conditions.[56-58] A similar pattern of results has been found in FCBT RCTs that have a minimal focus on parental anxiety management, with one supporting such parental involvement,[59] whereas others found it has few significant benefits over ICBT.[60-62] These studies investigated FCBTs that included a brief parent treatment component, such as psychoeducation about their own anxiety and/or restructuring anxiogenic thoughts. They did not, however, include a measure of parental anxiety. Therefore, these studies fail to provide a definitive conclusion concerning the effects of addressing parental anxiety on child anxiety outcomes when parents are actively involved in their children's treatment.

In a recent meta-analysis, Silverman and colleagues[54] were unable to find appreciable treatment gains in child anxiety interventions that included active parent involvement. Barmish and Kendall[33] suggested that the variability in the existing literature may be related to the presence of parental psychopathology, which may moderate the effectiveness of parental involvement on child outcomes. The following sections review all child anxiety studies in which parental symptoms were identified and/or addressed. The main findings of these studies are provided in **Table 2**.

Bottom-Up FCBT RCTs for Child Anxiety with Assessment of Parent Psychopathology

Wood and colleagues[24] conducted a bottom-up FCBT RCT for child anxiety and assessed for parental anxiety disorders at baseline, but did not directly address them in treatment. In the FCBT condition, parental goals were focused on decreasing anxiogenic parent–child interactions, improving communication skills, and implementing behavioral reward systems for their children. The FCBT intervention was found to be significantly more effective for reducing child anxiety than ICBT regardless of parental-anxiety status at baseline (based on parent and independent evaluator ratings, but not child-report). Children receiving FCBT treatment also experienced a more rapid decline in anxiety symptoms. Parental anxiety status at baseline did not impact any aspect of child treatment outcome. Change in parental anxiety over time, however, was not assessed. In addition, parents whose children received FCBT exhibited a greater decline in intrusive behavior on an observational task at post-treatment than parents whose children received ICBT.[63] Exploratory analyses suggested that this decrease in anxiogenic parental behavior may play a role in treatment outcomes for early adolescents, but not children. At 1-year follow-up, children who had been in FCBT still demonstrated less anxiety than children in ICBT. Although FCBT had promising results in this study, Barmish and Kendall[33] proposed that directly addressing parental anxiety as part of treatment may enhance child treatment outcomes.

Table 2
Bottom-up studies for treatment of child anxiety with assessment and/or management of parental psychopathology

Study, n, Child Age, Child Disorder	Anxiety-Related Parent Domains	Conditions	Parent Outcome	Child Outcome	Follow-Up
FCBT RCTs for Child Anxiety with Assessment of Parent Psychopathology					
Wood et al[24] n = 40; 6–13 y SAD, SOP, GAD	53% of parents had an AD (D)	FCBT vs ICBT; 12–16 sessions (stable medication allowed)	Not measured	FCBT > ICBT (PR; IE); FCBT = ICBT (D; CR); Parental AD unrelated to child outcome	Wood et al[63] Maintained at 1 year
FCBT RCTs for Child Anxiety with Assessment and Minimal Treatment of Parent Psychopathology					
Bodden et al[20] n = 128; 8–17 y SOP, SAD, GAD, SP, PD	39% of families had a father/mother had an AD (D)	ICBT vs FCBT vs WL; 13 sessions	Not measured	ICBT > FCBT > WL (D) CAO > C+PA (D) CAO: FCBT > ICBT (SR) C+PA: ICBT > FCBT (SR)	At 3 months: ICBT = FCBT > WL; Other results maintained
Kendall et al[23] n = 161; 7–14 y GAD, SAD, SOP	38% of mothers and 19% of fathers had an AD (D)	ICBT vs FCBT vs FESA; 16 sessions	ICBT = FCBT = FESA	ICBT = FCBT > FESA CAO > C+MA	Maintained at 1 year
Silverman et al[64] n = 119; 7–16 y GAD, SAD, SOP, SP, PD, OCD	40% of mothers had an AD (D, SR)	ICBT vs FCBT; 12–14 sessions	ICBT = FCBT	ICBT = FCBT	Maintained at 1 year

RCTs for Child Anxiety with Assessment and Adjunct Treatment of Parental Anxiety

Cobham et al[65] n = 60, 10–17 y GAD, SAD, OAD, SOP, SP, Agoraphobia	52% of the families with parent/s above anxiety symptom cutoff (SR)	GCBT (10 sessions) vs GCBT+PAM (10 sessions plus 4 sessions of PAM)	GCBT = CBT+PAM (SR)	GCBT = CBT+PAM CAO: GCBT+PAM = GCBT C+PA: GCBT+PAM > GCBT GCBT: CAO > C+PA CBT+PAM: CAO = C+PA	At 3 years: CAO: GCBT+PAM > GCBT C+PA: GCBT+PAM > GCBT GCBT: CAO = C+PA GCBT+PAM: CAO = C+PA
Creswell et al[55] n = 22, 6–12 y GAD, SAD, SOP, SP	55% of the mothers had an AD (D)	CFCBT (8 sessions) vs PICBT +CFCBT (8 sessions of PICBT and 8 sessions of CFCBT)	PICBT+CFCBT > CFCBT	CAO > C+PA C+PA: CFCBT = PICBT+CFCBT	N/A

Abbreviations: AD, anxiety disorder; CAO, child anxiety only; CFCBT, child-focused cognitive-behavioral therapy; C+MA, child plus maternal anxiety; C+PA, child plus parental anxiety; CR, child self-report; D, diagnostic; FAM, family anxiety management; FCBT, family cognitive-behavioral therapy; FESA, family education/support/attention; GAD, generalized anxiety disorder; GCBT, child group cognitive-behavioral therapy; ICBT, individual cognitive-behavioral therapy; IE, independent evaluator; OAD, overanxious disorder; OCD, obsessive–compulsive disorder; PAM, parental anxiety management; PD, panic disorder; PICBT, parent individual cognitive-behavioral therapy; PR, parent self-report; RCT, randomized controlled trial; SAD, separation anxiety disorder; SOP, social phobia; SP, specific phobia; SR, self-report; WL, waitlist.

Bottom-Up FCBT RCTs for Child Anxiety with Assessment and Minimal Management of Parent Psychopathology

Three FCBT RCTs that assessed parental anxiety included a minimal focus on parent anxiety management as part of FCBT:

1. Kendall and colleagues[23] randomly assigned children with anxiety diagnoses to FCBT, ICBT, or a family-based education/support/attention (FESA) active control condition. Parents receiving FCBT were provided with psychoeducation about child anxiety and strategies to respond to their child's anxious behavior. In addition to these goals, parents in FCBT received training on restructuring their maladaptive beliefs and expectations. They were also encouraged to apply the skills being taught in therapy to cope when they experienced their own anxiety. Child treatment gains were significantly greater in both treatment conditions than in FESA at post-treatment and 1-year follow-up; however, significant differences were not found between the two treatment conditions based on child diagnostic status and most self-report measures. Although no treatment was more effective in treating maternal anxiety, all three conditions had a minimal effect on mothers' diagnostic status. Across groups, 38% and 39% of maternal anxiety disorders were absent at post-treatment and follow-up, respectively. Thirty-nine percent of paternal anxiety diagnoses were absent at post-treatment; however missing data prevented further analyses of this variable among conditions. At 1-year follow-up, mothers' anxiety status was found to moderate child diagnostic outcome, as the children of mothers diagnosed with an anxiety disorder were significantly less likely than other children to have lost their anxiety diagnosis.

2. Silverman and colleagues[64] conducted a RCT in which FCBT targeted mother's behavior toward the child, mother–child conflict, and maternal anxiety when it was present. They also planned exposure tasks alongside their child, although this was always done in the context of treating the child's anxiety. Children were asked to appraise the level of conflict in their relationship with their parents as well as their parents' negative and positive behavior toward them. Children in both FCBT and ICBT experienced significant improvement; however, no treatment differences were found at post-treatment or 1-year follow-up. At the end of the study, maternal anxiety significantly improved in both conditions. This was maintained at follow-up. Child appraisal of the level of conflict in their relationship with their parents decreased significantly in FCBT, while both level of conflict and parental negative behavior decreased in ICBT. At follow-up, children who received FCBT reported increased improvement in both parent variables, while the ICBT findings remained the same. Unfortunately, this study did not report the impact of maternal diagnostic status on parental behavior or child anxiety outcomes.

3. FBCT for child anxiety has not always been associated with outcomes equivalent to ICBT for children whose parents have their own anxiety. Bodden and colleagues[20] divided children with anxiety diagnoses into two groups based on their parents' anxiety disorder status (present vs absent) and then randomly assigned them to FCBT and ICBT conditions. Within FCBT, therapists focused on family mechanisms thought to maintain child anxiety, such as parental anxiety, overcontrol, and accompanying dysfunctional beliefs. Parents and children were taught CBT skills together to reduce their coexisting anxiety. Other parental goals were directed at addressing parenting and communication skills and problematic familial interactions. Anxious children who received ICBT were found to be significantly more likely to be diagnosis free at post-treatment, as compared to children who received FCBT.[20] At 3-month follow-up, however, this difference was

no longer significant. The authors propose that the treatment conditions became equally effective only after parents have mastered the skills taught in treatment and began to transfer them to their children. Parents with anxiety disorders were found to have a negative impact on child outcome across conditions at post-treatment and follow-up. FCBT, however, did not offer significant improvements in diagnostic outcome for these children. Parent-report and self-report measures actually revealed an interaction effect of treatment by parental anxiety in which ICBT was more helpful for children with anxiety disordered parents and FCBT was more helpful for children who did not have anxious parents at post-treatment and follow-up. Unfortunately, parental anxiety was not assessed at post-treatment or follow-up.

Overall, among FCBT studies assessing and minimally addressing parental anxiety:

- Most did not find significant differences between FCBT and ICBT on child outcome.
- Parental anxiety was generally found to have a negative impact on child outcome, regardless of treatment condition.
- When parental outcomes were assessed over time, FCBT with minimal parent anxiety management was not more effective for parental anxiety than ICBT.
- The impact of including minimal parent anxiety management in FCBT on children was inconclusive.
- Only one study assessed parental behavior, did not focus on anxiogenic behavior specifically, and did not compare differences between FCBT and ICBT.[64] Therefore, the utility of addressing parental anxiogenic behavior in FCBT is unclear.

Research that examines the impact of providing both individual parent and child anxiety treatment may help to elucidate the association between treating parental anxiety and improving child outcomes.

Bottom-Up Studies for Child Anxiety with Assessment and Adjunct Treatment of Parental Anxiety

Two studies have been conducted that investigate the delivery of adjunct parental anxiety treatment in conjunction with CBT for child anxiety. Cobham and colleagues[21] divided children with anxiety diagnoses into two groups: children who had a parent with elevated anxiety symptoms and children who did not. Within these groups, participants were randomly assigned into two treatment conditions:

1. Child-focused group CBT
2. Child-focused group CBT plus four sessions of individual parent anxiety management (PAM) training (CBT+PAM).

PAM was designed to educate parents about the role of the family in the development and maintenance of child anxiety symptoms and to teach parents skills to manage their own anxiety, including cognitive restructuring, relaxation training, and contingency management.

At post-treatment, no difference was found in the percentage of diagnosis-free children in the CBT vs CBT+PAM condition.[21] There was a significant main effect demonstrating that children with anxious parents did worse in treatment than other children. A significant interaction was found between parental anxiety and treatment efficacy within the child-focused CBT group. Specifically, a significantly greater percentage of children without anxious parents were diagnosis free after receiving child CBT-only as compared to children with at least one anxious parent. This suggests that parental anxiety may impede a child's progress in child-focused CBT. Children in the CBT+PAM condition were equally likely to be diagnosis free, regardless of their parents' anxiety status. In addition, CBT+PAM was significantly more effective for children with anxious parents than child CBT-only but did not enhance treatment efficacy for children with nonanxious parents. While the addition of PAM was beneficial for children with an anxious parent, parental anxiety actually did not improve more in this condition than in child CBT-only. This suggests that another mechanism of change led to improvement in child outcome in the CBT+PAM condition. At 6-month follow-up, the majority of post-treatment results were maintained; however, the benefit of adding PAM for children of anxious parents was only a trend and no longer significant. All results at 1-year follow-up weakened even further.

Cobham and colleagues[65] then conducted a 3-year follow-up by repeating their child outcome measurement procedures, without reassessing parental anxiety. Unlike their previous findings, children with anxious parents were just as likely to be diagnosis free as those with nonanxious parents. They hypothesized that this was either due to anxious parents taking longer to recognize the shift in their child's anxiety or that these children's symptoms actually take longer to extinguish than those in children with nonanxious parents.

The inclusion of PAM was found to significantly increase the efficacy of child-focused CBT after three years, regardless of parental anxiety status.[65] In other words, the outcomes for all anxious children were improved by parental participation in PAM. This runs counter to Cobham and colleagues'[21] initial conclusion that the addition of a PAM component would be more beneficial only to children with anxious parents. The authors suggest that all parents in PAM were better able to help their children sustain treatment gains over time because this adjunct treatment addressed parents' anxiogenic behavior and taught them how to support and model effective anxiety management for their children. Unfortunately, the lack of measurement of parental behavior makes this explanation a possibility rather than a conclusive finding.

There were many other limitations to Cobham and colleagues'[21,65] study that restrict the validity of its results. First, there were mixed findings across outcome measures, and although diagnostic data resulted in significant treatment gains for children across conditions, this improvement was not supported by questionnaires or clinician ratings. Second, although the addition of PAM led to initial treatment gains for children of anxious parents, it did not significantly improve parental symptoms of anxiety more than the child-focused CBT-only condition. Therefore, the child outcome differences seen across treatment conditions are most likely not due to improvement in parental anxiety. Unfortunately, parental anxiety was not measured at 3-year follow-up, leaving no way to determine how changes in parental anxiety impacted child outcomes over time. The use of a parental diagnostic interview throughout the study may have more accurately measured the impact of treatment on parental anxiety and its influence on child outcome. Finally, although children were assigned to initial conditions based on one or both parents' anxiety status, no efforts were made to ensure that the parent with heightened anxiety actually attended the PAM sessions. This may also explain why PAM failed to significantly improve parental anxiety symptoms.

One pilot study subsequently assessed the impact of treating parental anxiety in the context of child anxiety treatment. Creswell and colleagues[55] assigned children to two treatment conditions based on their mother's diagnostic status (child-anxiety only vs child and maternal anxiety). Six of the 12 mothers who met diagnostic criteria for an anxiety disorder were then randomly selected to receive up to eight sessions of individual CBT tailored to their specific anxiety diagnosis. The remaining six mothers did not receive treatment. At the end of maternal anxiety treatment, five out of six treated mothers were anxiety diagnosis free. After this treatment, all mothers received eight sessions of individual CBT focused on helping their children learn to manage their anxiety. Specific skills learned included psychoeducation, identifying, monitoring, and restructuring children's anxious cognitions, promoting "brave" behavior, problem solving, social skills training, and relapse prevention. Children entered the fourth session to aid in the development of their fear hierarchy. They were also asked to give a brief presentation on a topic of choice with their mothers present to observe level of maternal overinvolvement and nonverbal expression of fear.

At the end of child-focused treatment, children whose mothers had a pretreatment anxiety diagnosis generally had poorer treatment outcomes than their peers.[55] Treatment of maternal anxiety, however, even when successful, did not significantly improve child outcomes. Maternal anxiety was also not significantly associated with level of maternal overinvolvement or nonverbal expression, although there was a trend in this direction. Of note, these anxiogenic maternal behaviors were significantly associated with child treatment outcomes. The authors suggest that maternal anxiety remission without improvement in maternal behavior may not lead to changes in child anxiety. Unfortunately, maternal behaviors were not assessed at baseline or over time, so any treatment-related behavioral changes are unknown. This study is also limited by its small sample size and lack of child involvement in treatment. In addition, no follow-up assessments were reported, which based on Cobham and colleagues'[65] follow-up study, appear to be an important factor in evaluating the effectiveness of treating parental anxiety in the context of child anxiety treatment.

Overall, among studies with assessment and adjunct treatment of parental anxiety:

- Findings are inconclusive about the effectiveness of delivering adjunct parent anxiety treatment in conjunction with CBT for child anxiety.
- Cobham and colleagues[21] revealed short-term benefits for anxious children whose anxious parents received PAM. At 3-year follow-up, however, these additional benefits were no longer observed and the addition of PAM was beneficial for child outcome regardless of parent anxiety status.[65] In addition, CBT+PAM did not significantly improve parental anxiety more than child-focused CBT only. Therefore, another mechanism of change, such as anxiogenic parental behavior, likely led to improvement in child outcome in the CBT+PAM condition. Unfortunately, parental behavior was not assessed.
- Creswell and colleagues[55] addressed many of the limitations of Cobham and colleagues'[21] study, as they assessed parental anxiety via diagnostic interview, ensured that mothers who met criteria for an anxiety disorder were the parents who actually received anxiety treatment, and offered more comprehensive maternal anxiety treatment. Counter to Cobham and colleagues'[21] findings, Creswell and colleagues[55] found that treating maternal anxiety offered no benefits to child outcome. Maternal anxiogenic behaviors were significantly associated with poorer child outcome. These behaviors may have to be ameliorated in addition to maternal anxiety to positively impact child anxiety. Small sample size, limited child involvement in treatment, lack of measures of maternal behaviors over time, and no follow-up data limited the conclusiveness of these findings.

OVERALL SUMMARY OF THE EXISTING LITERATURE

Overall, the preceding review leads to the following conclusions:

- Existing top-down studies assessing child anxiety and emotional constructs lend some support to the notion that successfully treating parental depression can improve child anxiety, although changes may take up to 1 year.
  - Only one top-down study included an assessment of child anxiety disorders[47] as opposed to an anxiety or emotional symptom measure, making it difficult to reach a definitive conclusion.
- Anxious parents whose symptoms were addressed in FCBT or an adjunct treatment did not improve more than anxious parents whose families received only child treatment.[21,23,64] Therefore, the impact of *effectively* treating parental anxiety in addition to child treatment has not been investigated.
  - One pilot study successfully treated maternal anxiety and provided child-focused treatment to parents; however, children did not receive their own treatment. Maternal remission was not associated with better child outcomes.[55] Parents and children with anxiety may both need to be treated directly.
- Teaching parents to manage their anxiogenic behavior may be associated with improvements in child anxiety. This conclusion is tentative, as only two studies have assessed parental behavior pre-FCBT and post-FCBT.[63,64]

Limitations

There are several limitations in the existing literature:

- Few top-down studies assessed the impact of parental psychopathology on child anxiety, with none focused on the effects of treating parental anxiety.
- Parental depression was not assessed or addressed in any of the bottom-up studies.
- Parental anxiety was not always evaluated at baseline or over time in FCBT RCTs.
- None of the bottom-up RCTs included a comprehensive psychosocial treatment for parental anxiety.
- Anxiogenic and depressogenic parental behaviors were typically not assessed.
- Although FCBT often targets anxiogenic parental behavior, lack of assessment at baseline or over time limits certainty of this mechanism of action between changes in parental psychopathology and child outcome.

IMPLICATIONS FOR RESEARCH
Assessment and Treatment of Parental Psychopathology

Results of this review provide several implications for improving the research on the assessment and treatment of parental psychopathology when children have anxiety:

1. First, top-down studies like STAR*D Child should be conducted with parents with an anxiety diagnosis to determine if treating parents alone may be a sufficient approach for improving child anxiety.
2. Second, due to poor outcomes in children with anxiety who also have a depressed parent, future bottom-up anxiety treatment studies should assess and treat parental depression. Regardless of the disorder targeted, reductions in parental psychopathology will be more likely after efficacious treatment as opposed to brief symptom management.

3. Third, child anxiety treatment studies that aim to address parental psychopathology should include assessments of parental diagnoses and symptoms over time to ensure that parents are actually improving. Long-term follow-up studies should also be conducted, as the benefits of parental remission on child anxiety may first appear only 1 year after baseline.[52,53]

Assessment and Treatment of Parental Behavior

Researchers should test the augmentation of treatment for parental psychopathology with intervention techniques targeting related anxiogenic and depressogenic parental behaviors, such as overinvolvement, expressions of fear, warmth and acceptance, and control.[55,66] Regardless of type of parental treatment, assessing changes in parental behaviors over time can help determine the mechanism of action between successful parent treatment of psychopathology and child outcome.[51] Longitudinal studies would also help determine if there is a lagged effect between changes in parental behavior and changes in child anxiety.

Assessment and Treatment of Parental Cognitions

Parental cognitions have been overlooked in this literature, yet likely also play a role. For example, if a child demonstrates concern about being accepted by peers, parents may have catastrophic thoughts about their child being rejected and become overinvolved during play dates. Future research should assess parental cognitions immediately after a parent–child interaction via a procedure such as video-mediated recall.[67] This assessment could be repeated over time to determine if change in parental cognitions serves as a mechanism of action between parental treatment and changes in anxiogenic/depressogenic parental behavior.

Directionality of Change between Parental Psychopathology and Child Anxiety

Future studies should also address the directionality of change between improvements in parental psychopathology and reductions in child anxiety. Although changes in child anxiety have been found to follow remission in parental psychopathology,[52] Silverman and colleagues[64] suggested there may be a more reciprocal relationship. Specifically, parent and child anxiety improved within the same time period, making directionality ambiguous; however, a significant lagged effect indicated that improvements in child anxiety preceded improvements in negative parental behavior. Similarly, Garber and colleagues[66] found concurrent improvements in parent and child depressive symptoms, with nonsignificant trends for lagged effects in both directions. Determining the directionality of change between parental psychopathology and child anxiety will help elucidate the need for both parent and child to engage in treatment.

Focusing on Anxiety and Depression in Families

Although research clearly indicates that parental anxiety and depression are associated with child anxiety, most studies reviewed did not assess both types of psychopathology, and no studies focused on both. Top-down studies assessing the effects of parental psychopathology on child outcome have treated only parental depression (not anxiety), and rarely include measures of child anxiety.[66,68] Similarly, child anxiety treatment studies assessing and/or treating parental psychopathology have focused on parental anxiety, but not depression. It is clearly not often possible to treat parent and child anxiety and depression in one study; however, future studies assessing the effects of treating parents on child outcomes should at minimum include assessments of parent and child anxiety as well as depression.

Future Methodological Designs

Several studies assessing the addition of treating parental psychopathology on child anxiety have already been conducted in this field, yet lack the methodological rigor necessary to determine the benefits of different combinations of parent and child treatment. Garber and colleagues[66] suggest conducting a 2 × 2 design whereby conditions would include parent treatment only, child treatment only, both parent and child treatment, and a no-treatment control. A similar design could also be conducted assessing the effects of treating parental psychopathology, anxiogenic/depressogenic parental behavior, or both, on child anxiety. Such studies would help to determine the most efficacious treatment approach for improving anxiety in children of parents with their own psychopathology.

IMPLICATIONS FOR CLINICAL PRACTICE

Owing to the need for further research disentangling the benefits of treating parental psychopathology in the context of child anxiety treatment, recommendations for clinical practice are difficult to provide. The potential benefits of conducting child and parent screenings for psychopathology, prevention programs for at-risk children, and the use of family-based models of treatment are discussed.

Importance of Screening Children When Parents Are in Treatment

Based on top-down findings that children of parents in treatment are at high risk for their own symptoms and often do not receive psychiatric services, screening children of these parents has been recommended.[69] Clinicians treating adults with children should inquire about their anxiety and functioning and discuss the benefits of bringing them in for assessment. Given that treating parents alone may take up to 1 year to positively impact child anxiety,[52] simultaneous child treatment should be encouraged.

Importance of Screening Parents at Child Evaluation and Engaging Them in Treatment

Because parental psychopathology has been shown to be associated with worse treatment outcomes for child anxiety, we also recommend that all parents be screened for anxiety and depressive symptoms at the time of their child's evaluation. Screening measures such as the Brief Symptom Inventory[70] and the PRIME-MD Patient Problem Questionnaire[71] have been feasible to use with parents in community mental health settings.[18,72]

Parents identified as having elevated symptom levels at the time of their child's evaluation should then be encouraged to enter into their own treatment. Engaging parents in treatment can be a complex task, and parents with their own symptoms often go untreated. For example, Swartz and colleagues[73] found that among mothers with an Axis I *DSM-IV-TR* diagnosis who were bringing their children to a mental health clinic, only 33% were currently receiving psychiatric treatment. Depressed parents have indicated several obstacles to attending their own treatment, including cost, transportation, and feeling uncomfortable discussing problems.[74] Utilizing a combination of motivational and ethnographic interviewing techniques has been found to be effective in helping parents with depression enter treatment.[75] It would also be helpful to educate parents about how their psychopathology can impact their child and how success in their own treatment could actually improve their child's well-being.

Prevention of Anxiety Disorders in Children at High Risk

Clinicians can focus on preventing anxiety in children of parents with psychopathology. CBT prevention programs for children of depressed parents have been found to be effective for reducing internalizing symptoms, yet typically focus on preventing depression.[76–79] Ginsburg[80] found that a cognitive-behavioral, family-based prevention program was effective for preventing anxiety in children of parents with anxiety disorders. The prevention program focused on addressing children's anxiety symptoms, dysfunctional cognitions, and deficits in problem-solving and coping skills as well as parent's modeling of anxiety, parental behaviors that enhance anxiety, and family conflict. At one year, children in the prevention group were significantly less likely to have developed an anxiety disorder than those on the waitlist. These studies demonstrate the potential benefits of providing preventive services to children of parents with anxiety and depression.

Family-Based Model for Treating Parental Psychopathology and Child Anxiety

In typical practice with families, clinicians recommend that parents go for their own treatment. Unfortunately, this often does not occur, or parents begin individual therapy that is completely separate from their child's treatment. Given that aspects of parental psychopathology and behavior may impact child anxiety, we think it is important to develop a family-based treatment paradigm that goes beyond FCBT to attend to parent and child needs equally. For example, parents may bring their children in for anxiety treatment, yet report their own symptoms of anxiety and depression. The children can begin either ICBT or FCBT. Parents can simultaneously engage in their own treatment with a dual focus on symptom reduction (via therapy and/or medication) and skills to manage their children effectively while struggling with their own functioning. The individual clinicians can form a collaborative team to develop a treatment plan that addresses how parent and child factors interact within the family system. Focusing on parental psychopathology in the context of child anxiety will likely generate the best outcomes.

ACKNOWLEDGMENTS

The authors thank Laura Scudellari and Jacquelyn Blocher for their assistance in the preparation of this article.

REFERENCES

1. Biederman J, Faraone SV, Hirshfeld-Becker DR, et al. Patterns of psychopathology and dysfunction in high-risk children of parents with panic disorder and major depression. Am J Psychiatry 2001;158(1):49–57.
2. Biederman J, Petty C, Faraone SV, et al. Parental predictors of pediatric panic disorder/agoraphobia: a controlled study in high-risk offspring. Depress Anxiety 2005;22(3):114–20.
3. Hammen C, Burge D, Burney E, et al. Longitudinal study of diagnoses in children of women with unipolar and bipolar affective disorder. Arch Gen Psychiatry 1990;47(12): 1112–7.
4. Lieb R, Isensee B, Höfler M, et al. Parental major depression and the risk of depression and other mental disorders in offspring: a prospective-longitudinal community study. Arch Gen Psychiatry 2002;59(4):365–74.

5. McClure EB, Brennan PA, Hammen C, et al. Parental anxiety disorders, child anxiety disorders, and the perceived parent-child relationship in an Australian high-risk sample. J Abnorm Child Psychol 2001;29(1):1–10.
6. Weissman MM, Warner V, Wickramaratne P, et al. Offspring of depressed parents: 10 years later. Arch Gen Psychiatry 1997;54(10):932–40.
7. Weissman MM, Wickramaratne P, Nomura Y, et al. Offspring of depressed parents: 20 years later. Am J Psychiatry 2006;163(6):1001–8.
8. Kramer RA, Warner V, Olfson M, et al. General medical problems among the offspring of depressed parents: a 10-year follow-up. J Am Acad Child Adolesc Psychiatry 1998;37(6):602–11.
9. Wolkind S. Mothers' depression and their children's attendance at medical facilities. J Psychosom Res 1985;29(6):579–82.
10. Silverman WK, Ginsburg GS. Anxiety disorders. In: Hersen M, Ollendick T, editors. Handbook of child psychopathology. New York: Plenum Press; 1998. p. 239–68.
11. Woodward LJ, Fergusson DM. Life course outcomes of young people with anxiety disorders in adolescence. J Am Acad Child Adolesc Psychiatry 2001;40(9):1086–93.
12. Pine DS, Cohen P, Gurley D, et al. The risk for early-adulthood anxiety and depressive disorders in adolescents with anxiety and depressive disorders. Arch Gen Psychiatry 1998;55(1):56–64.
13. Compton WM, Thomas YF, Stinson FS, et al. Prevalence, correlates, disability, and comorbidity of DSM-IV drug abuse and dependence in the United States: results from the national epidemiologic survey on alcohol and related conditions. Arch Gen Psychiatry 2007;64(5):566–76.
14. Boden JM, Fergusson DM, Horwood LJ. Anxiety disorders and suicidal behaviours in adolescence and young adulthood: findings from a longitudinal study. Psychol Med 2007;37(3):431–40.
15. Beidel DC, Turner SM. At risk for anxiety: I. Psychopathology in the offspring of anxious parents. J Am Acad Child Adolesc Psychiatry 1997;36(7):918–24.
16. Pilowsky DJ, Wickramaratne PJ, Rush AJ, et al. Children of currently depressed mothers: a STAR*D ancillary study. J Clin Psychiatry 2006;67(1):126–36.
17. Cooper PJ, Fearn V, Willetts L, et al. Affective disorder in the parents of a clinic sample of children with anxiety disorders. J Affect Disord 2006;93(1–3):205–12.
18. Vidair HB, Reyes JA, Shen S, et al. Screening parents during child evaluations: exploring parent and child psychopathology in the same clinic. J Am Acad Child Adolesc Psychiatry 2011;50(5):441–50.
19. Berman SL, Weems CF, Silverman WK, et al. Predictors of outcome in exposure-based cognitive and behavioral treatments for phobic and anxiety disorders in children. Behav Ther 2000;31:713–31.
20. Bodden DH, Bögels SM, Nauta MH, et al. Child versus family cognitive-behavioral therapy in clinically anxious youth: an efficacy and partial effectiveness study. J Am Acad Child Adolesc Psychiatry 2008;47(12):1384–94.
21. Cobham VE, Dadds MR, Spence SH. The role of parental anxiety in the treatment of childhood anxiety. J Consult Clin Psychol 1998;66(6):893–905.
22. Cooper PJ, Gallop C, Willetts L, et al. Treatment response in child anxiety is differentially related to the form of maternal anxiety disorder. Behav Cogn Psychother 2008;36:41–8.
23. Kendall PC, Hudson JL, Gosch E, et al. Cognitive-behavioral therapy for anxiety disordered youth: a randomized clinical trial evaluating child and family modalities. J Consult Clin Psychol 2008;76(2):282–97.
24. Wood JJ, Piacentini JC, Southam-Gerow M, et al. Family cognitive behavioral therapy for child anxiety disorders. J Am Acad Child Adolesc Psychiatry 2006;45(3):314–21.

25. Southam-Gerow MA, Kendall PC, Weersing VR. Examining outcome variability: correlates of treatment response in a child and adolescent anxiety clinic. J Clin Child Psychol 2001;30(3):422–36.
26. Rapee RM. Group treatment of children with anxiety disorders: outcome and predictors of treatment response. Austral J Psychol 2000;52:125–9.
27. Liber JM, van Widenfelt BM, Goedhart AW, et al. Parenting and parental anxiety and depression as predictors of treatment outcome for childhood anxiety disorders: has the role of fathers been underestimated? J Clin Child Adolesc Psychol 2008;37(4): 747–58.
28. Crawford AM, Manassis K. Familial predictors of treatment outcome in childhood anxiety disorders. J Am Acad Child Adolesc Psychiatry 2001;40(10):1182–9.
29. Thienemann M, Moore P, Tompkins K. A parent-only group intervention for children with anxiety disorders: pilot study. J Am Acad Child Adolesc Psychiatry 2006;45(1): 37–46.
30. Victor AM, Bernat DH, Bernstein GA, et al. Effects of parent and family characteristics on treatment outcome of anxious children. J Anxiety Disord 2007;21(6):835–48.
31. Toren P, Wolmer L, Rosental B, et al. Case series: brief parent-child group therapy for childhood anxiety disorders using a manual-based cognitive-behavioral technique. J Am Acad Child Adolesc Psychiatry 2000;39(10):1309–12.
32. Gunlicks ML, Weissman MM. Change in child psychopathology with improvement in parental depression: a systematic review. J Am Acad Child Adolesc Psychiatry 2008;47(4):379–89.
33. Barmish AJ, Kendall PC. Should parents be co-clients in cognitive-behavioral therapy for anxious youth? J Clin Child Adolesc Psychol 2005;34(3):569–81.
34. Creswell C, Cartwright-Hatton S. Family treatment of child anxiety: outcomes, limitations and future directions. Clin Child Fam Psychol Rev 2007;10(3):232–52.
35. Ginsburg GS, Schlossberg MC. Family-based treatment of childhood anxiety disorders. Int Rev Psychiatry 2002;14:143–54.
36. Goodman SH, Gotlib IH. Risk for psychopathology in the children of depressed mothers: a developmental model for understanding mechanisms of transmission. Psychol Rev 1999;106(3):458–90.
37. Murray L, de Rosnay M, Pearson J, et al. Intergenerational transmission of social anxiety: the role of social referencing processes in infancy. Child Dev 2008;79(4): 1049–64.
38. Whaley SE, Pinto A, Sigman M. Characterizing interactions between anxious mothers and their children. J Consult Clin Psychol 1999;67(6):826–36.
39. Dumas JE, LaFreniere PJ, Serketich WJ. "Balance of power": a transactional analysis of control in mother-child dyads involving socially competent, aggressive, and anxious children. J Abnorm Psychol 1995;104(1):104–13.
40. Leib R, Wittchen H, Hofler M, et al. Parental psychopathology, parenting styles, and the risk of social phobia in offspring: a prospective, longitudinal community study. Arch Gen Psychiatry 2000;57:859–66.
41. Chorpita BF, Albano AM, Barlow D. Cognitive processing in children: relation to anxiety and family influences. J Clin Child Psychol 1996;25(2):170–6.
42. Hibbs ED, Hamburger SD, Lenane M, et al. Determinants of expressed emotion in families of disturbed and normal children. J Child Psychol Psychiatry 1991;32(5): 757–70.
43. Kashani JH, Vaidya AF, Soltys SM, et al. Correlates of anxiety in psychiatrically hospitalized children and their parents. Am J Psychiatry 1990;147(3):319–23.
44. Modell JD, Modell PJG, Wallander J, et al. Maternal ratings of child behavior improve with treatment of maternal depression. Fam Med 2001;33(9):691–5.

45. Byrne C, Browne G, Roberts J, et al. Changes in children's behavior and costs for service use associated with parents' response to treatment for dysthymia. J Am Acad Child Adolesc Psychiatry 2006;45(2):239–46.
46. Forman DR, O'Hara MW, Stuart S, et al. Effective treatment for postpartum depression is not sufficient to improve the developing mother-child relationship. Dev Psychopathol 2007;19(2):585–602.
47. Weissman MM, Pilowsky DJ, Wickramaratne PJ, et al. Remissions in maternal depression and child psychopathology: a STAR*D-child report. JAMA 2006;295(12): 1389–98.
48. Fava M, Rush AJ, Trivedi MH, et al. Background and rationale for the sequenced treatment alternatives to relieve depression (STAR*D) study. Psychiatr Clin North Am 2003;26(2):457–94, x.
49. Rush AJ, Trivedi M, Fava M. Depression, IV: STAR*D treatment trial for depression. Am J Psychiatry 2003;160(2):237.
50. Rush AJ, Fava M, Wisniewski SR, et al. Sequenced treatment alternatives to relieve depression (STAR*D): rationale and design. Control Clin Trials 2004;25(1):119–42.
51. Foster CE, Webster MC, Weissman MM, et al. Remission of maternal depression: relations to family functioning and youth internalizing and externalizing symptoms. J Clin Child Adolesc Psychol 2008;37(4):714–24.
52. Pilowsky DJ, Wickramaratne P, Talati A, et al. Children of depressed mothers 1 year after the initiation of maternal treatment: findings from the STAR*D-Child Study. Am J Psychiatry 2008;165(9):1136–47.
53. Wickramaratne P, Gameroff MJ, Pilowsky DJ, et al. Children of depressed mothers 1 year after remission of maternal depression: findings from the STAR*D-Child study. Am J Psychiatry 2011;168(6):593–602.
54. Silverman WK, Pina AA, Viswesvaran C. Evidence-based psychosocial treatments for phobic and anxiety disorders in children and adolescents. J Clin Child Adolesc Psychol 2008;37(1):105–30.
55. Creswell C, Willetts L, Murray L, et al. Treatment of child anxiety: an exploratory study of the role of maternal anxiety and behaviours in treatment outcome. Clin Psychol Psychother 2008;15(1):38–44.
56. Mendlowitz SL, Manassis K, Bradley S, et al. Cognitive-behavioral group treatments in childhood anxiety disorders: the role of parental involvement. J Am Acad Child Adolesc Psychiatry 1999;38(10):1223–9.
57. Spence SH, Donovan C, Brechman-Toussaint M. The treatment of childhood social phobia: the effectiveness of a social skills training-based, cognitive-behavioural intervention, with and without parental involvement. J Child Psychol Psychiatry 2000; 41(6):713–26.
58. Ost LG, Svensson L, Hellström K, et al. One-Session treatment of specific phobias in youths: a randomized clinical trial. J Consult Clin Psychol 2001;69(5):814–24.
59. Barrett PM, Dadds MR, Rapee RM. Family treatment of childhood anxiety: a controlled trial. J Consult Clin Psychol 1996;64(2):333–42.
60. Barrett PM. Evaluation of cognitive-behavioral group treatments for childhood anxiety disorders. J Clin Child Psychol 1998;27(4):459–68.
61. Heyne D, King NJ, Tonge BJ, et al. Evaluation of child therapy and caregiver training in the treatment of school refusal. J Am Acad Child Adolesc Psychiatry 2002;41(6): 687–95.
62. Nauta MH, Scholing A, Emmelkamp PM, et al. Cognitive-behavioral therapy for children with anxiety disorders in a clinical setting: no additional effect of a cognitive parent training. J Am Acad Child Adolesc Psychiatry 2003;42(11):1270–8.

63. Wood JJ, McLeod BD, Piacentini JC, et al. One-year follow-up of family versus child CBT for anxiety disorders: exploring the roles of child age and parental intrusiveness. Child Psychiatry Hum Dev 2009;40(2):301–16.
64. Silverman WK, Kurtines WM, Jaccard J, et al. Directionality of change in youth anxiety treatment involving parents: an initial examination. J Consult Clin Psychol 2009;77(3): 474–85.
65. Cobham VE, Dadds MR, Spence SH, et al. Parental anxiety in the treatment of childhood anxiety: a different story three years later. J Clin Child Adolesc Psychol 2010;39(3):410–20.
66. Garber J, Ciesla JA, McCauley E, et al. Remission of depression in parents: links to healthy functioning in their children. Child Dev 2011;82(1):226–43.
67. Ohr PS, Vidair HB, Gunlicks-Stoessel M, et al. Maternal mood, video-mediated cognitions, and daily stress during home-based, family interactions. J Fam Psychol 2010;24(5):625–34.
68. Swartz HA, Frank E, Zuckoff A, et al. Brief interpersonal psychotherapy for depressed mothers whose children are receiving psychiatric treatment. Am J Psychiatry 2008; 165(9):1155–62.
69. Jellinek MS, Bishop SJ, Murphy JM, et al. Screening for dysfunction in the children of outpatients at a psychopharmacology clinic. Am J Psychiatry 1991;148(8):1031–6.
70. Derogatis L, Savitz K. The SCL-90–R and Brief Symptom Inventory (BSI) in primary care. Handbook of psychological assessment in primary care settings. Mahwah (NJ): Erlbaum; 2000. p. 297–334.
71. Spitzer RL, Kroenke K, Williams JB. Validation and utility of a self-report version of PRIME-MD: the PHQ primary care study. Primary Care Evaluation of Mental Disorders. Patient Health Questionnaire. JAMA 2009;282(18):1737–44.
72. Ferro T, Verdeli H, Pierre F, et al. Screening for depression in mothers bringing their offspring for evaluation or treatment of depression. Am J Psychiatry 2000;157(3): 375–9.
73. Swartz HA, Shear MK, Wren FJ, et al. Depression and anxiety among mothers who bring their children to a pediatric mental health clinic. Psychiatr Serv 2005; 56(9):1077–83.
74. Vidair HB, Boccia AS, Johnson JG, et al. Depressed parents' treatment needs and children's problems in an urban family medicine practice. Psychiatr Serv 2011;62(3): 317–21.
75. Swartz HA, Zuckoff A, Grote NK, et al. Engaging depressed parents in psychotherapy: Integrating techniques from motivational interviewing and ethnographic interviewing to improve treatment participation. Prof Psychol Res Pract 2007;38(4): 430–9.
76. Garber J, Clarke GN, Weersing VR, et al. Prevention of depression in at-risk adolescents: a randomized controlled trial. JAMA 2009;301(21):2215–24.
77. Beardslee WR, Gladstone TR, Wright EJ, et al. A family-based approach to the prevention of depressive symptoms in children at risk: evidence of parental and child change. Pediatrics 2003;112(2):e119–31.
78. Clarke GN, Hornbrook M, Lynch F, et al. A randomized trial of a group cognitive intervention for preventing depression in adolescent offspring of depressed parents. Arch Gen Psychiatry 2001;58(12):1127–34.
79. Compas BE, Forehand R, Keller G, et al. Randomized controlled trial of a family cognitive-behavioral preventive intervention for children of depressed parents. J Consult Clin Psychol 2009;77(6):1007–20.
80. Ginsburg GS. The Child Anxiety Prevention Study: intervention model and primary outcomes. J Consult Clin Psychol 2009;77(3):580–7.

Index

Note: Page numbers of article titles are in **boldface** type.

A

Age
  as factor in selective mutism, 623
  as factor in social phobia, 623
Agoraphobia, **593–600**
  described, 594–596
  DSM-V changes related to, 596–597
  panic disorder and, 594–600
Amitriptyline
  for anxiety in pediatric medical setting, 650
Amygdala
  attentional modulation of, 506–507
  in PTSD
    neuroimaging of, 581
Antidepressant(s)
  tricyclic
    for anxiety in pediatric medical setting, 650
    for SAD, 532
Anxiety
  age-appropriate
    vs. pathologic anxiety, 644
  in children
    parental psychopathology and, **669–689**. *See also* Parental psychopathology, child anxiety related to
    described, 457–458
  parental
    as risk factor for anxiety disorders, 467–468
  pathologic
    vs. age-appropriate anxiety, 644
  in pediatric medical setting, **643–653**
    age-appropriate *vs.* pathologic, 644
    assessment of, 647–648
    FSSs, 647
    physical disease and, 644–647
      psychosomatic considerations, 646–647
      somatopsychic considerations, 645
    treatment of, 648–650
      pharmacotherapy in, 649–650
      psychotherapy in, 648–649
  prevalence of
    variance in estimates of, 459–460

Child Adolesc Psychiatric Clin N Am 21 (2012) 691–702
http://dx.doi.org/10.1016/S1056-4993(12)00064-8
1056-4993/12/$ – see front matter © 2012 Elsevier Inc. All rights reserved.

childpsych.theclinics.com

Moving?

Make sure your subscription moves with you!

To notify us of your new address, find your **Clinics Account Number** (located on your mailing label above your name), and contact customer service at:

Email: journalscustomerservice-usa@elsevier.com

800-654-2452 (subscribers in the U.S. & Canada)
314-447-8871 (subscribers outside of the U.S. & Canada)

Fax number: 314-447-8029

Elsevier Health Sciences Division
Subscription Customer Service
3251 Riverport Lane
Maryland Heights, MO 63043

*To ensure uninterrupted delivery of your subscription, please notify us at least 4 weeks in advance of move.

Printed and bound by CPI Group (UK) Ltd, Croydon, CR0 4YY

08/06/2025

01896870-0019